Cranial Nerves: Anatomy, Pathology, Imaging

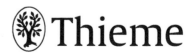

Cranial Nerves: Anatomy, Pathology, Imaging

Devin K. Binder, MD, PhD
Research Assistant Professor
Division of Biomedical Sciences
University of California
Riverside, California

Clinical Assistant Professor
UCR-UCLA Thomas Haider Program in Biomedical Sciences

D. Christian Sonne, MD
Clinical Assistant Professor of Radiology
University of California—San Francisco
San Francisco, California

Nancy J. Fischbein, MD
Associate Professor of Radiology
Stanford University Medical Center
Stanford, California

Thieme
New York • Stuttgart

Thieme Medical Publishers, Inc.
333 Seventh Ave.
New York, NY 10001

Editorial Director: Michael Wachinger
Executive Editor: Kay D. Conerly
Editorial Assistant: Lauren Henry
International Production Director: Andreas Schabert
Production Editor: Donald Whitehead, MPS Content Services
Vice President, International Marketing and Sales: Cornelia Schulze
Chief Financial Officer: James Mitos
President: Brian D. Scanlan
Compositor: MPS Content Services, A Macmillan Company
Printer: King Printing Co., Inc.

Library of Congress Cataloging-in-Publication Data

Binder, Devin K.
  Cranial nerves : anatomy, pathology, imaging / Devin K. Binder, D.
Christian Sonne, Nancy J. Fischbein.
     p. ; cm.
  Includes index.
  ISBN 978-1-58890-402-7 (alk. paper)
  1. Nerves, Cranial—Pathophysiology—Handbooks, manuals, etc. 2. Nerves,
Cranial—Pathophysiology—Atlases. 3. Nerves, Cranial—Handbooks, manuals,
etc. 4. Nerves, Cranial—Atlases. I. Sonne, D. Christian. II. Fischbein,
Nancy. III. Title.
  [DNLM: 1. Cranial Nerves—pathology—Handbooks. 2. Cranial
Nerves—anatomy & histology—Handbooks. 3. Cranial Nerve
Diseases—diagnosis—Handbooks. 4. Diagnostic Imaging—Handbooks. WL 39
B612c 2010]
  RC410.B56 2010
  616.8′56—dc22
                              2009039889

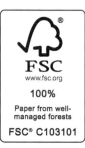

FSC
www.fsc.org
100%
Paper from well-managed forests
FSC® C103101

Printed in the United States of America

5 4 3 2

ISBN 978-1-58890-402-7

To Bill Dillon and others whose teachings have imparted to us knowledge and appreciation of the cranial nerves.

Contents

Foreword

I have had an intellectual affair with cranial nerves since my days as a neuroradiology fellow at University of California, San Francisco. Cranial nerves tie together two of my loves: the brain and the anatomy of the face and neck. Many neuroradiologists and other practitioners shy away from the complexity of the cranial nerves, as assessing and imaging the cranial nerves leads them by necessity into difficult anatomy at and below the skull base. Few neurosurgeons, in my experience, appreciate fully the myriad neurological manifestations of extracranial disease of the cranial nerves.

It is with these needs in mind that three of the most talented physicians I know, world-class neurosurgeon Devin K. Binder, MD, PhD, and superb neuroradiologists Nancy Fischbein, MD, and Christian Sonne, MD, collaborated to produce *Cranial Nerves: Anatomy, Pathology, and Imaging.* Their work beautifully summarizes the functional anatomy and pathology of the 12 cranial nerves, complete with bullet-point summaries and gorgeous illustrations highlighting case studies. This contribution combines the surgical perspective of an experienced neurosurgeon and the imaging knowledge of two talented neuroradiologists to provide to the broad community of clinical neuroscientists and practitioners a better understanding of complex cranial nerve anatomy and pathology.

They have exceeded my expectations and produced a wonderful addition to my library that will become a classic.

William P. Dillon, MD
Professor and Chief of Neuroradiology
University of California, San Francisco
San Francisco, California
June 2009

Preface

This book is intended for medical practitioners with varying levels of knowledge, from the medical student beginning to study the cranial nerves to house officers and physicians whose clinical practice involves cranial nerves. Specialists in neurology, neurosurgery, neuroradiology, otolaryngology, ophthalmology, maxillofacial surgery, radiation oncology, and emergency medicine would, of course, be expected to have an interest in cranial nerves. The anatomy and pathology of cranial nerves, however, may in fact be of interest to a broad variety of physicians at many levels, as well as to other health sciences professionals, including nurses and physician assistants in the fields listed above. Students and practitioners of dentistry, speech pathology, audiology, physical and health education, and rehabilitation sciences may also find this book useful in their clinical practice.

We wrote this book because there is currently no cranial nerve atlas that combines normal anatomy with case studies and pathology illustrated with modern cross-sectional techniques. The shift in medical education from didactic to problem-based learning is paralleled in this book. Over the past few years, advances in imaging have enabled improved visualization of structures and pathologies that could not be previously identified noninvasively. Pathology affecting every cranial nerve can now be assessed routinely with high-resolution computed tomography and magnetic resonance imaging.

Following a general introduction to the cranial nerves, each chapter explores one of the 12 cranial nerves. Anatomical information regarding origin, course, and function is presented first. This is followed by normal imaging anatomy, a differential diagnosis of various pathologies affecting the nerve (organized from proximal to distal), and, finally, a series of illustrative clinical cases with detailed annotated imaging. Information is presented in bulleted outline format that eliminates superfluous text and facilitates information retrieval. Where appropriate, boxes with more detail on specific pathologies accompany the text. Clinical and imaging pearls abound throughout. The Appendices provide more detailed information on brainstem anatomy, pupil and eye movement control, parasympathetic ganglia, and cranial nerve reflexes.

Drawing on our years of experience in teaching residents and fellows in neurosurgery and neuroradiology, we bring to this book a wealth of case-based learning. We are pleased to have the opportunity to share with you our teaching file of high-quality images of numerous cranial nerve pathologies with clinical correlation. We hope that this book will serve as a frequently referenced learning tool for all levels of interested healthcare professionals. We will have succeeded in our goals if we have fired the interest of our readers in this important topic and if we have contributed to patient care.

Devin K. Binder, MD, PhD
D. Christian Sonne, MD
Nancy J. Fischbein, MD

Introduction to the Cranial Nerves

- The 12 cranial nerves control motor and sensory functions of the head and neck, including innervation of voluntary and involuntary muscles and reception of general and special sensory information.
- A thorough understanding of cranial nerve anatomy, function, and imaging is crucial to the evaluation of cranial neuropathies.
- Cranial nerves carry fibers subserving six different types of functions (**Table 0.1**).
- **Table 0.2** summarizes the functions of the individual cranial nerves.
- As all the cranial nerves lie at the base of the brain, it is important to become familiar with the soft tissue and bony anatomy of the skull base (**Figs. 0.1, 0.2, Tables 0.3, 0.4**).
- Cranial nerve nuclei lie in the brainstem (see Appendix A) and are organized from medial to lateral and top to bottom as follows (**Fig. 0.3**):
  - Somatomotor nuclei lie close to the midline.
    - Oculomotor nucleus (III)
    - Trochlear nucleus (IV)
    - Abducens nucleus (VI)
  - Hypoglossal nucleus (XII)
  - Visceromotor nuclei (the origin of preganglionic parasympathetic fibers) lie more laterally.
    - Edinger-Westphal nucleus (preganglionic parasympathetics to the sphincter pupillae and ciliary muscles)
    - Lacrimal nucleus (preganglionic parasympathetics to the lacrimal gland)
    - Superior salivatory nucleus (preganglionic parasympathetics to the submandibular and sublingual glands)
    - Inferior salivatory nucleus (preganglionic parasympathetics to the parotid gland)
    - Dorsal motor nucleus of the vagus (preganglionic parasympathetics forming the vagus nerve proper)
  - Branchial motor nuclei lie still more laterally.
    - Motor nucleus of the trigeminal nerve (V, muscles of mastication)
    - Nucleus of the facial nerve (VII, muscles of facial expression)
    - Nucleus ambiguus (IX and X, muscles of the pharynx and larynx)

Table 0.1 Cranial Nerve Modalities

Category	Function	Cranial Nerves
General somatic efferent (GSE) (somatic motor)	Innervate muscles that develop from somites	III, IV, VI, XII
Special visceral efferent (SVE) (branchial motor)	Innervate muscles that develop from the branchial arches	V, VII, IX, X, XI
General visceral efferent (GVE) (visceral motor)	Innervate the viscera, glands, and smooth muscle (parasympathetic autonomic innervation)	III, VII, IX, X
General somatic afferent (GSA) (general sensory)	Transmit somatic sensation from the head, neck, sinuses, and meninges	V, VII, IX, X
Visceral afferent (VA) (visceral sensory)	Transmit visceral information but not pain impulses	IX, X
Special afferent (SA) (special sensory)	Transmit smell, vision, taste, balance, and hearing information	I, II, VII, VIII, IX

Note: Somite—one of the paired cell masses formed from early embryonic paraxial mesoderm. *Branchial arch*—also "gill arch." Typically six in vertebrates; in lower vertebrates give rise to gills; in higher vertebrates appear transiently then give rise to specialized structures in head and neck. *Efferent*—away from the central nervous system (CNS; motor). *Afferent*—toward the CNS (sensory).

Table 0.2 Cranial Nerve Functions

Nerve	Name	Functions
I	Olfactory	Special sensory (SA) for smell
II	Optic	Special sensory (SA) for vision
III	Oculomotor	Somatic motor (GSE) to SR, IR, MR, IO muscles
		Visceral motor (GVE, parasympathetic) to sphincter pupillae and ciliary muscles
IV	Trochlear	Somatic motor (GSE) to SO muscle
V	Trigeminal	Branchial motor (SVE) to muscles of mastication (temporalis, masseter, lateral and medial pterygoids), mylohyoid, tensor tympani, tensor veli palatini, anterior belly of digastric muscle
		General sensory (GSA) from face, oral cavity, nasal cavity, sinuses, anterior two thirds of tongue, dura of anterior and middle cranial fossae
VI	Abducens	Somatic motor (GSE) to LR muscle
VII	Facial	Branchial motor (SVE) to muscles of facial expression (including orbicularis oculi, orbicularis oris, zygomaticus major, levator anguli oris, depressor anguli oris, buccinator, corrugator supercilii, and platysma), stapedius, posterior belly of digastric
		Visceral motor (GVE, parasympathetic) to lacrimal gland (via GSPN), oral and nasal mucosa (via GSPN), and submandibular and sublingual glands (via chorda tympani)
		General sensory (GSA) from external auditory meatus, lateral pinna, mastoid, mucosa of pharynx, nose, and palate
		Special sensory (SA) for taste from anterior two thirds of tongue (via chorda tympani)
VIII	Vestibulocochlear	Special sensory (SA) for balance (via superior and inferior vestibular nerves) and hearing (via cochlear nerve)
IX	Glossopharyngeal	Branchial motor (SVE) to stylopharyngeus muscle
		Visceral motor (GVE, parasympathetic) to parotid gland (via LSPN)
		General sensory (GSA) from posterior external ear, tragus, posterior one third of the tongue, soft palate, nasopharynx, tympanic membrane, eustachian tube, mastoid region
		Visceral sensory (VA) from carotid body (O_2, CO_2 chemoreceptors) and carotid sinus (baroreceptors)
		Special sensory (SA) for taste from posterior one third of tongue
X	Vagus	Branchial motor (SVE) to pharyngeal and laryngeal muscles, including palatoglossus
		Visceral motor (GVE, parasympathetic) to smooth muscles and glands of pharynx (via pharyngeal plexus), larynx, heart, esophagus, stomach, other thoracoabdominal viscera down to the splenic flexure
		General sensory (GSA) from ear, external auditory meatus, external surface of the tympanic membrane, dura of posterior cranial fossa, larynx
		Visceral sensory (VA) from pharynx, larynx, trachea, lungs, heart, esophagus, stomach, other thoracoabdominal viscera down to the splenic flexure, aortic arch baroreceptors, aortic body chemoreceptors
		Special sensory (SA) for taste from the epiglottis, hard and soft palates and pharynx
XI	Spinal accessory	Branchial motor (SVE) to sternocleidomastoid and trapezius muscles
XII	Hypoglossal	Somatic motor (GSE) to all the intrinsic muscles of the tongue (longitudinal, transverse, and vertical muscles) and all of the extrinsic muscles of the tongue (hyoglossus, genioglossus, styloglossus, geniohyoid) except palatoglossus (innervated by X)

Abbreviations: GSA, general somatic afferent; GSE, general somatic efferent; GSPN, greater superficial petrosal nerve; GVE, general visceral efferent; IO, inferior oblique; IR, inferior rectus; LR, lateral rectus; LSPN, lesser superficial petrosal nerve; MR, medial rectus; SA, special afferent; SO, superior oblique; SR, superior rectus; SVE, special visceral efferent.

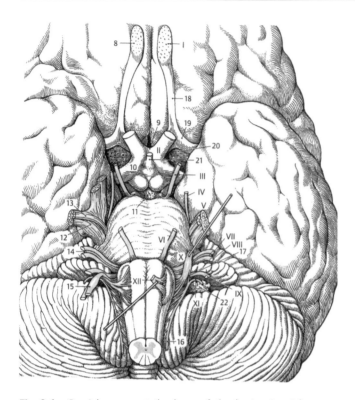

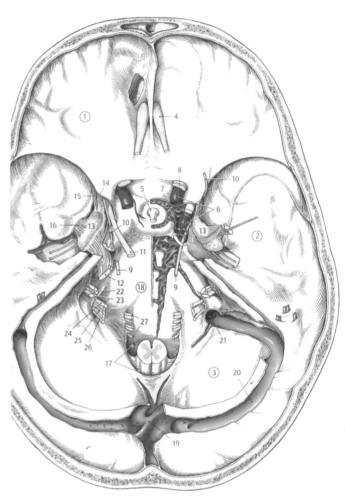

Fig 0.1 Cranial nerves at the base of the brain. Cranial nerves (I–XII) are labeled with Roman numerals. Associated structures include: 8—olfactory bulb, 9—optic chiasm, 10—optic tract, 11—interpeduncular fossa, 12—sensory root (portio major) of the trigeminal nerve and trigeminal (semilunar, gasserian) ganglion, 13—motor root (portio minor) of the trigeminal nerve, 14—nervus intermedius, 15—superior ganglion of the vagus nerve, 16—spinal root of the accessory nerve, 17—internal branch (fibers traversing accessory nerve to vagus nerve), 18—olfactory tract, 19—lateral olfactory stria, 20—anterior perforated substance, 21—hypophyseal stalk, 22—choroid plexus.

Fig 0.2 The skull base from above. 1—anterior cranial fossa, 2—middle cranial fossa, 3—posterior cranial fossa, 4—olfactory bulb, 5—hypophysis (pituitary gland), 6—internal carotid artery, 7—cavernous sinus, 8—optic nerve, 9—abducens nerve, 10—trochlear nerve, 11—oculomotor nerve, 12—trigeminal nerve, 13—trigeminal (semilunar, gasserian) ganglion, 14—ophthalmic nerve (V_1), 15—maxillary nerve (V_2), 16—mandibular nerve (V_3), 17—foramen magnum, 18—clivus, 19—torcular Herophili (confluence of sinuses), 20—transverse sinus, 21—internal jugular vein, 22—facial nerve, 23—vestibulocochlear nerve, 24—glossopharyngeal nerve, 25—vagus nerve, 26—accessory nerve, 27—hypoglossal nerve.

Table 0.3 Skull Base Foramina and Cranial Nerve Exit Points

Nerve	Name	Skull base foramen
I	Olfactory	Cribriform plate
II	Optic	Optic canal
III	Oculomotor	Superior orbital fissure
IV	Trochlear	Superior orbital fissure
V_1	Ophthalmic division of trigeminal	Superior orbital fissure
V_2	Maxillary division of trigeminal	Foramen rotundum
V_3	Mandibular division of trigeminal	Foramen ovale
VI	Abducens	Superior orbital fissure
VII	Facial	Internal auditory meatus
VIII	Vestibulocochlear	Internal auditory meatus
IX	Glossopharyngeal	Jugular foramen
X	Vagus	Jugular foramen
XI	Spinal Accessory	Jugular foramen
XII	Hypoglossal	Hypoglossal canal

Table 0.4   Skull Base Foramina/Spaces and Their Contents

Foramen/Space	Contents
Cribriform plate	Olfactory nerve (I)
	Anterior and posterior ethmoidal arteries and nerves
Optic canal	Optic nerve (II)
	Ophthalmic artery
Superior orbital fissure	Oculomotor nerve (III)
	Trochlear nerve (IV)
	Ophthalmic nerve (V_1) (nasociliary, frontal, and lacrimal branches)
	Abducens nerve (VI)
	Orbital branch of middle meningeal artery
	Recurrent meningeal branch of lacrimal artery
	Superior ophthalmic vein
Cavernous sinus	Oculomotor nerve (III)
	Trochlear nerve (IV)
	Ophthalmic nerve (V_1)
	Maxillary nerve (V_2)
	Abducens nerve (VI)
	Internal carotid artery
	Sympathetic plexus
Foramen rotundum	Maxillary nerve (V_2)
	Artery of foramen rotundum (branch of internal maxillary artery)
	Emissary veins
Foramen ovale	Mandibular nerve (V_3)
	LSPN
	Accessory meningeal branch of maxillary artery
	Emissary veins
Meckel's cave	Trigeminal (gasserian, semilunar) ganglion
Foramen lacerum	Meningeal branches of ascending pharyngeal artery; *not* ICA
Foramen spinosum	Meningeal (recurrent) branch of V_3
	Middle meningeal artery
	Middle meningeal vein
Vidian canal (pterygoid canal)	Vidian nerve (GSPN + deep petrosal nerve)
	Vidian artery and vein
Supraorbital foramen	Supraorbital nerve (of V_1) and vessels
Infraorbital canal and foramen	Infraorbital nerve (of V_2) and vessels
Inferior orbital fissure	Infraorbital nerve (of V_2)
	Zygomatic nerve (of V_2)
	Infraorbital artery and vein
	Inferior ophthalmic vein
Greater palatine foramen	Greater palatine nerve (of V_2) and vessels
Lesser palatine foramen	Lesser palatine nerve (of V_2) and vessels
Sphenopalatine foramen	Nasopalatine nerve (of V_2)
	Nasal nerve (of V_2)
	Sphenopalatine artery
Incisive foramen	Nasopalatine nerve (of V_2) and vessels
Mandibular foramen	Inferior alveolar nerve (of V_3)
Mental foramen	Mental nerve (of V_3)
Foramen cecum	Emissary vein from the superior sagittal sinus to frontal sinus and nose and anterior falcine artery (located between frontal crest and crista galli)

Table 0.4   Skull Base Foramina/Spaces and Their Contents (*continued*)

Foramen/Space	Contents
Pterygopalatine fossa	Maxillary nerve (V$_2$)
	Pterygopalatine ganglion
	Vidian nerve
	Maxillary artery
	Vidian artery and vein
Infratemporal fossa	Mandibular nerve (V$_3$) and branches
	Chorda tympani nerve (of VII)
	Otic ganglion
	Maxillary artery
	Pterygoid venous plexus
	Temporalis and medial and lateral pterygoid muscles
Petrotympanic fissure	Chorda tympani (of VII)
Greater petrosal foramen	GSPN
Lesser petrosal foramen	LSPN
Carotid canal	Internal carotid artery
	Sympathetic plexus
Dorello's canal	Abducens nerve (VI)
Internal acoustic meatus	Facial nerve (VII)
	Nervus intermedius
	Vestibulocochlear nerve (VIII)
	Labyrinthine artery (branch of AICA)
Stylomastoid foramen	Facial nerve (VII)
Jugular foramen	*Pars nervosa*
	Glossopharyngeal nerve (IX)
	Jacobson's nerve (tympanic branch of IX)
	Pars venosa
	Vagus nerve (X)
	Spinal accessory nerve (XI)
	Arnold's nerve (auricular branch of X)
	Posterior meningeal artery (from vertebral)
	Internal jugular vein/jugular bulb
Hypoglossal canal	Hypoglossal nerve (XII)
	Anterior meningeal artery
Foramen magnum	Spinal cord
	Spinal root of accessory nerve (XI)
	Vertebral arteries
	Anterior spinal artery
	Posterior spinal arteries
	Anterior and posterior meningeal arteries

Abbreviations: AICA, anterior inferior cerebellar artery; GSPN, greater superficial petrosal nerve; ICA, internal carotid artery; LSPN, lesser superficial petrosal nerve

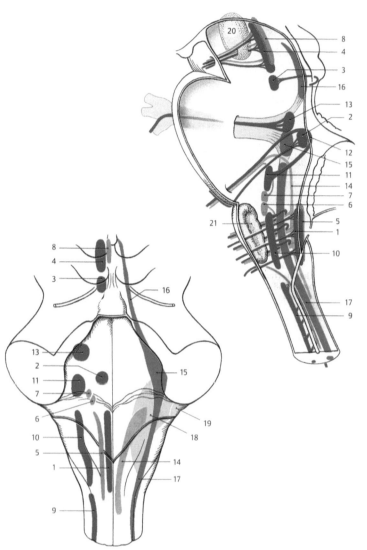

Fig 0.3 Cranial nerve nuclei (dorsal and lateral views). *Somatomotor nuclei.* 1—hypoglossal nucleus, 2—abducens nucleus, 3—trochlear nucleus, 4—oculomotor nucleus. *Visceromotor nuclei.* 5—dorsal motor nucleus of the vagus, 6—inferior salivatory nucleus, 7—superior salivatory nucleus, 8—Edinger-Westphal nucleus. *Branchial motor nuclei.* 9—spinal nucleus of the accessory nerve, 10—nucleus ambiguus, 11—facial nucleus, 12—internal genu of the facial nerve, 13—motor nucleus of the trigeminal nerve. *Viscerosensory and special sensory nuclei.* 14—nucleus of the tractus solitarius, 15—principal sensory (pontine) nucleus of the trigeminal nerve, 16—mesencephalic nucleus of the trigeminal nerve, 17—spinal nucleus of the trigeminal nerve, 18—vestibular nuclei, 19—cochlear nuclei.

- Spinal nucleus of the accessory nerve (XI, sternocleidomastoid and trapezius muscles)
  ○ Viscerosensory and special sensory nuclei are located most laterally, including:
    - Mesencephalic nucleus of the trigeminal nerve (V, proprioception)
    - Principal sensory (pontine) nucleus of the trigeminal nerve (V, light touch)
    - Spinal nucleus of the trigeminal nerve (V, pain and temperature)
    - Nucleus of the tractus solitarius (rostral portion [gustatory nucleus] receives special sensory taste fibers from VII, IX, and X; caudal portion [cardiorespiratory nucleus] receives viscerosensory information from IX and X)
    - Vestibular nuclei (VIII, balance)
    - Cochlear nuclei (VIII, auditory information)

Cranial Nerve Pathology

- It is very useful to classify cranial nerve pathology by site of the lesion (e.g., brainstem, cisternal, or more peripheral) and also by type of pathology (e.g., neoplasm, vascular, trauma) (**Table 0.5**).

Cranial Nerve Imaging

- The ability of modern magnetic resonance imaging (MRI) to demonstrate detailed anatomy of the brainstem, basal cisterns, and skull base has aided the evaluation of cranial neuropathies.
- MRI is generally the study of choice for imaging cranial nerves (**Table 0.6**).

Table 0.5   General Categories of Cranial Nerve Pathology

Site of Pathology	Types of Pathology
Brainstem	Ischemia/infarction
	Demyelinating disease
	Neoplasm
	Trauma (shear injury or contusion)
	Hemorrhage/vascular malformation
	Infection (encephalitis, abscess)
Cisternal	Vascular (aneurysm, compressive vascular loop)
	Neoplasm (neural tumor, compressive mass, leptomeningeal spread of tumor)
	Infection (basilar meningitis, viral neuritis)
	Ischemic (microvascular infarction of nerve)
	Miscellaneous (brain herniation with neural compression, sarcoidosis, siderosis)
Cavernous (III, IV, V_1, V_2, VI)	Neoplasm (sellar, paracavernous)
	Vascular (aneurysm, fistula, dissection)
	Inflammation (pseudotumor, sarcoidosis)
	Infection (cavernous sinus thrombophlebitis)
Orbital (II, III, IV, V_1, V_2, VI)	Trauma
	Inflammation (e.g., viral neuritis)
	Demyelination (e.g., optic neuritis)
	Infection
	Neoplasm
	Pseudotumor
Internal auditory canal (VII, VIII)	Neoplasm (schwannoma, hemangioma)
	Trauma (temporal bone fracture)
	Inflammation (neuritis)
	Infection (skull base osteomyelitis)
	Vascular loop
Foraminal (V_3, IX, X, XI, XII)	Neoplasm (schwannoma, meningioma, paraganglioma, perineural spread of disease, bony tumors)
	Vascular (pseudoaneurysm, dural fistula)
	Infection (skull base osteomyelitis)
	Trauma (skull base fracture)
Extracranial	Neoplasm (schwannoma, squamous cell carcinoma, lymphoma, perineural tumor)
	Inflammation (abscess)
	Vascular (dissection, pseudoaneurysm)
	Trauma

- It is essential to cover the entire course of the nerve so as not to overlook pathology. This includes the brainstem (cranial nerve nucleus), cisternal or subarachnoid segment of the nerve, cavernous and/or foraminal segment of the nerve (depending on its course), and the extracranial portion of the nerve to the level of its target organ.
- If symptoms suggest a supranuclear origin for cranial nerve dysfunction (e.g., "central" facial palsy versus "peripheral" facial palsy), then the whole brain must be studied. Another example is certain visual deficits (notably homonymous hemianopsia), which require study of the whole brain rather than optic nerves or chiasm only.

- Proximity of certain cranial nerves to one another may result in multiple cranial neuropathies caused by a single pathologic process. This provides useful localizing information (e.g., cavernous sinus for nerves III, IV, VI, V_1, V_2, and sympathetics) and may help focus imaging studies.
- Keep in mind certain key "can't miss" pathologies:
  - Cranial nerve III: posterior communicating artery aneurysm
  - Cranial nerve V: perineural spread of tumor
  - Cranial nerve VII: parotid malignancy
  - Cranial nerve XII: "pseudomass" of denervation change

Table 0.6   Utility of Specific MR Sequences for Cranial Nerve Imaging

MR Sequence	Characteristics/Advantages
T1WI: sagittal, axial, coronal	Sensitive to infiltration of fat planes and loss of normal marrow signal
	Anatomical definition
	Parotid gland lesions well seen
T2WI: axial and/or coronal FSE with fat saturation	Lesion characterization
	Patency of CSF spaces
	Denervation changes
Post-gadolinium T1WI: axial, coronal with fat saturation	Enhancement of characteristics of lesion
	Sensitive to perineural spread of tumor, meningeal infiltration, metastatic foci
MR angiogram/venogram	Vascular lesions
	Pulsatile tinnitus, vascular loops
MPGR	Meningeal hemosiderin (e.g., superficial siderosis)
	Parenchymal hemorrhage
FIESTA	Cisternal course of cranial nerves
	Assessment of neurovascular compression
3-D FSE T2 orbits	Globe pathology (e.g., retinoblastoma)

Abbreviations: 3-D, three-dimensional; CSF, cerebrospinal fluid; FIESTA, fast imaging employing steady-state acquisition; FSE, fast spin echo; MPGR, multiplanar gradient-recalled; T1WI, T1-weighted image; T2WI, T2-weighted image.

1 Olfactory Nerve

Functions

- Special afferent (SA) for sense of smell

Anatomy

- The olfactory system (**Fig. 1.1**) consists of the olfactory epithelium, olfactory bulbs (**Fig. 1.2**), olfactory striae, and a variety of target brain areas partly though not exclusively devoted to processing olfactory information (**Fig. 1.3**).
- The olfactory nerves, like the optic nerves (II), differ from other cranial nerves in that they are really central nervous system (CNS) tracts. Both are composed of secondary sensory axons rather than primary sensory axons, and both have cellular constituents like the CNS and therefore demonstrate CNS rather than peripheral nervous system (PNS) pathologies (e.g., astrocytomas rather than schwannomas).

Olfactory Epithelium

- The *olfactory epithelium* has multiple cellular components, including the following:
  - *Olfactory cells*. Bipolar neurons (~100 million) in the olfactory epithelium in the upper posterior nasal cavity.

These cells have cilia projecting into mucus secreted by *Bowman glands* and express specific membrane receptor proteins to detect odorants (1 in **Fig. 1.2**).
  - *Sustentacular cells*. Support the olfactory cells.
  - *Basal cells*. The stem cells for new olfactory cells, which undergo constant replacement throughout life.

Olfactory Bulb and Tract

- Olfactory cells send bundles of unmyelinated axons (*olfactory nerves* proper) across the cribriform plate of the ethmoid bone to synapse on the second-order neurons in the *olfactory bulb* (**Fig. 1.2**).
- *Mitral cells* and *tufted cells* are the two types of secondary olfactory neurons in the olfactory bulb. At points of synapse with mitral and tufted cells, clusters of fibers called *olfactory glomeruli* are formed (**Fig. 1.2**). *Granule cells* (inhibitory interneurons) in the olfactory bulbs have no axons but form dendrodendritic synapses with mitral cells.
- The *olfactory tract* includes the axons of mitral and tufted cells and travels posteriorly in the olfactory sulcus between the gyrus rectus medially and the orbitofrontal gyrus laterally. It splits into lateral, medial, and intermediate *olfactory striae* at the *anterior perforated substance*.

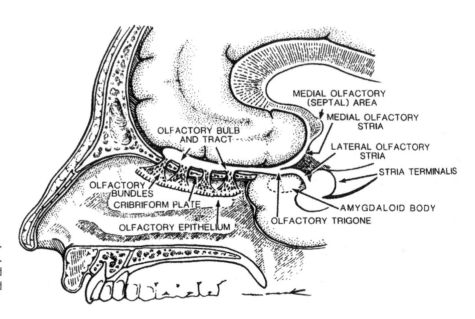

Fig. 1.1 Olfactory system (sagittal view). See text for details. (From Harnsberger HR. Handbook of Head and Neck Imaging (2nd ed.) St. Louis, MO: Mosby, 1995. Reprinted with permission.)

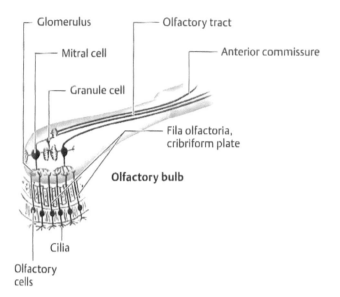

Fig. 1.2 Olfactory bulb. 1, olfactory epithelial cells (primary neurons); 2, cribriform plate; 3, olfactory bulb; 4, mitral cell; 5, glomerulus; 6, olfactory tract; 7, anterior olfactory nucleus.

Olfactory Striae

- The *olfactory trigone* (**Fig. 1.3**) is the triangle formed by the lateral and medial striae.
- *Lateral olfactory stria* projects to the
  - *Anterior olfactory nucleus* (**Figs. 1.2, 1.3**). Located between the olfactory bulb and tract, it receives fibers from the tufted cells and sends axons to either (1) cross in the *anterior commissure* to the contralateral anterior olfactory nucleus and olfactory bulb or (2) the ipsilateral olfactory cortical areas.
  - Amygdala (**Fig. 1.3**).
  - Primary olfactory cortex = the *piriform* (L., "pear-shaped") *cortex* (**Fig. 1.3**) (lateral olfactory gyrus from lateral olfactory stria to amygdala) as well as the *periamygdaloid cortex.* This is the primary olfactory pathway.
- Fibers then travel from the piriform cortex (primary olfactory cortex) to the following:
  - Entorhinal cortex (**Fig. 1.3**) (secondary olfactory cortex) to the hippocampus, insula, and frontal lobe by way of the *uncinate fasciculus.*
  - Amygdala, lateral preoptic hypothalamus, and the nucleus of the diagonal band.
  - Mediodorsal (MD) thalamic nucleus to the orbitofrontal cortex (for conscious analysis of odor, a phylogenetically newer pathway).
- *Medial olfactory stria.* Projects to the septal area (subcallosal area and the paraterminal gyrus) (also termed the *medial olfactory area*). This phylogenetically older pathway mediates the emotional/autonomic response to odors with its limbic connections.
- *Intermediate olfactory stria.* Projects to the anterior perforated substance (intermediate olfactory area) between the *olfactory trigone* (triangle formed by lateral and medial striae) and the optic tract.
- *Rhinencephalon* ("smell brain"). Olfactory bulbs, tracts, striae, and anterior olfactory nucleus and piriform cortex.
- *Anterior perforated substance.* Bounded by the medial and lateral olfactory striae anteriorly, optic tract medially, and posteriorly by the diagonal band of Broca. Transmits perforating vessels.
- *Diagonal band of Broca.* White matter tract connecting septal nuclei to amygdala, connects all three olfactory areas (medial, intermediate, and lateral).
- Efferent fibers from the olfactory areas travel in
  - The *medial forebrain bundle (*MFB) from all three olfactory areas to the hypothalamus and brainstem reticular formation.
  - The *stria medullaris thalami* from the olfactory areas to the habenular nucleus (epithalamus).
  - The *stria terminalis* from the amygdala to the anterior hypothalamus and preoptic area. The hypothalamus sends the olfactory information to the reticular formation, superior and inferior salivatory nuclei (for salivation in response to odors), and dorsal motor nucleus of X (to cause acceleration of peristalsis and increased gastric secretion).

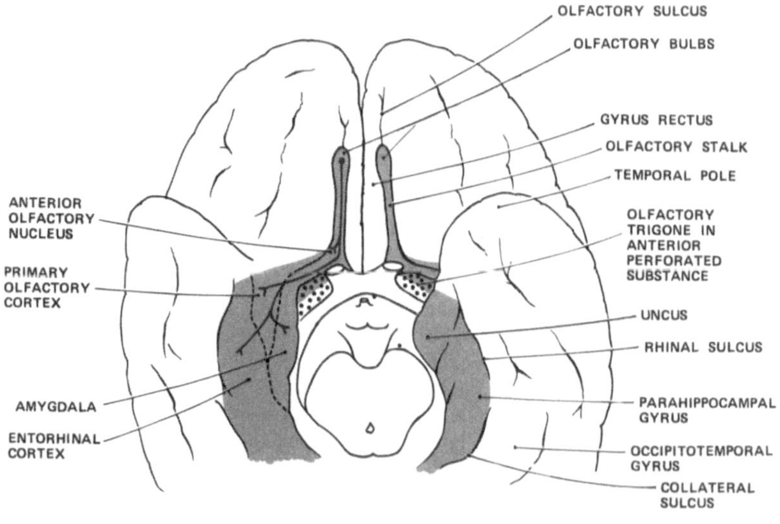

Fig. 1.3 Olfactory system (basal view). Together, the olfactory bulbs, tracts ("stalks"), striae, anterior olfactory nucleus, and piriform cortex make up the primary olfactory pathway. See text for details. (From Gilman S, Newman SW. Manter and Gatz's Essentials of Clinical Neuroanatomy and Neurophysiology [10th ed.]. Philadelphia: F.A. Davis Publishers, 2003. Reprinted with permission.)

Olfactory Nerve: Normal Images (Figs. 1.4, 1.5, 1.6)

Olfactory System Lesions

- Loss of smell (*anosmia*) can be produced by a lesion anywhere along the olfactory pathway, from the olfactory epithelium, olfactory bulb, olfactory tracts, and/or central structures (posterior orbitofrontal, subcallosal, anterior temporal, or insular cortex).
- Unilateral anosmia suggests an olfactory lesion proximal to the piriform cortex (which has bilateral representation.

Types

Lesions Causing Anosmia

- Infectious/inflammatory
  - Sinonasal inflammatory disease (rhinitis, sinusitis, sinonasal polyposis). Congestion prevents odorants from accessing receptors.
  - Viral infections (e.g., influenza) (presumably due to mucosal edema)
  - Basilar meningitis
  - Neurosarcoidosis
- Toxic (e.g., chronic smoking)

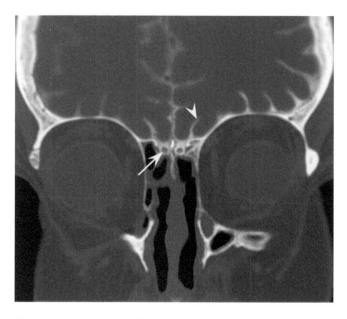

Fig. 1.5 Coronal image from a CT cisternogram demonstrates bilateral and symmetric olfactory bulbs (*arrow*) surrounded by contrast material in the subarachnoid space. Note the normal morphology of the olfactory sulcus (*arrowhead*).

- Traumatic
  - Due to closed head injury with or without cribriform plate fracture. Olfactory axon filaments can be sheared by trauma at the point where they pass through the cribriform plate.

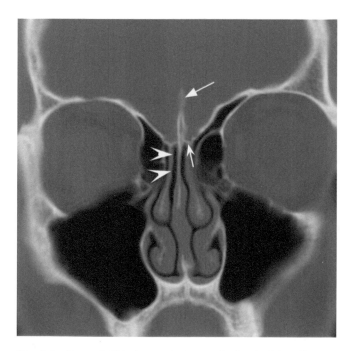

Fig. 1.4 Coronal CT in bone window at the level of the olfactory bulbs shows a normal well-aerated olfactory recess (*arrowheads*). Also indicated is the cribriform plate (*concave arrow*), inferior and lateral to the crista galli (*straight arrow*). The crista galli is the site of attachment of the anterior falx cerebri.

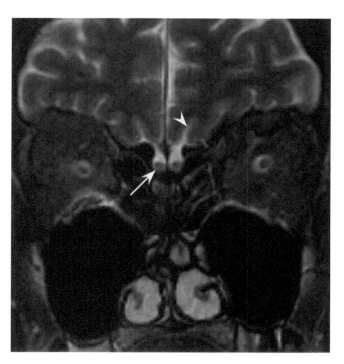

Fig. 1.6 Coronal fast spin echo T2-weighted MR image with fat saturation shows normal olfactory bulbs (*arrow*) and olfactory sulcus (*arrowhead*).

- Congenital
  - Congenital absence of odorant receptors
  - Kallmann syndrome—familial, anosmia with hypogonadotrophic hypogonadism (anosmia due to agenesis of olfactory bulbs)
- Neurodegenerative disease
  - Alzheimer disease
  - Huntington disease
  - Parkinson disease
  - Down syndrome
  - Korsakoff syndrome (due to mediodorsal [MD] thalamic lesion)
- Neoplastic
  - Mass lesions of the anterior cranial fossa (especially meningiomas)
  - Esthesioneuroblastomas (olfactory neuroblastomas) arise in upper nasal cavity, present with anosmia, nasal obstruction, epistaxis
- Iatrogenic
  - After radiation therapy
  - After anterior skull base surgery or temporal lobectomy surgery

Lesions Causing Parosmia and Cacosmia

- *Parosmia* is perversion of smell, whereas *cacosmia* is the perception of unpleasant odors. These are usually seen after closed head injury or in the setting of psychiatric disease (olfactory hallucinations) or complex partial seizures.
- *Hyperosmia* (increased sense of smell) may occur with migraine or adrenal cortical insufficiency (Addison's disease).
- *Zinc* and *vitamin A* deficiency may cause hyposmia (reduced sense of smell) and parosmia in addition to hypogeusia (reduced taste perception) and dysgeusia (distorted taste perception).

Olfactory Hallucinations

- Caused by temporal lobe seizures (*uncinate fits*), schizophrenia, and depression

Olfactory Nerve: Pathologic Images

Case 1.1

A 40-year-old female presents with anosmia, epistaxis, and nasal congestion (**Figs. 1.7, 1.8**).

Diagnosis

Olfactory neuroblastoma (esthesioneuroblastoma)

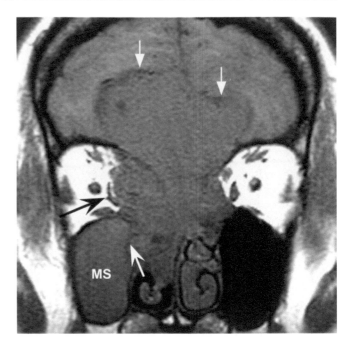

Fig. 1.7 Coronal T1-weighted MR image demonstrates a large homogeneous mass centered in the upper nasal cavity with intracranial extension and displacement of the frontal lobes superiorly (*straight white arrows*). The olfactory bulbs cannot be identified. Orbital extension displaces the right medial rectus muscle (*black arrow*). Secretions within the right maxillary sinus (MS) are secondary to obstruction by tumor in the region of the sinus ostium (*white concave arrow*).

Differential Diagnosis

- Meningioma (more broad dural base, often with dural "tail")
- Other primary paranasal sinus tumors, including squamous cell carcinoma, sinonasal undifferentiated carcinoma (SNUC), malignant minor salivary gland tumor (pathology is usually necessary to distinguish among these tumors)
- Lymphoma (may be indistinguishable, but often a more infiltrative growth pattern with less of a bulky dominant mass)

Esthesioneuroblastoma

- *Epidemiology.* Rare tumor. Accounts for ~3% of all intranasal tumors. Approximately equal M:F distribution. Bimodal age distribution, larger peak in late adulthood (>50 years).
- *Clinical presentation.* Arises from the basal cells of the olfactory mucosa at the cribriform plate and typically presents with nasal congestion, epistaxis, anosmia, and headache. Tumors are generally large at time of presentation. Gross intracranial spread occurs in ~30% of cases, but microscopic involvement of the dura overlying the cribriform plate is almost always present. Cervical lymph node and distant metastases may occur during

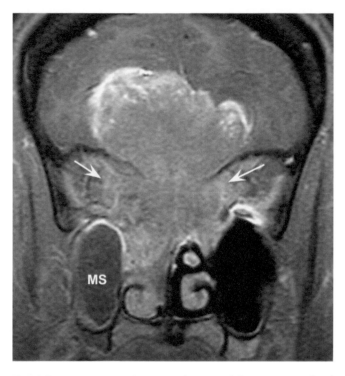

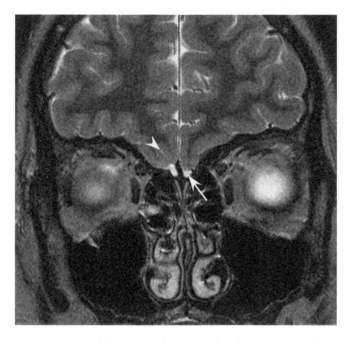

Fig. 1.8 A more posterior coronal post-gadolinium T1-weighted MR image with fat saturation demonstrates fairly homogeneous enhancement of this large soft tissue mass, as well as bilateral orbital involvement (*white arrows*). The trapped right maxillary sinus (MS) secretions do not enhance. Esthesioneuroblastoma.

Fig. 1.9 Coronal fast spin echo T2-weighted MR image with fat saturation in this patient with Kallmann syndrome demonstrates absence of the olfactory bulbs (*arrow* indicates "empty" olfactory groove). The right olfactory sulcus is shallow (*arrowhead*), while the left is absent.

the course of the disease but are uncommon at initial presentation.

- *Imaging.* Typically intermediate signal on both T1- and T2-weighted images. Post-gadolinium, there is generally intense and homogeneous enhancement.
- *Pathology.* Member of the family of primitive neuroectodermal tumors (PNETs). Densely cellular with small round cells. Homer-Wright rosettes (around central granulofibrillar material with radially arranged nuclei) and pseudorosettes (around blood vessels) are typical.
- *Treatment.* Surgery (anterior skull base resection) and radiation therapy are the mainstay of treatment, though some advocate chemotherapy and radiation therapy. Favorable prognosis with total resection and adjunctive treatment.

Case 1.2

A 15-year-old male presents for evaluation of delayed puberty and is found to have anosmia (**Fig. 1.9**).

Diagnosis

Kallmann syndrome

Kallmann Syndrome
- *Epidemiology.* 1 in 10,000 men and 1 in 50,000 women.
- *Clinical presentation.* Hypogonadotrophic hypogonadism and anosmia/hyposmia. Patients present with delayed puberty, infertility, cryptorchidism, anosmia/hyposmia, and occasionally other associated congenital abnormalities.
- *Imaging.* Coronal magnetic resonance imaging (MRI) best demonstrates aplasia or hypoplasia of the olfactory bulbs, tracts, and sulci. Occasional soft tissue masses between the forebrain and upper nasal vault can be seen, presumably representing masses of dysplastic arrested neurons.
- *Pathology.* X-linked developmental disorder causing abnormal development and migration of olfactory nerves and supporting cells.
- *Treatment.* Replacement hormones can be given to ameliorate hypogonadism.

Case 3.3

A 50-year-old female presents with personality change, anosmia, and right-sided visual loss. Examination reveals right-sided anosmia and optic atrophy and left-sided papilledema (**Figs. 1.10, 1.11, 1.12, 1.13**).

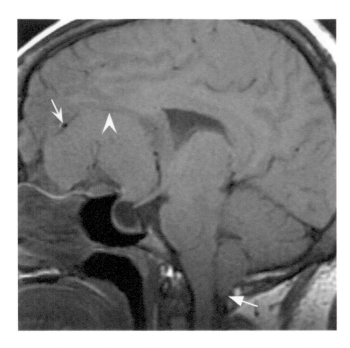

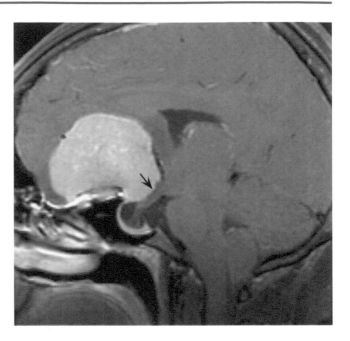

Fig. 1.10 Sagittal pre-gadolinium T1-weighted MR image demonstrates a large isotense mass arising from the floor of the anterior cranial fossa. The frontal lobes (*arrowhead*) are displaced superiorly and vessels are displaced peripherally (*concave arrow*), as is typical of an extraaxial lesion. Note the incidental low-lying cerebellar tonsil (*straight arrow*) at the foramen magnum.

Fig. 1.11 Sagittal fat-saturated post-gadolinium T1-weighted MR image demonstrates intense and homogeneous enhancement of the mass. Posteriorly, the mass abuts the optic chiasm and pituitary stalk (*black arrow*).

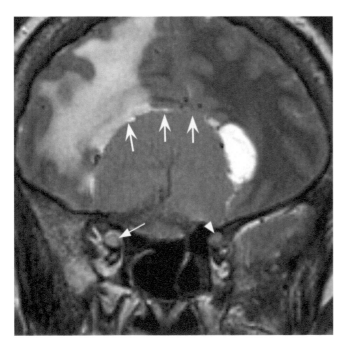

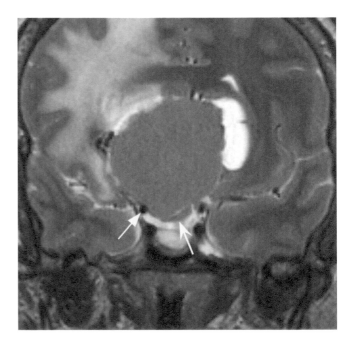

Fig. 1.12 Coronal fast spin echo T2-weighted MR image at the level of the orbital apex and planum sphenoidale shows an intermediate signal intensity mass with associated vasogenic edema within the right frontal white matter. The frontal lobes are displaced superiorly (*concave arrows*). The skull base is markedly thickened due to hyperostosis. The right optic nerve (*straight arrow*) is abnormally bright compared with the normal left optic nerve (*arrowhead*), consistent with injury that is most likely due to ischemia or infarction.

Fig. 1.13 More posteriorly, the mass abuts the right supraclinoid carotid artery (*straight arrow*) and severely compresses the right side of the optic chiasm (*concave arrow*). Olfactory groove meningioma.

Diagnosis

Olfactory groove meningioma with Foster-Kennedy syndrome

Foster-Kennedy Syndrome
- Caused by olfactory groove or sphenoid ridge masses (especially meningiomas)
- Consists of the following:
  - Ipsilateral anosmia (pressure on olfactory bulb or tract)
  - Ipsilateral optic atrophy (injury of ipsilateral optic nerve)
  - Contralateral papilledema (secondary to raised intracranial pressure due to mass lesion)

Case 3.4

A 36-year-old male with a history of remote head trauma presents for evaluation of inflammatory paranasal sinus disease and is noted to have anosmia (**Figs. 1.14, 1.15**).

Diagnosis

Encephalomalacia secondary to remote traumatic injury to olfactory apparatus and inferior frontal lobes

Traumatic Brain Injury
- *Epidemiology.* At least 1.4 million cases of traumatic brain injury (TBI)/year in United States causing 50,000 deaths/year and lifelong disability to 80,000–90,000/year. Bimodal age distribution (15–24 and >75 years more common).
- *Clinical presentation.* Immediate sequelae can include skull fracture, intraparenchymal hematoma (IPH), epidural hematoma (EDH), subdural hematoma (SDH), diffuse axonal injury (DAI), subarachnoid hemorrhage (SAH), intraventricular hemorrhage (IVH), cerebral edema, and intracranial hypertension. Delayed sequelae from prior TBI can include encephalomalacia, posttraumatic epilepsy, postconcussive syndrome, pneumocephalus, intracranial hypotension, cranial nerve palsies, hydrocephalus, and long-term personality or cognitive changes. TBI in the anterior cranial fossa is particularly associated with posttraumatic anosmia due to olfactory nerve injury as well as cerebrospinal fluid (CSF) leak secondary to cribriform plate or other anterior skull base fractures.
- *Imaging.* Depends on type and severity of TBI. Common sites of injury include inferior frontal and anterior temporal lobes. Common acute findings include extraaxial collections, parenchymal contusions, and skull fractures. If the trauma is remote, then nonspecific encephaloma-

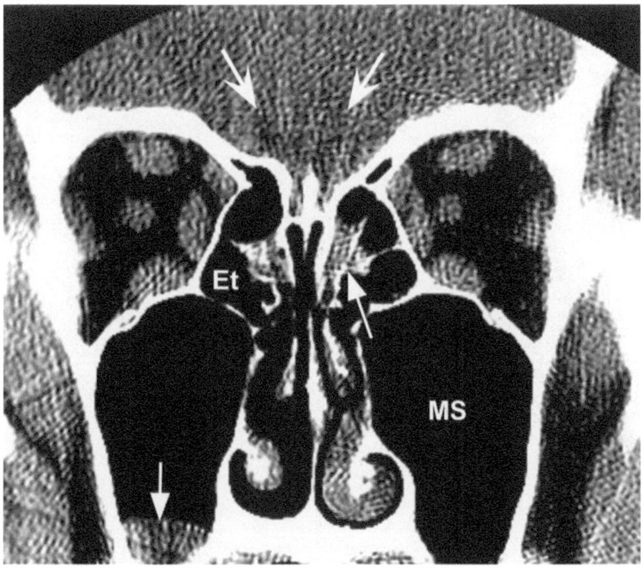

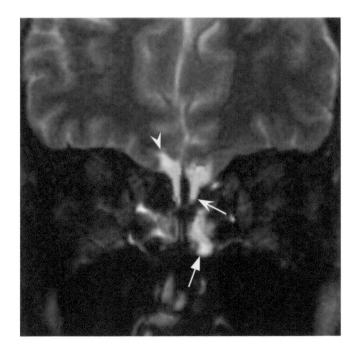

Fig. 1.14 A coronal CT scan of the paranasal sinuses was performed to evaluate inflammatory sinus disease. A coronal image presented in soft tissue window shows a small amount of right maxillary sinus (MS) and ethmoid (Et) mucosal thickening (*straight arrows*), as well as faint low attenuation (*concave arrows*) in the inferior frontal lobes suggesting posttraumatic encephalomalacia.

Fig. 1.15 Follow-up MR with coronal fast spin echo T2-weighted image with fat saturation demonstrates absence of the olfactory bulbs and tracts (expected location indicated by *concave arrow*), consistent with prior traumatic injury to the olfactory nerves. Encephalomalacia of the gyri recti (*arrowhead*) is seen as well, with prominence of basal CSF spaces. Bright signal within the ethmoids represents mucosal thickening with secretions (*straight arrow*).

lacia is seen. For posttraumatic anosmia, coronal MRI is the best imaging study for evaluation of injury to the olfactory apparatus and inferior frontal lobes. CSF leak is best evaluated by direct coronal thin-section computed tomography (CT) imaging using a bone algorithm. The presence and site of CSF leak may be confirmed using intrathecal contrast instillation or a nuclear medicine radioisotope study.

- *Pathology.* Cortical contusions result in localized hemorrhage and tissue necrosis. Shear injury (DAI) to axons leads to formation of axon retraction balls, followed by Wallerian degeneration. Intracranial hypertension, posttraumatic seizures, and metabolic derangements can lead to secondary neuronal injury.
- *Treatment.* No treatment for posttraumatic anosmia. Cognitive, physical, and speech therapy as needed for other deficits.

2 Optic Nerve

Functions

• Special afferent (SA) for vision.

Anatomy (Figs. 2.1, 2.2)

Retina

• Divided into four quadrants by horizontal and vertical meridians (superior/inferior and nasal/temporal)
• *Phototransduction* occurs by photoreceptors (rods and cones), which contain light-sensitive pigments. Rods are

absent from macula and optic disc (blind spot). Cones (color vision, three types: R, G, B) (~7 million cones) are tightly packed in the macula (100,000), which is at the posterior pole 4 mm lateral to optic disc and accounts for most visual acuity.
• Flow of information in retina is from photoreceptors to *bipolar cells* to *ganglion cells*. Other cell types in retina include *horizontal cells* (neurons), *amacrine cells* (neurons) and *Müller cells* (glial cells) that are thought to modulate the signal (e.g., surround inhibition).
• The axons of retinal ganglion cells form the *optic nerve* at the optic disc. Note that, like the olfactory nerve and unlike other cranial nerves, the optic nerve is really a CNS tract.

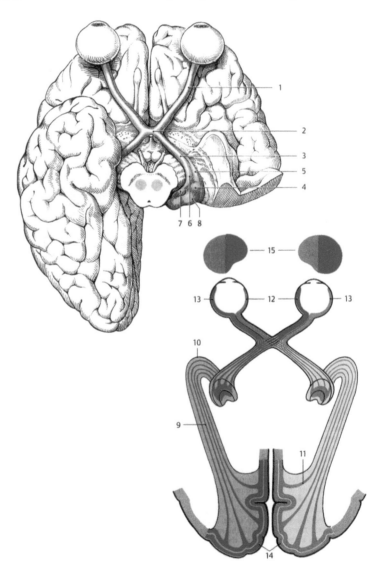

Fig. 2.1 Visual pathway and adjacent structures. 1, optic nerve; 2, optic chiasm; 3, optic tract; 4, lateral geniculate nucleus [LGN]; 5, lateral root of optic tract [to LGN]; 6, medial root of optic tract [to superior colliculus and pretectum]; 7, medial geniculate nucleus [part of auditory pathway]; 8, pulvinar [thalamic nucleus]; 9, optic radiation; 10, temporal genu; 11, occipital genu; 12, nasal retina [fibers cross at chiasm]; 13, temporal retina [fibers remain ipsilateral]; 14, striate cortex [primary visual cortex]; 15, visual fields.

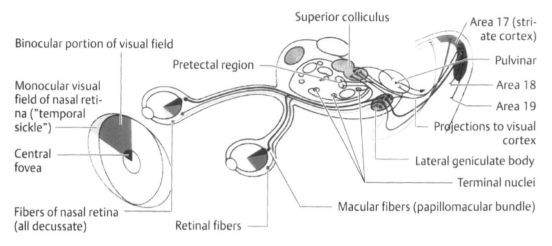

Fig. 2.2 Slightly more detailed view of visual pathway demonstrates the retinocollicular and retinopretectal tracts as well as the retinogeniculate pathway. Not shown is the retinohypothalamic tract (to suprachiasmatic nucleus (SCN) of hypothalamus) (see text).

Optic Nerves and Optic Chiasm

- Optic nerve (**Figs. 2.3, 2.4**) contains 1 million fibers (comparison: cochlear nerve 50,000 fibers). Macular fibers are on the temporal side of the optic disc and the adjacent optic nerve and move to the central part of the nerve as the papillomacular bundle for most of the distal pathway. The larger nonmacular fibers are on the periphery.
- Optic nerve is 50 mm long and has four portions:
  1. Intraocular (1 mm) (also called optic nerve head). Axons become myelinated.
  2. Intraorbital (25 mm). From back of globe to optic canal.

3. Intracanalicular (9 mm). Traverses optic canal with ophthalmic artery and sympathetic plexus.
4. Intracranial (4 to 16 mm). Lies superior to the internal carotid artery (ICA) as ICA exits cavernous sinus and gives off ophthalmic artery. The sphenoid sinus is inferomedial, whereas the anterior cerebral artery (ACA) (A1 segment), gyrus rectus, olfactory tract, and anterior perforated substance lie superior.
- See **Table 2.1** for a summary of vascular supply of the visual pathway.
- The two optic nerves converge at the *optic chiasm* where the nasal axons from the nasal retina decussate and the axons from the temporal retina remain ipsilateral.

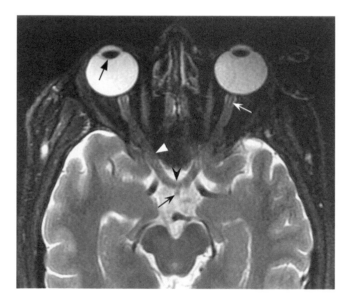

Fig. 2.3 Axial T2-weighted image demonstrates high signal intensity fluid within the ocular globes. The right lens is well seen (*black straight arrow*). Normal optic nerve (*white concave arrow*) is seen surrounded by perioptic fluid in the optic sheath. More posteriorly, the nerves traverse the optic canal (*white arrowhead*) to meet at the optic chiasm (*black arrowhead*) in the midline. Note that the pituitary stalk (*small black curved arrow*) is located just posterior to the optic chiasm.

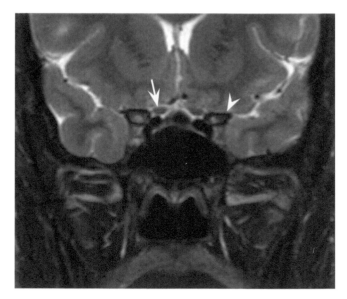

Fig. 2.4 Coronal T2-weighted image shows normal optic nerves entering the optic canals. The right optic nerve is indicated (*arrow*). The nerves lie medial to the anterior clinoid processes (*arrowhead*) and just above the flow void of the internal carotid artery.

Table 2.1 Vascular Supply of Visual Pathway

Structure	Vascular Supply
Retina	• The ophthalmic artery branches from the supraclinoid ICA and lies below and lateral to CN II in the optic canal. Five to 15 mm from the globe it gives off *central retinal artery* (CRA) which pierces CN II and continues forward in its core to divide into superior and inferior branches at the optic disc. Second-order nasal and temporal branches supply nerve fiber layer and inner retina (including ganglion cells). Infarction in territory of CRA may be caused by emboli, thrombi, hypercoagulable states, migraine, and arteritis.
	• Ophthalmic artery also gives off dural branches (anterior falcine and recurrent meningeal arteries), orbital branches, short posterior ciliary arteries (outer retinal layers, sclera, rods, cones) and long posterior ciliary arteries (ciliary body and iris), which form the anastomotic network, supply some of the optic disc, and 50% supply the macula.
Optic nerve	• Proximal part supplied by small branches of ophthalmic artery (pial plexus)
	• Distal (posterior) part supplied by small branches from ICA and ACA
Optic chiasm	• Superior part supplied by perforators from ACommA
	• Inferior part supplied by perforators from ICA, PCommA, PCA
Optic tract	• Supplied by branches of PCommA, PCA, anterior choroidal artery
Lateral geniculate nucleus	• Lateral part supplied by anterior choroidal artery
	• Medial part supplied by lateral posterior choroidal artery
Optic radiations	• Upper (parietal) supplied by MCA branches
	• Lower (temporal) supplied by PCA branches
Visual cortex	• Supplied by PCA calcarine branch, and MCA anastomoses via angular or posterior temporal arteries

Abbreviations: ACA, anterior cerebral artery; ACommA, anterior communicating artery; CN, cranial nerve; CRA, central retinal artery; ICA, internal carotid artery; MCA, middle cerebral artery; PCA, posterior cerebral artery; PCommA, posterior communicating artery.

• Positioning of the optic chiasm: The *prefixed chiasm* (9%) lies over the tuberculum sellae, 80% over the sella turcica (L., "Turkish saddle"); the *postfixed chiasm* (11%) lies over the dorsum sellae.
• The optic chiasm (**Fig. 2.5**) is located below the suprachiasmatic recess of the third ventricle, lamina terminalis, and anterior commissure; the pituitary stalk is immediately posterior.

Retinal Targets

• There are four brain regions that directly receive visual information from the retina (**Fig. 2.2**):
  1. *Retinogeniculate pathway.* Primary pathway for visual information; to lateral geniculate nucleus (LGN) of thalamus for conscious vision
  2. *Retinopretectal tract.* Retina to *pretectal area* of midbrain for pupillary light reflex (see Appendix B)
  3. *Retinocollicular tract.* To *superior colliculus* for eye movement reflexes (e.g., conjugate eye movements in response to head movements)
  4. *Retinohypothalamic tract.* To bilateral *suprachiasmatic nuclei* (SCN) of hypothalamus for circadian rhythms and neuroendocrine function

Optic Tracts

• Extend from chiasm posterolaterally around hypothalamus, around cerebral peduncles to lateral geniculate nuclei

• Vascular relationships: Posterior communicating artery (PCommA) located inferior to optic tracts in suprasellar cistern, posterior cerebral artery (PCA) and basal vein of Rosenthal apposed to optic tracts in perimesencephalic cistern

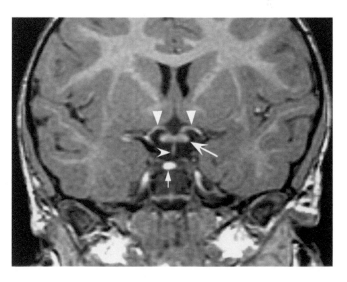

Fig. 2.5 Coronal thin-section spoiled gradient echo (SPGR) image demonstrates a normal optic chiasm (*concave arrow*) beneath the anterior cerebral arteries (*straight arrowheads*) and above the pituitary stalk (*concave arrowhead*). Note the posterior pituitary "bright spot" (*small straight arrow*).

Lateral Geniculate Nucleus (Fig. 2.6)

- In the inferolateral thalamus lateral to the upper midbrain
- Contains tertiary neurons that form the optic radiations to the primary visual cortex surrounding the calcarine fissure
- Contains six laminae (I–VI). I, IV, VI from contralateral eye; II, III, V from ipsilateral eye

Optic Radiations (Geniculocalcarine Tracts) (Figs. 2.1, 2.2, 2.7)

- Formed by axons of LGN neurons projecting to calcarine cortex of occipital lobe.
- Sweep posteriorly around lateral and posterior portion of lateral ventricles.
- *Parietal lobe optic radiations* start in the medial LGN and take a direct, nonlooping course over the top of the inferior horn of the lateral ventricle and then travel posteriorly through the parietal white matter to the superior calcarine cortex (subserve *inferior* visual fields).
- *Temporal lobe optic radiations* start in the lateral LGN, course anteriorly toward the temporal pole before turning posteriorly in a sharp loop (*Meyer's loop*) to course around the lateral wall of the inferior horn of the lateral

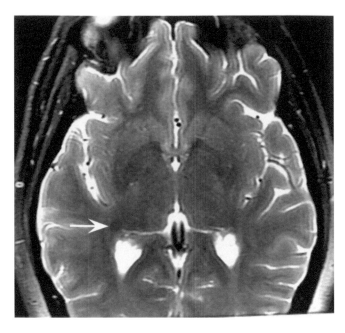

Fig. 2.6   Axial T2-weighted image at the level of the third ventricle shows the lateral geniculate nucleus (*arrow*) as a faint, relatively low signal focus at the lateral margin of the posterior thalamus.

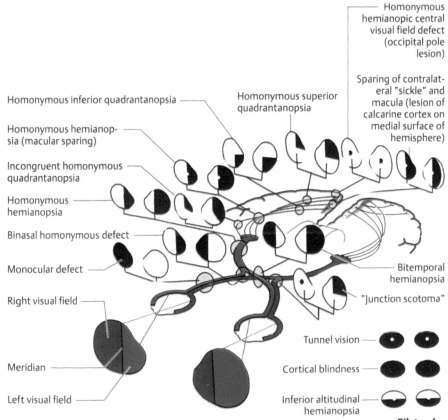

Types and localization of visual field defect

Fig. 2.7   Sites of lesions in the visual pathway and their associated visual field deficits.

ventricle then posteriorly to the inferior calcarine cortex (subserve *superior* visual fields). They account for *contralateral superior quadrantanopsia* following temporal lobectomy.
- Ventral optic radiations are closely associated with the posterior limb of the internal capsule.

Visual Cortex and Visual Association Areas

- Primary visual cortex (area 17) in walls and floor of calcarine sulcus in medial occipital lobe.
- Geniculocalcarine afferent input to layer IV of six-layered neocortex.
- On cross-section, white matter stria (*stria of Gennari*, thick white matter band in layer IV) can be seen with naked eye (thus *striate* cortex).
- Macula projects to posterior one third of the calcarine cortex (occipital pole). Macula represented posteriorly, peripheral retina anteriorly (fovea at occipital pole), upper field inferior, right field on left.
- Primary visual cortex projects to secondary visual areas (peristriate cortex) V2 (area 18) and V3 (area 19) in adjacent occipital lobe cortex.

Optic Nerve: Normal Images (Figs. 2.3, 2.4, 2.5, 2.6)

Optic Pathway Lesions

- The most common visual disorders are pathologies of the globe and vary by age:
  - Children: nearsightedness (myopia)
  - Adults: farsightedness (hyperopia)
  - Elderly: cataracts, glaucoma, retinal hemorrhages/detachment, macular degeneration
- Episodic visual loss in early adulthood is usually caused by migraines and in late adulthood by transient ischemic attacks (TIAs).

Nonneurologic Causes of Visual Loss (related to abnormal light transmission through the eye)

- *Cornea.* Scarring, deposits, infection, ulceration, and trauma.
- *Anterior chamber.* Hemorrhage, infection, open-angle glaucoma (90% of glaucoma cases; drainage pathway is partially open, there is gradual visual loss, and the eye looks normal), closed-angle glaucoma (increased intraocular pressure, red and painful eye).
- *Lens.* Cataracts, traumatic dislocation, diabetes (sorbitol accumulation), Wilson disease, Down syndrome, and spinocerebellar ataxia.
- *Vitreous humor.* Hemorrhage from retinal or ciliary vessels due to trauma, arteriovenous malformation (AVM),

or aneurysm (*Terson syndrome,* usually from *ruptured anterior communicating artery (ACommA) aneurysm*). "Floaters" are opacities in the vitreous humor. A sudden increase in floaters with a flash of light occurs with retinal detachment.
- *Uveitis.* Inflammation of the uvea (consists of iris, ciliary body, and choroid layer); accounts for ~10 to 15% of all cases of total blindness in the United States and has many causes, including inflammatory disease (e.g., systemic lupus erythematosis, sarcoidosis, rheumatoid arthritis, ulcerative colitis, Behçet disease), infection (e.g., cytomegalovirus [CMV], tuberculosis [TB], *Toxoplasma, Histoplasma*), and autoimmune disease (e.g., multiple sclerosis [MS]).

Types

Retinal Pathologies

- *Diabetic retinopathy.* Associated with microaneurysms, arteriovenous (A-V) nicking, "dot and blot" hemorrhages, exudates, and neovascularization. Leading cause of blindness in the United States.
- *Hypertensive retinopathy.* Associated with arteriolar narrowing, A-V nicking, hemorrhage and "cotton wool" exudates, and copper- or silver-wiring.
- *Senile macular degeneration.* Leading cause of blindness in the elderly. The hereditary form may also occur in children and young adults. Usually spares the peripheral retina.
- *Retinal detachment.* Fluid collects between the sensory retina and the retinal pigment epithelium.
- *Amaurosis fugax.* Sudden onset of transient monocular blindness usually from a *small fibrin embolus.*
- *Retinitis pigmentosa.* Begins in childhood and adolescence, male preponderance. Autosomal recessive (AR) or autosomal dominant (AD) inheritance on chromosome 3. Degeneration of all retinal layers (neuroepithelium and pigment epithelium) with foveal sparing. Starts with impairment of twilight vision (*nyctalopia*) progressing to blindness.
  - *Usher syndrome.* AR, retinitis pigmentosa with congenital hearing loss as well.
  - *Lawrence-Moon-Biedl syndrome.* AR, retinitis pigmentosa, obesity, congenital heart disease, developmental delay, polydactyly, renal disease, diabetes insipidus.
  - *Cockayne syndrome.* AR, retinitis pigmentosa, cataracts, photosensitivity, pendular nystagmus, ataxia, severe cerebellar atrophy, striatocerebellar calcifications, prognathism, anhidrosis, poor lacrimation.
  - *Stargardt disease.* Onset at 6 to 20 years of age; causes slow macular degeneration, especially of the central cones (opposite of retinitis pigmentosa).
  - *Leber hereditary optic neuropathy (LHON).* Congenital mitochondrial disorder associated with painless unilateral central vision loss.

- *Retinopathy of prematurity (retrolental fibroplasia).* Vascular proliferative disease of the retina originally related to oxygen therapy to premature infants. Risk factors are low birth weight and prematurity.
- *Retinoblastoma.* Congenital malignant retinal tumor. Presents with leukocoria (white pupil).
- *Subarachnoid hemorrhage (SAH).* Associated with hemorrhage between the internal limiting membrane and the vitreous fibers (subhyaloid or preretinal hemorrhages).
- *Roth spot.* A pale spot in the retina from the accumulation of white blood cells (WBC) and fibrin, associated with subacute bacterial endocarditis (SBE) or embolic plaques.

Optic Nerve Pathologies

- *Optic disc edema.*
  - *Bilateral.* Papilledema (90% of cases), papillitis, optic neuritis, ischemic optic neuropathy, neuroretinitis (disc edema with an inflammatory macular star), inflammatory disease, infiltrative disease.
  - *Unilateral.* Optic neuritis, asymmetric papilledema, ischemic optic neuropathy, inflammatory disease, infiltrative disease, Foster-Kennedy syndrome (ipsilateral disc edema and contralateral disc atrophy caused by frontal masses), neuroretinitis.
- *Papillitis* is optic disc edema associated with inflammatory or demyelinating diseases.
- *Papilledema* is optic disc edema associated with increased intracranial pressure. Causes enlarged visual blind spot and constricted visual field without visual acuity change. Develops as increased cerebrospinal fluid (CSF) pressure in the optic sheath compresses nerve fibers, resulting in axonal swelling and leaking. Unilateral papilledema can occur with optic nerve tumors. Visual acuity and pupillary light reflexes are usually normal (especially early).
- *Optic neuritis.* Inflammation, infection, and/or demyelination of the optic nerve. Presents with rapid partial or total loss of vision in one or both eyes. It usually occurs in young adults with scotoma in macular area and blind spot (cecocentral scotoma), may be associated with retrobulbar neuritis or papillitis, and local tenderness or pain is present with eye movements. Magnetic resonance imaging (MRI) may reveal T2 prolongation and gadolinium enhancement associated with the involved nerve(s). It is the first symptom of MS in 15% of cases. Vision returns to normal within a few weeks in two thirds of cases. Steroids speed the recovery (intravenous methylprednisolone followed by oral prednisone). Dyschromatopsia is a common persistent problem. In children, it is more frequently bilateral and of a viral or post-viral etiology. Differential diagnosis includes MS, acute disseminated encephalomyelitis (ADEM), syphilis, Lyme disease, vasculitis, neurosarcoidosis, and prior radiation.
- *Ischemic optic neuropathy.* Most common cause of *painless monocular blindness* in patients older than 50 years. It has abrupt onset and is caused by occlusion of the central retinal artery. Produces an *altitudinal field deficit*, flame hemorrhage, and edema with disc atrophy. One third of cases are bilateral, and are usually associated with diabetes or hypertension.
- *Toxic and nutritional optic neuropathies.* Cause bilateral, *symmetric central* or *centrocecal scotomas* (unlike demyelinating disease) with normal peripheral fields. Caused by B vitamin deficiencies, ethanol (EtOH), methanol, and other toxins. Patients do well if treated early.
- *Traumatic optic neuropathy.* Can occur at any point from posterior globe to optic chiasm, but usually occurs at the level of the optic canal. Can result from direct nerve injury or vascular compromise. Optic canal fractures are frequently associated with concomitant ICA injury with the risk of developing a carotid-cavernous fistula (CCF).
- *Optic nerve glioma.* Presents in children (usually <10 years of age) with visual dysfunction, hypothalamic dysfunction, and potentially obstructive hydrocephalus; associated with neurofibromatosis type 1 (NF-1) (see Case 2.5 below).

Visual Field Deficits (Fig. 2.7)

- *Hemianopia.* Blindness in half the visual field.
- *Homonymous.* Same field is involved in each eye (left or right).
- *Concentric visual field constriction* (tunnel vision). May be psychogenic or caused by glaucoma, papilledema, and retinitis pigmentosa. If psychogenic, the field does not change with distance.
- *Prechiasmatic lesion deficits.*
  - Monocular blindness (if entire nerve involved).
  - *Scotoma.* An island of decreased vision surrounded by normal vision. *Central* scotoma involves a fixation point and *cecocentral* is a fixation point connected to the blind spot.
  - Visual loss extending out to the periphery.
- *Chiasmatic lesion deficits.*
  - *Junctional scotoma.* Caused by a lesion at the optic nerve/chiasm border, resulting in ipsilateral central scotoma and a contralateral superior temporal quadrantanopsia ("*pie in the sky*").
  - *Bitemporal hemianopsia.* Due to sellar and suprasellar masses, sarcoidosis, aneurysms, and Langerhans cell histiocytosis.
- *Retrochiasmatic lesion deficits.*
  - Homonymous deficits.
  - Congruous deficits. Means an identical field defect in each eye. Lesions closer to the cortex create more congruous deficits.
  - *Meyer's loop.* Temporal lobe lesion involving fibers from the superior field causes a *pie in the sky* deficit (contralateral superior quadrantanopsia).
  - *Macular sparing.* Caused by a PCA stroke with the occipital pole being supplied by middle cerebral artery (MCA) collaterals.

○ *Bilateral central scotomas.* Caused by occipital pole strokes.

○ *Homonymous altitudinal hemianopsias.* Caused by bilateral occipital strokes. Monocular altitudinal deficits are usually caused by ischemic optic neuropathies.

• See **Table 2.2** for differential diagnosis of lesions affecting the visual pathway.

Optic Nerve: Pathologic Images

Case 2.1

A 3-month-old girl was found to have leukocoria in the left eye (**Figs. 2.8, 2.9**).

Diagnosis

Retinoblastoma

Table 2.2 Imaging Differential Diagnosis of Visual Pathway Lesions

Location	Lesions
Prechiasmatic	Retina
	Retinoblastoma
	Retinal detachment
	Optic nerve/sheath tumors
	Optic glioma
	Optic nerve sheath meningioma
	Inflammatory lesions of optic nerve/sheath
	Optic neuritis
	Orbital pseudotumor
	Sarcoidosis
	Orbital masses extrinsic to optic nerve
	Hemangioma
	Lymphangioma
	Graves disease (enlarged extraocular muscles)
	Pseudotumor (may or may not involve muscles)
	Malignant tumor
	Metastatic tumor
	Lymphoma
	Rhabdomyosarcoma
Chiasmatic	Pituitary adenoma
	Rathke cleft cyst
	Optic glioma
	Craniopharyngioma
	Parasellar meningioma
	Aneurysm (ICA, ophthalmic, ACA, ACommA)
Retrochiasmatic	Infarction (*e.g.* anterior choroidal artery, PCA)
	Neoplasm, either primary glial or metastatic
	Multiple sclerosis/ADEM (demyelinating disease)
	AVM
	Temporal lobectomy

Abbreviations: ACA, anterior cerebral artery; ACommA, anterior communicating artery; ADEM, acute disseminated encephalomyelitis; ICA, internal carotid artery; PCA, posterior cerebral artery.

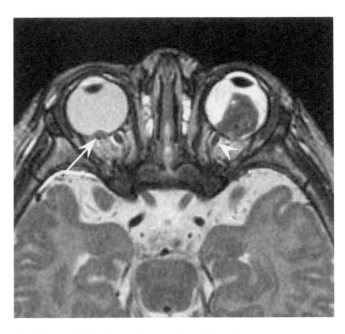

Fig. 2.8 Axial 3-D fast spin echo T2-weighted image shows a large mass within the left globe extending to the level of the optic disc and nerve (*arrowhead*). Note the smaller retinal-based mass (*arrow*) within the right globe near the macula in this patient with bilateral retinoblastoma.

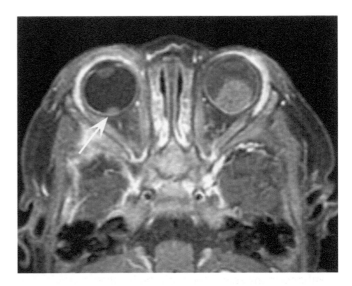

Fig. 2.9 Postcontrast fat-saturated T1-weighted image of the same patient as in **Fig. 2.8** shows homogeneous enhancement of both large and small (*arrow*) masses.

Retinoblastoma

• *Epidemiology.* Most common malignant extracranial solid tumor in children. Ninety percent occur before 5 years of age. Genetic predisposition due to loss of the *Rb* tumor suppressor gene (chromosome 13q), then a spontaneous mutation of *Rb* on the other (normal) chromosome ("two-hit" hypothesis).

- *Clinical presentation.* Leukocoria (white pupil), squint (strabismus), red/painful eye, secondary glaucoma. Most present by age 2 years; 75% unilateral, 25% bilateral.
- *Imaging.* Intraocular retinal-based mass. May be multifocal. Ninety percent show calcification on computed tomography (CT). MRI shows dark T2 signal and usually uniform enhancement. Thin-section three-dimensional (3-D) fast spin echo (FSE) T2 may be most sensitive for small retinal lesions.
- *Pathology.* Member of the PNET (primitive neuroectodermal tumor) family of tumors. Small round cells with Homer-Wright rosettes and Flexner-Wintersteiner rosettes (sheets of cells forming rosettes around an empty lumen). *Trilateral retinoblastoma* is bilateral retinoblastoma with pineoblastoma (another intracranial PNET).
- *Treatment.* Surgery (enucleation) or chemotherapy; 90% survival rate with early treatment. Genetic counseling is essential.

Case 2.2

A 7-year-old boy presents with blindness and weakness following Epstein-Barr virus (EBV) infection 1 month earlier (**Figs. 2.10, 2.11**).

Diagnosis

Right optic neuritis secondary to ADEM

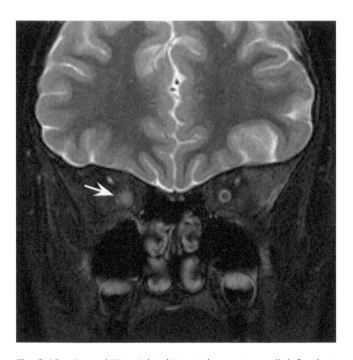

Fig. 2.10 Coronal T2-weighted image demonstrates ill-defined enlargement and high signal intensity of the right optic nerve-sheath complex (*arrow*). It may be difficult to distinguish the optic nerve and sheath on noncontrast images in the setting of pathologic involvement. The normal optic nerve and surrounding high signal of the sheath are clearly visible on the left.

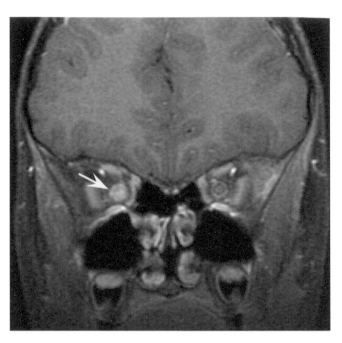

Fig. 2.11 Postcontrast fat-saturation image shows homogeneous enhancement of the enlarged right optic nerve-sheath complex (*arrow*). The homogeneous high signal intensity on T2WI and the diffuse, homogeneous enhancement postcontrast are consistent with optic neuritis in this patient with ADEM.

Acute Disseminated Encephalomyelitis
- *Epidemiology.* Monophasic demyelination that typically occurs after a viral illness or vaccination (smallpox, rabies, varicella, rubella).
- *Clinical presentation.* Acute focal neurologic deficits related to CNS demyelination, often including headache, meningeal signs, and seizures. Unilateral or bilateral optic neuritis (painful change/loss in vision) is common.
- *Imaging.* Orbital imaging may demonstrate edema and/or enhancement of the optic nerve(s) or chiasm. Abnormal brain/spinal cord findings include multifocal areas of T2 hyperintensity in the white matter, with variable enhancement. Imaging findings may mimic MS and clinical correlation is required for diagnosis.
- *Pathology.* Perivenous demyelination with axonal sparing and mononuclear infiltration. Thought to be an autoimmune response to a CNS antigen possibly similar to a viral epitope (molecular mimicry).
- *Treatment.* Steroids. In isolated cases intravenous immunoglobulin (IVIG) and plasmapheresis have been used. Most recover without persistent neurologic deficits, though deficits may persist. In some cases the process may be relapsing.

Case 2.3

A 41-year-old male had presented previously with complaints of sudden onset, red proptotic eye for 1 to 2 weeks.

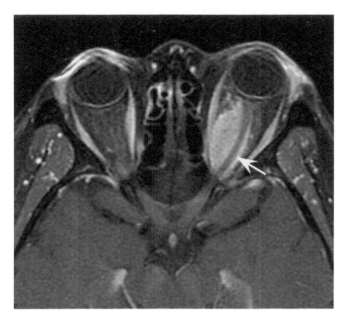

Fig. 2.12 Axial postcontrast fat-saturated T1-weighted MR image demonstrates a large well-circumscribed enhancing intraorbital mass surrounding a normal appearing left optic nerve (*arrow*).

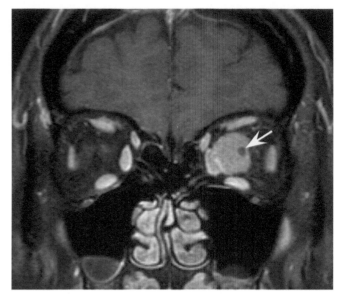

Fig. 2.13 A coronal postcontrast fat-saturated T1-weighted MR image clearly shows the encasement of the optic nerve (*arrow*) by this unusually large and eccentric optic nerve sheath meningioma.

CT scan showed intraorbital mass, hyperdense on precontrast images and homogeneously enhancing. The patient then developed significant loss of visual acuity over a 24-hour period, which prompted emergent biopsy (**Figs. 2.12, 2.13**).

Diagnosis

Unilateral (left) optic nerve sheath meningioma

Meningioma
- *Epidemiology.* Fifteen percent of primary intracranial tumors; peak at age 40 to 60 years, and females are more commonly affected. Incidence increased by prior radiation and the presence of genetic syndromes such as neurofibromatosis type 2 (NF-2).
- *Clinical presentation.* Headache, seizures, and/or focal neurologic deficit related to tumor location.
- *Imaging.* MR typically demonstrates a well-circumscribed extraaxial mass that is isointense on T1-weighted imaging (T1WI), iso/hyperintense on T2WI, and shows intense and homogeneous enhancement and often a dural tail. Associated vasogenic edema (best seen on T2 or fluid-attenuated inversion recovery [FLAIR]) in the brain parenchyma may be present, and bony hyperostosis may be appreciated. CT often best demonstrates associated calcifications or adjacent bony hyperostosis. Catheter angiography is often performed for preoperative embolization.
- *Pathology.* Originate from *arachnoid cap cells.* Blood supply is typically from carotid artery (ECA) branches, but meningiomas may parasitize pial vessels from the internal carotid circulation, especially around the skull base. Often involve adjacent dura and bone. Rarely metastasize. Several different pathologic types (three basic types: meningothelial, fibroblastic, and transitional) have been described. Grading: Grade I, benign; Grade II, atypical; Grade III, anaplastic/malignant.
- *Treatment.* Surgery with or without preoperative embolization. Radiation therapy may be indicated for residual and/or recurrent disease. Prognosis is generally good. Recurrence is dependent on grade and postoperative tumor residual volume.

Imaging Pearl

- Meningiomas of the optic nerve sheath may show peripheral linear enhancement along the sheath known as tramtracking.

Case 2.4

A 57-year-old female presented with progressive left vision loss and no specific diagnosis was made. She then re-presented nine years later with progressive right vision loss (**Figs. 2.14, 2.15**).

Diagnosis

Bilateral optic nerve sheath meningiomas

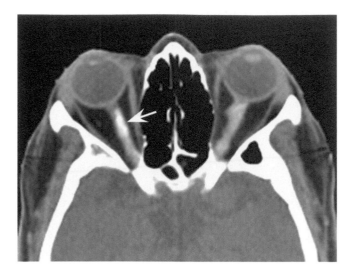

Fig. 2.14   Axial CT demonstrates irregular thickening and increased density along both intraorbital optic nerves, with areas of clear-cut calcification on the right (*arrow*).

Case 2.5

A 5-year-old female with neurofibromatosis type 1 (NF-1) presented with subacute onset of visual loss (**Figs. 2.16, 2.17**).

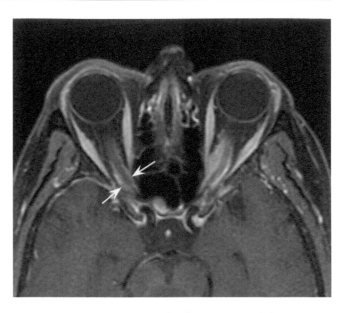

Fig. 2.15   Postcontrast T1-weighted MR image with fat saturation in the same patient as in **Fig. 2.14** shows enhancing tissue encasing both right and left optic nerves. The enhancing tissue is more mass-like on the left and more subtle on the right. The more linear enhancement along the right optic nerve sheath seen on post-gadolinium T1-weighted MRI is known as tram-tracking (*arrows*). Bilateral optic nerve sheath meningioma.

Diagnosis

Optic glioma

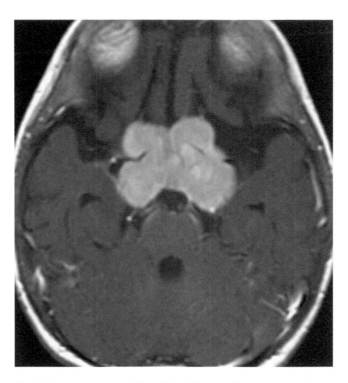

Fig. 2.16   Postcontrast T1-weighted image demonstrates a large homogeneously enhancing suprasellar extraaxial mass centered in the expected location of the optic chiasm, compatible with an optic glioma.

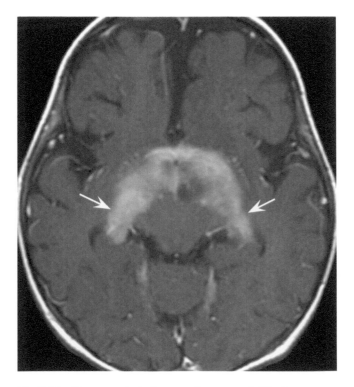

Fig. 2.17   More superiorly, the mass has a more infiltrating appearance as it extends posterolaterally along the expected course of both optic tracts (*arrows*).

Optic Glioma

- *Epidemiology.* Account for ~3 to 6% of pediatric brain tumors, peak age <10 years, female predominance, associated with NF-1. When bilateral, the lesions are almost always associated with NF-1.
- *Clinical presentation.* Visual dysfunction, hypothalamic dysfunction, obstructive hydrocephalus (when mass is large), occasionally diencephalic syndrome.
- *Imaging*: Diffuse fusiform enlargement of the optic nerve, chiasm, and/or tracts. May also appear as a more discrete suprasellar mass. Typically T1 hypointense and T2 hyperintense on MRI. Variable enhancement though usually moderate to marked. Other intracranial manifestations include plexiform neurofibromas, nonenhancing bright T2 lesions within white matter and deep gray nuclei thought to represent myelin vacuolization, sphenoid wing dysplasia, supratentorial and/or brainstem astrocytomas.
- *Pathology.* Optic gliomas in children are typically low-grade (World Health Organization [WHO] Grade 1, juvenile pilocytic astrocytoma). Unlike other juvenile pilocytic astrocytomas (Grade 1 gliomas), however, they tend to be noncystic in the optic pathway. Contain loose cells and eosinophilic Rosenthal fibers. May be higher-grade lesions in children. In adults, optic gliomas are typically high-grade lesions.
- *Treatment.* Most extend in the chiasm and along the optic tract and are therefore not surgically resectable; therefore they are usually observed, with chemotherapy and/or radiation therapy for progressive disease. Subtotal resection of large or exophytic lesions is sometimes considered, and resection of prechiasmatic lesions (confined to the optic nerve) can be curative. Primary rationale for chemotherapy is to delay the need for irradiation in children <5 years of age. Hormone replacement may be required for endocrine dysfunction.

Case 2.6

A 38-year-old female presents with bitemporal hemianopsia (**Figs. 2.18, 2.19, 2.20, 2.21**).

Diagnosis

Pituitary macroadenoma

Pituitary Adenomas

- *Epidemiology.* Account for 15% of intracranial tumors, most common suprasellar masses in adults. There is a *female predominance* with prolactin- and adrenocorticotrophic hormone (ACTH)-secreting tumors and a *male predominance* with growth hormone (GH)-secreting tumors. Twenty-five percent of tumors are nonsecreting.
- *Clinical presentation.* Varies by tumor type. Prolactin-secreting tumors present with *amenorrhea/galactorrhea* in women and decreased libido or impotence in men.

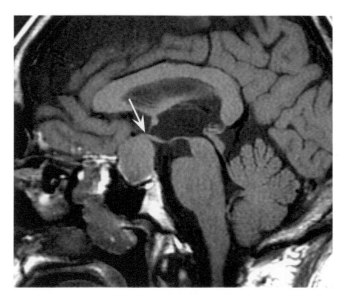

Fig. 2.18 Sagittal T1-weighted image of the sella demonstrates a soft tissue mass arising from and enlarging the sella. Note the suprasellar extension that elevates the optic chiasm (*arrow*).

GH-secreting tumors cause *acromegaly* in adults and *gigantism* in children. ACTH-secreting tumors cause *Cushing disease*. Visual changes occur when the mass grows large enough to impinge upon the optic apparatus.

- *Imaging.* CT shows sellar expansion with bony remodeling. Most are homogeneous and isodense but may be hyperdense if hemorrhagic. Macroadenomas are typically intermediate signal intensity on both T1- and T2WI and show homogeneous enhancement post-gadolinium,

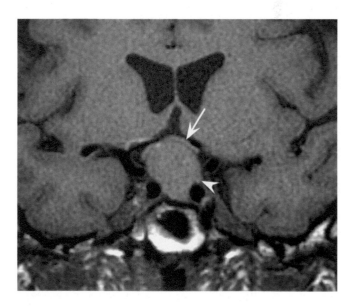

Fig. 2.19 Coronal T1-weighted image clearly shows thinning of the superiorly displaced optic chiasm (*arrow*) as it drapes over the sellar and suprasellar mass. The mass extends superolaterally over the left cavernous internal carotid artery (*arrowhead*), suggesting possible invasion into the cavernous sinus.

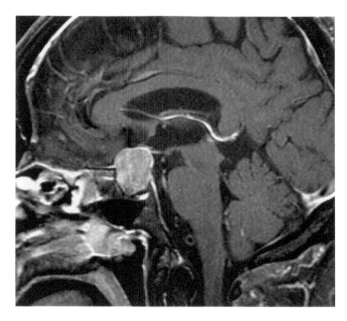

Fig. 2.20 Following contrast administration the mass enhances homogeneously. The imaging appearance is most consistent with pituitary macroadenoma.

though there may be areas of cystic or necrotic change and/or hemorrhage. Cavernous sinus compression or invasion may occur. Posterior pituitary is typically hyperintense on T1 ("bright spot") and may be displaced by the mass. In patients presenting with diabetes insipidus, the bright spot may be absent. Microadenomas typically show delayed and *decreased enhancement* on dynamic

contrast-enhanced imaging as compared with normal pituitary gland.

- *Pathology.* Diffuse pattern of monotonous polygonal cells. Hematoxylin-eosin (H&E) staining reveals acidophils, basophils, or chromophobes (null cells) depending on tumor type.
- *Treatment.* Surgery (transsphenoidal resection). Consider dopamine agonist (e.g., bromocriptine) for prolactinomas, octreotide (somatostatin analog) for GH-secreting tumors. Radiation therapy may be used for residual or recurrent disease. Pituitary apoplexy due to intratumoral infarction and/or hemorrhage is a surgical emergency usually treated with steroids and prompt surgical decompression.

Case 2.7

A 50-year-old male complains of headache, progressive visual loss, and reduced libido (**Figs. 2.22, 2.23**).

Diagnosis

Craniopharyngioma

Craniopharyngiomas
- *Epidemiology.* Account for 2 to 5% of primary intracranial tumors. There is no gender predominance. Bimodal age distribution with a peak at <20 years of age and a second peak at 50 years.

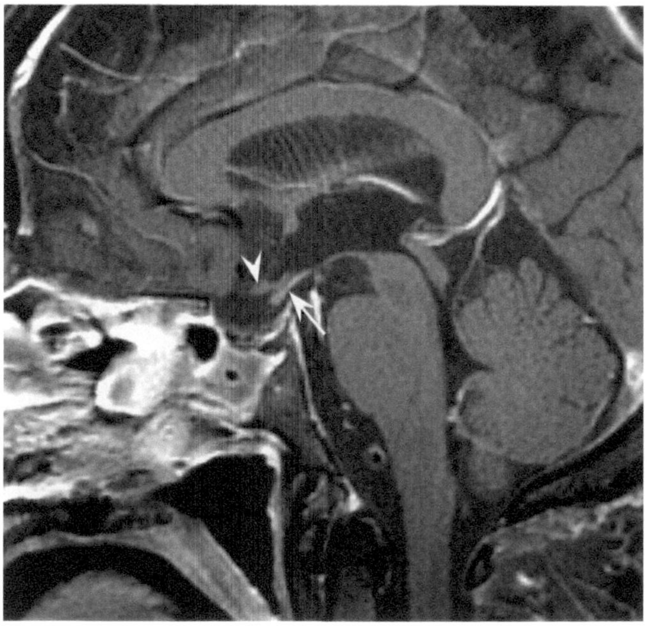

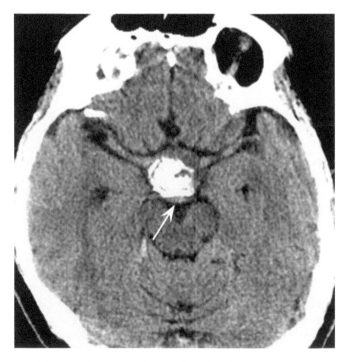

Fig. 2.21 Postcontrast T1-weighted image after transsphenoidal surgery with gross total resection of the mass. Note the return to normal position of the optic chiasm (*arrowhead*) and pituitary stalk (*arrow*). The sella remains enlarged.

Fig. 2.22 Axial CT image shows a densely calcified suprasellar mass which displaces the optic chiasm (*arrow*) posteriorly.

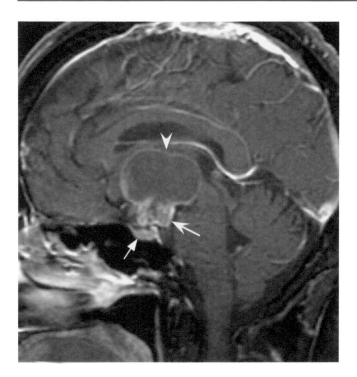

Fig. 2.23 Sagittal postcontrast fat-saturated T1-weighted MR image in the same patient as in **Fig. 2.22** shows a large heterogeneous suprasellar mass, with a more inferior solid enhancing component (*concave arrow*) and a more superior rim-enhancing cystic component (*arrowhead*). The more inferior solid component was calcified on the CT scan. This is consistent with craniopharyngioma. Note the normally enhancing pituitary gland (*small straight arrow*) within the sella inferiorly.

- *Clinical features.* Present with headache, endocrine abnormalities (hypopituitarism) from pituitary compression, and visual abnormalities from optic chiasm compression. Hydrocephalus and papilledema may be present.
- *Imaging.* Heterogeneous, mixed solid and cystic, often calcified, suprasellar mass with variable intrasellar extension. Enhancement of solid components and periphery of cystic components is typical. Cysts are usually heterogeneous on CT and MRI due to variable protein content and/or hemorrhage.
- *Pathology.* Derived from squamous cells from *Rathke pouch* (a diverticulum that arises from the roof of the primitive oral cavity). The cyst is typically filled with *"machine oil" fluid* and cholesterol crystals that can elicit a granulomatous reaction. Nearly always contains *calcification.*
- *Treatment.* Surgery is the treatment of choice, but involvement of hypothalamus/pituitary stalk results in high morbidity due to radical surgery; this combined with high recurrence rates has led to the concept of subtotal resection followed by postoperative radiotherapy. Adjunctive therapies include stereotactic cyst aspiration and cyst sclerotherapy.

Case 2.8

A 17-year-old male presents with acute left homonymous hemianopsia following a motor vehicle accident. He complains of neck pain and is found to have a vertebral artery dissection (**Figs. 2.24, 2.25, 2.26**).

Diagnosis

Occipital lobe infarction due to vertebral artery dissection and embolus to PCA

Acute Ischemic Stroke (PCA Distribution)

- *Epidemiology.* Stroke is the third leading cause of death in the United States after heart disease and cancer. Posterior circulation (vertebrobasilar) stroke is much less common than anterior circulation (ICA/MCA/ACA). Stroke in the young (as in this case) has a distinct epidemiology, with main contributing factors including trauma (cervical arterial dissection), vascular disease (e.g., fibromuscular dysplasia, moyamoya disease), inflammatory disease (vasculitides), hypercoagulable states (e.g., protein C and S deficiencies, antithrombin III deficiency), or genetic or cardiac abnormalities.
- *Clinical presentation.* As the PCAs supply the inferomedial temporal lobes and medial occipital lobes (see **Table 2.1**), the clinical symptoms depend on precise location of the infarction. Acute contralateral homonymous hemianopsia with macular sparing (the macula has bilateral blood supply) is most common. Potential associated findings include alexia, anomia (especially color), and impaired

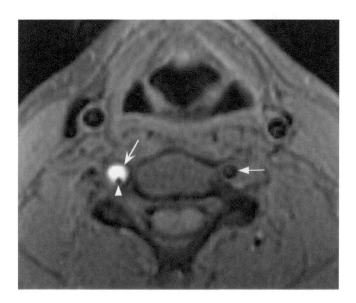

Fig. 2.24 Axial T1-weighted image with fat saturation (no contrast) demonstrates a peripheral "crescent" of bright signal (*concave arrow*) peripheral to the right vertebral artery flow void, compatible with arterial dissection and intramural hematoma. The narrowed residual right vertebral artery flow void (*arrowhead*) and the normal left vertebral artery flow void (*straight arrow*) can be compared.

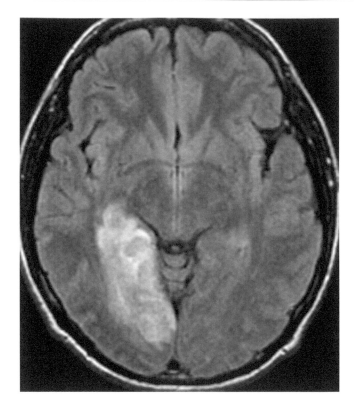

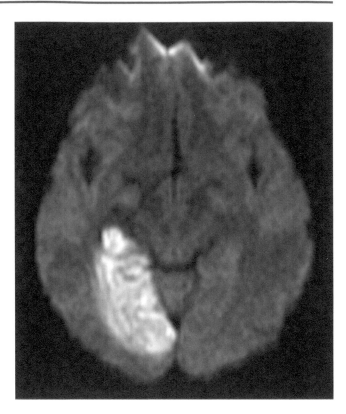

Fig. 2.25 Axial FLAIR image shows swelling and cytotoxic edema within the right posteromedial temporal lobe and paramedian occipital lobe consistent with an acute infarct in the right PCA territory.

Fig. 2.26 A corresponding axial diffusion-weighted image in the same patient as in **Fig. 2.25** shows hyperintensity, which confirms acute ischemia.

Table 2.3 CT and MR Imaging Features of Ischemic Stroke

Time after Stroke	Pathophysiology	MRI	CT
Immediate	Vessel occlusion Perfusion deficit	• Absent flow void on spin echo MRI • No flow-related enhancement on MRA • Hyperintense vessel on FLAIR • Arterial enhancement distal to stenosis (due to collaterals, delayed washout) • Perfusion defects: delayed MTT	• Hyperdense MCA • Stenosis/occlusion on CTA • Arterial enhancement distal to stenosis (due to collaterals, delayed washout) • Perfusion defects: delayed MTT

Minutes to Hours	Cell death—Infarction	• Reduction in diffusion (low ADC)
		• High signal on T2/FLAIR
		• Low CBF and CBV
			• Hypodense tissue
			  ◦ "Insular ribbon" sign
			  ◦ Basal ganglia hypodensity
			• Mass effect
			  ◦ Sulcal effacement
			• Low CBF and CBV

Hours to Days	Blood–brain barrier defects	• Vasogenic edema • Increasing mass effect • Petechial hemorrhage • Contrast enhancement	• Vasogenic edema • Increasing mass effect • Petechial hemorrhage • Contrast enhancement
Weeks to Months	Encephalomalacia	• Resolving mass effect and enhancement • Focal volume loss • Residual T2 prolongation (gliosis) • Facilitated diffusion (high ADC)	• Resolving mass effect and enhancement • Focal volume loss • Residual low attenuation (gliosis)

Abbreviations: ADC, apparent diffusion coefficient; CBF, cerebral blood flow; CBV, cerebral blood volume; CT, computed tomography; CTA, CT angiography; FLAIR, fluid-attenuated inversion recovery; MCA, middle cerebral artery; MRA, magnetic resonance angiography; MRI, magnetic resonance imaging; MTT, mean transit time.

memory. Bilateral PCA occlusion can cause cortical blindness, central scotomas (from bilateral poles), altitudinal defects, and/or prosopagnosia (inability to name faces, localization is occipitotemporal or "fusiform" gyrus).

- *Imaging.* See **Table 2.3** for details of stroke imaging. In cases of dissection, computed tomography angiography (CTA) or magnetic resonance angiography (MRA) may demonstrate focal luminal narrowing of the involved vessel. Axial T1WI with fat saturation best identify intramural hematoma in the subacute stage (few days to weeks), seen as a crescent of T1 hyperintensity within the vessel wall. Conventional angiography may show an intimal flap, but it is usually unnecessary for the diagnosis.
- *Pathology.* Stroke pathology changes as the lesion evolves. By 6 hours, there is microvacuolation (dilated mitochondria) and shrunken hyperchromatic cells. By 12 to 24 hours there is neuronal necrosis and pyknosis. By 1 to 2 days polymorphonuclear leukocytes (PMNs) accumulate. At 2 to 5 days there is blood–brain barrier breakdown and edema. At 5 to 7 days macrophage infiltration occurs. At 10 to 20 days there is astrocytosis around the infarct, and enhancement begins secondary to neovascularization. After 3 months there is a cystic space (coagulation necrosis) with surrounding astrocytosis (glial scar).
- *Treatment.* Thrombolysis (with intravenous tissue plasminogen activator) may be considered in the acute stage. Anticoagulation (e.g., with warfarin) and/or antiplatelet agents (e.g., aspirin) may help to prevent further strokes. A variety of devices for endovascular mechanical thrombectomy are under study. Treatment of dissection includes anticoagulation but can require endovascular occlusion, particularly in the setting of trauma.

3 Oculomotor Nerve

Functions

- General somatic efferent (GSE). Somatic motor innervation to
  - Inferior rectus (IR). Depresses eye.
  - Superior rectus (SR). Elevates eye.
  - Medial rectus (MR). Adducts eye.
  - Inferior oblique (IO). Elevates eye when eye adducted; extorts (laterally rotates) eye when eye abducted.
  - Levator palpebrae superioris (LPS). Raises eyelid.
- General visceral efferent (GVE). Parasympathetic innervation to
  - Sphincter pupillae. Constricts pupil (miosis).
  - Ciliary muscles. Contraction causes lens to bulge (accommodation).

Anatomy

- The oculomotor *nuclear complex* is in the midbrain at the level of the superior colliculus, ventral to the cerebral aqueduct (separated by periaqueductal gray matter, PAG) and dorsal to the medial longitudinal fasciculus (MLF) (**Figs. 3.1, 3.2, 3.3**).

- Subnuclei supply individual muscles. Lateral subnuclei supply the ipsilateral IR, IO, and MR muscles. Medial subnucleus supplies contralateral SR (via decussating axons). Central subnucleus in the midline supplies the LPS bilaterally.
- The Edinger-Westphal nucleus is in the rostral portion of the oculomotor nuclear complex and supplies preganglionic parasympathetic innervation.

Nerve Course

- *Fascicular portion.* Lower motor nerve (LMN) axons (with parasympathetic fibers located dorsal and superficial to somatic motor axons) course through the tegmentum of the midbrain, traversing the MLF and decussating fibers of the superior cerebellar peduncle (SCP), the red nucleus (RN), and the medial aspect of the cerebral peduncles to exit the midbrain and enter the interpeduncular cistern at the midbrain–pons junction.
- *Subarachnoid portion (in cistern).* Nerve passes between posterior cerebral artery (PCA) and superior cerebellar artery (SCA), courses forward inferolateral to the posterior communicating artery (PCommA) and medial to the uncus, pierces the dura lateral to posterior clinoid

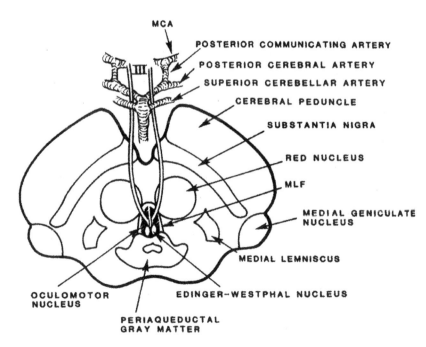

Fig. 3.1 Cross-section of midbrain at the level of the superior colliculus demonstrating oculomotor nucleus, Edinger-Westphal nucleus, and course of CN III (see text). (MCA, middle cerebral artery.) (MLF, medial longitudinal fasciculus.) (From Harnsberger HR. Handbook of Head and Neck Imaging [2nd ed.] St. Louis, MO: Mosby, 1995. Reprinted with permission.)

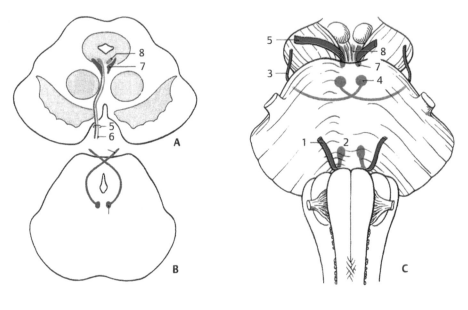

Fig. 3.2 Comparison of nuclear regions and exits of oculomotor, trochlear, and abducens nerves. **(A)** Midbrain at the level of the superior colliculus. **(B)** Midbrain at the level of the inferior colliculus. **(C)** Ventral view of brainstem. (1, abducens nerve; 2, abducens nucleus; 3, trochlear nerve; 4, trochlear nucleus; 5, oculomotor nerve; 6, visceromotor (parasympathetic) fibers; 7, oculomotor nucleus; 8, Edinger-Westphal nucleus.)

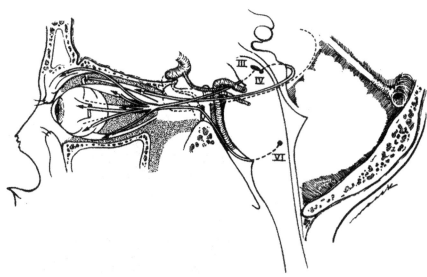

Fig. 3.3 Comparison of origins and courses of oculomotor, trochlear, and abducens nerves. The oculomotor and trochlear nerves originate in the midbrain, whereas the abducens nerve originates in the lower pons. All three nerves ultimately exit the cranial base into the eye via the superior orbital fissure (see text for details). (From Harnsberger HR. Handbook of Head and Neck Imaging [2nd ed.] St. Louis, MO: Mosby, 1995. Reprinted with permission.)

process, and enters the "oculomotor triangle" (formed by dural folds from tentorium cerebelli attachments) in the posterior roof of the cavernous sinus to wind up in the superolateral wall of the *cavernous sinus* (superior to cranial nerve [CN] IV) (**Fig. 3.4**).

- After traversing the cavernous sinus, CN III reaches the *superior orbital fissure* (SOF), where it divides into superior and inferior divisions, both of which pass into the *orbit* through the annulus of Zinn. The superior division ascends lateral to the optic nerve to supply SR and LPS; the inferior division supplies IR, IO, MR, and the presynaptic parasympathetics (**Fig. 3.5**).

- Presynaptic parasympathetic fibers terminate in the ciliary ganglion near the apex of the extraocular muscle cone. Postganglionic fibers form six to 10 *short ciliary nerves* that travel with *nasociliary nerve* (of CN V$_1$) forward between the choroid and sclera to reach the ciliary body and iris. These control *sphincter pupillae* muscle to

cause pupillary constriction and *ciliary muscles* to cause lens accommodation (**Fig. 3.5**).

Oculomotor Nerve: Normal Images (Figs. 3.6, 3.7, 3.8, 3.9, 3.10, 3.11, 3.12, 3.13)

Oculomotor Nerve Lesions

- Oculomotor palsies may be categorized as isolated (only CN III affected) or complex (multiple cranial neuropathies including CN III).

- Most common causes of isolated CN III palsies in adult are ischemia, mass effect due to aneurysm, uncal herniation, and neoplasm.

- Complex palsies affecting CN III are usually due to brainstem lesions affecting other tracts/nerves or meningeal

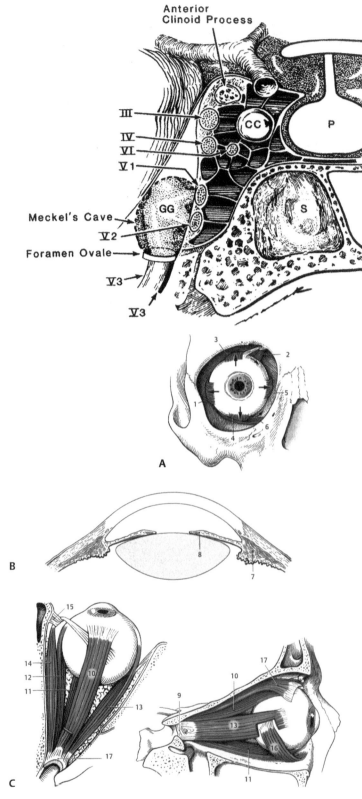

Fig. 3.4 Coronal view through the cavernous sinus demonstrates CN III, IV, VI, and V_1 and V_2 in the lateral wall of the cavernous sinus and CN VI within the cavernous sinus adjacent to the cavernous portion of the internal carotid artery. Note that CN V_3 does not enter the cavernous sinus but rather leaves the cranial base through the foramen ovale. (CC, cavernous segment of internal carotid artery; GG, Gasserian ganglion; P, pituitary gland; S, sphenoid sinus.) (From Harnsberger HR. Handbook of Head and Neck Imaging [2nd ed.] St. Louis, MO: Mosby, 1995. Reprinted with permission.)

or skull base pathologies that affect adjacent CNs (e.g., cavernous sinus, SOF, orbital apex).

- CN III palsy may be complete or incomplete, with the pupil variably involved or spared.
- In complete oculomotor palsy, the eye is depressed and abducted ("down-and-out") due to unopposed action of the SO and LR muscles.
- Pupillomotor (parasympathetic) fibers are situated peripherally in the nerve, so ischemia is thought to prefer-

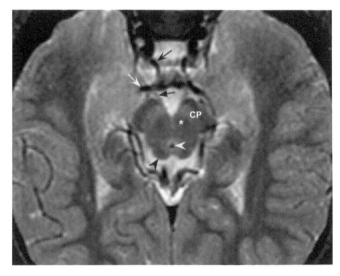

Fig. 3.5 Schematic of extraocular and intraocular muscles. **(A)** Anterior view. (1, LR muscle; 2, SO muscle; 3, SR muscle; 4, IR muscle; 5, MR muscle; 6, IO muscle.) **(B)** Intraocular muscles. (7, ciliary muscle; 8, sphincter pupillae muscle.) **(C)** Superior (left) and lateral (right) views. (9, common annular tendon [annulus of Zinn]; 10, SR muscle; 11, IR muscle; 12, MR muscle; 13, LR muscle; 14, SO muscle; 15, trochlea; 16, IO muscle; 17, LPS muscle.)

Fig. 3.6 Axial fast spin echo T2 at the level of the midbrain demonstrates normal cerebral peduncles (CP) and red nuclei (*asterisk*) and superior colliculi (*black arrowhead*). The oculomotor nuclei are located just anterior to the cerebral aqueduct of Sylvius (*white arrowhead*). Note both CN III exiting anteriorly into the interpeduncular fossa. The right CN III (*black straight arrow*) passes adjacent to the right PCA (*white curved arrow*) and PCommA (*black concave arrow*).

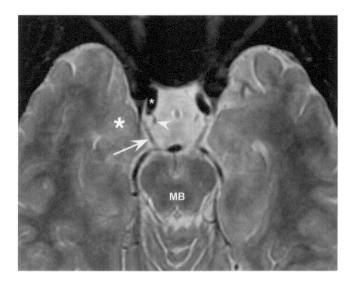

Fig. 3.7 Axial fast spin echo T2-weighted image demonstrates both CN III (*arrow* on right CN III) exiting the midbrain (MB) and traversing the subarachnoid space to the posterior margin of the cavernous sinus. CN III passes lateral to the PCommA (*arrowhead*) as it exits the right supraclinoid carotid artery (*white asterisk*) and medial to the adjacent uncus of the temporal lobe (*black asterisk*).

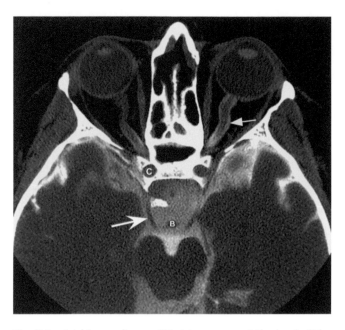

Fig. 3.8 Axial image from a CT cisternogram at the level of the midbrain shows the cisternal segment of CN III (*concave arrow*) traversing the subarachnoid space. In addition, there is subarachnoid contrast within the optic sheath (*straight arrow*) along the left optic nerve. Note the (B) basilar artery and (C) carotid canal.

entially affect somatic motor fibers in the interior of the nerve (supplied by the *vasa nervorum*), whereas compressive lesions preferentially (or first) affect the more superficial pupillomotor fibers. If parasympathetic fibers are involved, the pupil is "fixed and dilated" (mydriatic and unresponsive to light due to dysfunction of pupillary sphincter) and there is paralysis of lens accommodation (ciliary muscle dysfunction).

- Imaging evaluation of patients with nuclear CN III lesions should include magnetic resonance imaging (MRI) (brainstem to orbit) and MR angiography (MRA) (to evaluate the posterior circulation).

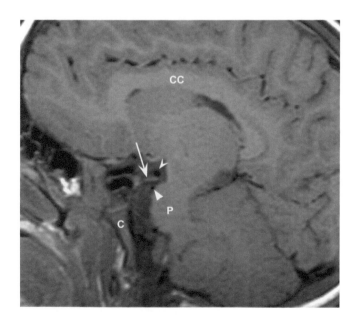

Fig. 3.9 Sagittal T1-weighted image demonstrates CN III (*arrow*) passing between the PCA (*concave arrowhead*) and SCA (*straight arrowhead*) as it exits the midbrain. Note the pons (P), clivus (C) and corpus callosum (CC) on this midsagittal image.

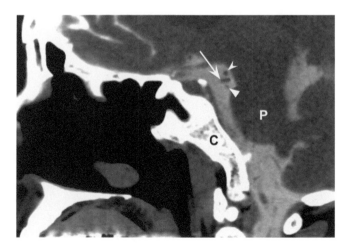

Fig. 3.10 Reconstructed sagittal image from a CT cisternogram shows CN III (*arrow*) passing between the PCA (*concave arrowhead*) and SCA (*straight arrowhead*) nicely outlined by contrast within the subarachoid space. Note the pons (P) and clivus (C).

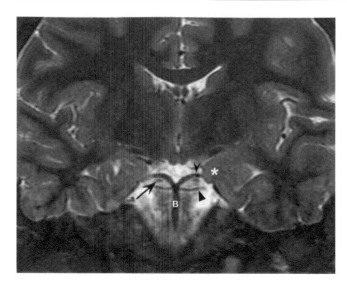

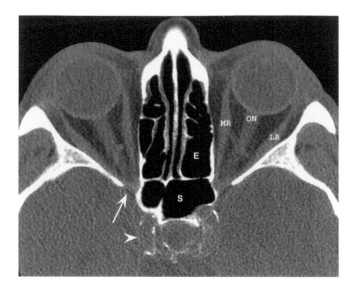

Fig. 3.11 Coronal fast spin echo T2-weighted image demonstrates CN III (*arrow*) passing between the PCA (*concave arrowhead*) and SCA (*straight arrowhead*), distal branches of the basilar artery (B). Note the close relationship of the uncus (*asterisk*) to CN III.

Fig. 3.12 Axial CT image of the orbits with soft tissue window shows a normal superior orbital fissure (*arrow*). Note the thin mural calcifications along the cavernous segment of the internal carotid artery (*arrowhead*). Note the normal MR and LR muscles, and optic nerve-sheath complex (ON). Normal aeration is seen within the sphenoid sinus (S) and ethmoid air cells (E).

Types

Brainstem Lesions (Nucleus or Fascicular Segment of Nerve)

- Congenital CN III palsies are rare but make up 20 to 43% of oculomotor palsies in children (secondary to maldevelopment, birth trauma, or intrauterine insult).
- Ischemia.

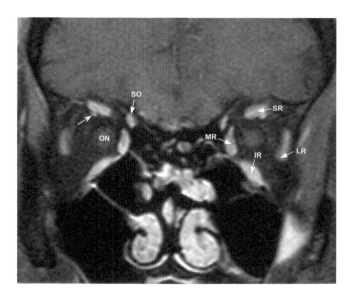

Fig. 3.13 Coronal postcontrast fat-saturated T1-weighted image shows the normal orbital anatomy. Note the normal enhancement of the extraocular muscles including the SR/LPS (levator palpebrae superioris) complex, MR, LR, IR, and SO. Enhancement of the right superior ophthalmic vein (SOV, *arrow*) is seen just inferior to the SR muscle. The normal optic nerve-sheath complex (ON) does not significantly enhance.

- Neoplasm.
- Infectious/inflammatory.
- Demyelinating disease.
- A pure nuclear lesion is rare but characteristically results in unilateral oculomotor palsy with weakness of the ipsilateral and contralateral SR and LPS (with bilateral incomplete ptosis due to bilateral innervation of the SR and LPS).
- Nuclear CN III lesion associated with ataxia, nystagmus, and altered mental status should prompt consideration of Wernicke encephalopathy (thiamine deficiency with neuronal loss and gliosis in ocular motor nuclei, usually with bilateral ophthalmoparesis).
- Specific named midbrain syndromes:
  1. *Weber syndrome.* Ventral midbrain lesion affecting CN III (ipsilateral oculomotor palsy) and cerebral peduncle (contralateral hemiparesis/hemiplegia).
  2. *Claude syndrome.* Lesion of midbrain tegmentum affecting CN III (ipsilateral oculomotor palsy), RN (contralateral tremor), and SCP (ipsilateral ataxia).
  3. *Benedikt syndrome.* Lesion of midbrain tegmentum affecting CN III (ipsilateral oculomotor palsy), RN (contralateral tremor), SCP (ipsilateral ataxia), and the cerebral peduncle (contralateral hemiparesis/hemiplegia).
  4. *Nothnagel syndrome.* Lesion of midbrain tectum affecting CN III and SCP, causing unilateral or bilateral oculomotor palsy, gaze paralysis, and ipsilateral ataxia.

Lesions in the Subarachnoid Space (Cisternal Segment of Nerve)

- *Ischemia.* Isolated oculomotor palsy with *pupillary sparing* is usually indicative of ischemic oculomotor palsy (caused by diabetes, hypertension, atherosclerosis). Diabetic third nerve palsy is usually painful, develops over a few hours, and has a good prognosis for recovery. Imaging is not indicated in the clinical setting of a classic diabetic oculomotor palsy.
- *Compression by aneurysm* (see **Table 3.1**). Usually due to PCommA aneurysm. Extrinsic compression preferentially affects outer pupillomotor (parasympathetic) fibers early, resulting in a fixed and dilated (mydriatic) pupil.
- *Uncal herniation.* As with aneurysmal compression, compression of CN III by the uncus leads to an ipsilateral fixed and dilated pupil.
- Compression by tumor (typically schwannoma or meningioma).
- Leptomeningeal spread of tumor.
- Demyelinating disease (Miller-Fisher variant of Guillain-Barré syndrome includes ophthalmoplegia, ataxia, and areflexia).
- Inflammation/meningitis with secondary neuritis.
- Ophthalmoplegic migraine.
- Radiation injury (abrupt onset, usually 1–2 years after radiation therapy, enhancement along CN common).

Lesions in the Cavernous Sinus (Cavernous Segment of Nerve)

- Contents of cavernous sinus: CN III, IV, VI, V_1, V_2, sympathetic fibers, and the cavernous segment of the internal carotid artery (ICA). CN III palsy caused by a cavernous sinus lesion is often associated with other cranial neuropathies.
- Complete *cavernous sinus syndrome* involves CN III, IV, VI, V_1, V_2 and ICA sympathetics (total unilateral ophthalmoplegia, V_1/V_2 pain/paresthesias/sensory loss). Pupil is fixed and at midposition due to loss of both sympathetics and parasympathetics.
- Specific pathologies:
  1. Neoplasm (compression, e.g., meningioma, vs. infiltration, e.g., lymphoma).
  2. Vascular (carotid-cavernous fistula [CCF], giant ICA aneurysm)—most often affects CN VI first. Direct (high-flow) CCF can produce pulsatile exophthalmos, chemosis, ophthalmoplegia, vision loss, and an orbital bruit; whereas indirect (low-flow) CCFs are dural fistulae and can present with more subtle findings of conjunctival injection and/or venous stasis retinopathy.
  3. Inflammatory (e.g., sarcoidosis, Tolosa-Hunt syndrome).
  4. Infection (e.g., often due to bacterial or fungal sphenoid sinusitis with extension to the cavernous sinus). *Cavernous sinus thrombosis* is due usually to direct trauma or extension of an orbital or facial infection

Table 3.1 Nonhemorrhagic Clinical Presentations of Cerebral Aneurysms

Presenting Finding	Type of Aneurysm and Mechanism
Visual loss	• Usually due to compression of optic nerve or chiasm by proximal ICA, carotid-ophthalmic, or ACommA large (>10 mm) or giant (>25 mm) aneurysms • Symptoms include fluctuating but progressive visual loss (can be misdiagnosed as optic neuritis but much slower in onset) • Inferior nasal quadrantanopsia or junctional scotoma (ipsilateral central scotoma and contralateral superior temporal quandrantanopsia): ipsilateral carotid-ophthalmic aneurysm (due to pressure on optic nerve from overlying falciform ligament, the dural fold between the anterior clinoid processes) • Bitemporal hemianopsia: superior hypophyseal artery, A1 or ACommA aneurysm compressing the optic chiasm • Homonymous hemianopia: (rare) retrochiasmal optic tract compression by distal supraclinoid ICA aneurysm
Oculomotor palsy	• Most common neuroophthalmologic sign of aneurysm mass effect • Usually due to PCommA aneurysm compressing CN III in subarachnoid space • May also be caused by intracavernous, basilar artery, SCA, and PCA aneurysms • Ninety percent of patients with PCommA aneurysms have symptoms before rupture • Pupillary involvement occurs early, other signs late • Distinguish from ischemic oculomotor neuropathy (e.g., from diabetes, HTN) which is pupil-sparing and tends to affect an older population
Trochlear palsy	• Intracavernous carotid aneurysm can compress trochlear nerve (CN IV) in cavernous sinus • Usually obscured by combined CN III and/or VI palsies • SCA aneurysms may compress CN IV in ambient cistern
Abducens palsy	• Intracavernous carotid aneurysm can compress abducens nerve (CN VI) in cavernous sinus • Often associated with ipsilateral Horner syndrome (ptosis, miosis, anhidrosis) • Presence of ipsilateral CN V_1 pain/sensory loss (cornea, forehead) is an important localizing sign
Seizures	• Usually MCA aneurysm with mass effect on temporal lobe; may also be laterally directed supraclinoid ICA aneurysm, may see associated temporal lobe edema
Diabetes insipidus	• Usually ACommA aneurysm due to compression of the pituitary stalk or hypothalamus

Abbreviations: ACommA, anterior communicating artery; CN, cranial nerve; HTN, hypertension; ICA, internal carotid artery; MCA, middle cerebral artery; PCA, posterior cerebral artery; SCA, superior cerebellar artery.

and presents with retroorbital pain, proptosis, chemosis, eyelid edema, and ophthalmoplegia.

5. Pituitary apoplexy (acute enlargement of the pituitary gland leads to acute cavernous sinus compression).

6. Radiation injury (e.g., following radiosurgery for cavernous sinus meningiomas).

Lesions in the Superior Orbital Fissure

- Contents of superior orbital fissure: CN III, IV, VI, V_1, superior ophthalmic vein.
- Complete *superior orbital fissure* syndrome involves CN III, IV, VI, V_1, and superior ophthalmic vein (total ophthalmoplegia, V_1 pain/paresthesias/sensory loss, proptosis/chemosis/lid edema). Pupil is fixed and mydriatic due to preferential loss of parasympathetics.
- The superior and inferior divisions of CN III can be affected separately here as they divide and enter the orbit.
- Pathology of individual lesions is similar to the cavernous sinus (above) but also can include bony lesions (e.g., fibrous dysplasia, osseous metastases).

Lesions of the Orbit

- Although lesions of the orbit may impair extraocular muscle function, a true CN III palsy does not usually result from orbital lesions. Myasthenia gravis may present with ophthalmoparesis and mimic CN III palsy.
- In situations of orbital invasion by tumor (e.g., squamous cell carcinoma, melanoma, basal cell carcinoma), consider the possibility of perineural spread of disease along CN III back to the superior orbital fissure/cavernous sinus.

Treatment

- Correction of diplopia following CN III injury may require prism therapy and/or strabismus surgery. Correction should not be undertaken until recovery is complete; in most cases the deficit stabilizes within ~6 months.

Oculomotor Nerve: Pathologic Images

Case 3.1

A 55-year-old female with breast carcinoma presents with acute onset of a left CN III palsy (**Figs. 3.14, 3.15**).

Diagnosis

Breast cancer metastasis to left midbrain

Metastatic Tumors to the Nervous System

- *Epidemiology.* More common than all other intracranial tumors combined. Occur in 10 to 30% of all patients with systemic cancer.
- *Clinical presentation.* Present with headache, back pain, focal neurologic deficit, and/or seizures depending on location.

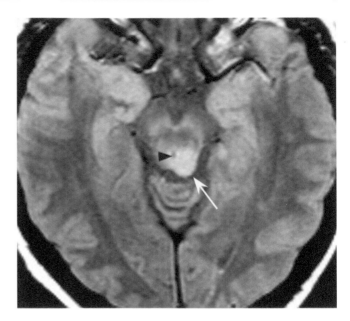

Fig. 3.14 Axial proton density-weighted image demonstrates a focal high signal intensity in the dorsal left midbrain with slight mass effect upon the cerebral aqueduct (*arrowhead*) and expansion of the left superior colliculus (*arrow*).

- ○ *Skull.* Breast, lung, prostate, and multiple myeloma are most common.
- ○ *Dural.* Breast and lung are most common.
- ○ *Leptomeningeal.* Breast, lung, melanoma, leukemia/lymphoma are particularly common. Leptomeningeal carcinomatosis is diffuse seeding of the leptomeninges by tumor, usually causing cranial neuropathies and cerebrospinal fluid (CSF) obstruction. CSF analysis typi-

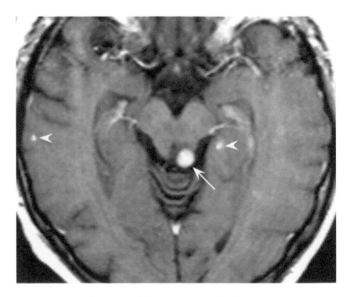

Fig. 3.15 Axial post-gadolinium T1-weighted image at the same level demonstrates a round, intensely enhancing mass centered on the left superior colliculus (*arrow*). Mild peripheral hypointensity is compatible with adjacent vasogenic edema. Additional enhancing punctate lesions (*arrowheads*) are present. This patient was subsequently found to have diffuse metastatic breast cancer.

cally shows increased protein and normal or decreased glucose, and CSF cytology may show neoplastic cells.

- ○ *Parenchymal* (accounts for 30% of brain tumors; mean survival is 3–6 months). Lung, breast, melanoma, renal cell, and colon adenocarcinoma are the most common primary malignancies (in order of decreasing relative frequency). Site specificity: cerebrum > cerebellum > brainstem > spinal cord.
- *Imaging. Parenchymal disease:* enhancing lesion(s) often with extensive surrounding vasogenic edema. Though usually multiple, solitary metastases may be found in approximately one quarter to one third of cases. They typically occur at the *gray–white junction* and are round and well-circumscribed. Hemorrhage is especially common with hypervascular tumors, in particular *melanoma, renal cell carcinoma, papillary thyroid carcinoma,* and *choriocarcinoma.* Melanoma may be hyperintense on pre-gadolinium T1-weighted image (T1WI) due to melanin or hemorrhage. *Leptomeningeal disease:* focal or diffuse leptomeningeal enhancement may be seen on postcontrast imaging.
- *Treatment.* Surgery for large symptomatic metastases, otherwise radiotherapy (RT) ± radiosurgery ± chemotherapy.

Case 3.2

A 55-year-old male presents with acute onset of a right CN III palsy. He has a complete right oculomotor palsy, but he also has paresis of left upgaze and bilateral incomplete ptosis (**Figs. 3.16, 3.17, 3.18**).

Diagnosis

Right midbrain infarction affecting CN III nucleus and fascicles

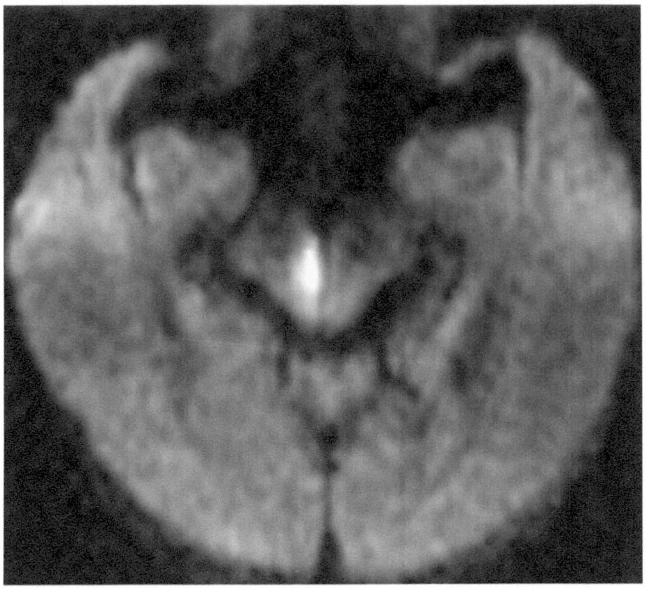

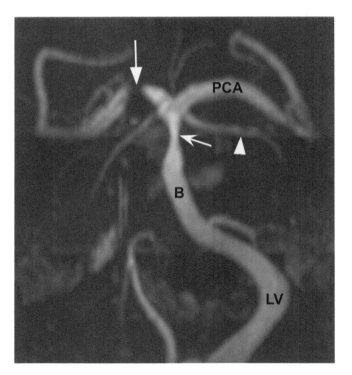

Fig. 3.17 Axial diffusion-weighted image in the same patient as in **Fig. 3.16** shows corresponding hyperintensity, consistent with reduced diffusion in the setting of acute infarction.

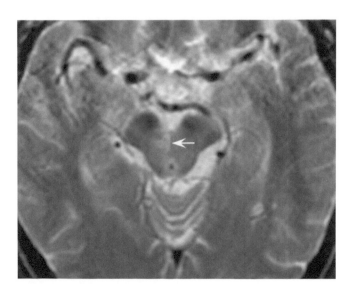

Fig. 3.16 Axial fast spin echo T2-weighted image demonstrates a focus of hyperintensity (*arrow*) in the right paramedian midbrain along the course of the exiting fibers of CN III. Note the sharply defined margin with respect to the midline, which is typical of a perforator infarct.

Fig. 3.18 An anterior projection of the vertebrobasilar system from a 3-D time-of-flight MRA in this patient with a dominant left vertebral artery (LV) and tortuous basilar artery (B) demonstrates a focal occlusion of the right posterior cerebral artery (*straight arrow*) (PCA labeled on left) as well as severe stenosis of the distal basilar artery (*concave arrow*), proximal to the take-off of the superior cerebellar artery (*straight arrowhead*). Atherosclerotic change and occlusion of a perforator artery arising from the right PCA were felt to be the etiology of the infarct.

Clinical Pearls

- Posterior circulation (vertebrobasilar) ischemia may manifest as transient ischemic attacks (TIAs) consisting of vertigo, dizziness, alteration in consciousness, loss of vision, dysarthria, weakness, and/or other specific CN findings
- Crossed deficits (motor or sensory deficit on one side of the face and the opposite side of the body) signify brainstem dysfunction.
- Brainstem infarction is associated with CN deficits appropriate for the level of the brainstem affected (midbrain, pons, or medulla) (see Appendix A).
- An oculomotor nuclear lesion in the midbrain will lead to ipsilateral oculomotor palsy but also affect the contralateral LPS and SR muscles due to bilateral innervation. Associated findings such as contralateral hemiparesis or ataxia help localize the lesion and constitute named midbrain stroke syndromes (e.g., Weber, Claude, Benedikt, Nothnagel; see text above).

Imaging Pearls

- Difficult to evaluate the posterior fossa and brainstem with computed tomography (CT), typically need MRI.
- Acute infarction is associated with reduced (bright) diffusion.
- Brainstem perforator infarcts typically respect the midline.

Case 3.3

A 34-year-old female presents with intermittent diplopia. On clinical examination she is found to have a right CN III palsy (**Figs. 3.19, 3.20**).

Diagnosis

Schwannoma of right CN III

Schwannoma (Also Known as Neurilemmoma)
- *Epidemiology.* Accounts for 7% of intracranial tumors. Five percent are multiple, usually with *neurofibromatosis type 2* (NF-2). Benign, no gender predominance, mean age 40 to 50 years (although onset by 20 years with NF-2).
- *Clinical presentation.* Pain and/or focal neurologic deficit depending on location. Occur intracranially and along the spinal cord at the root entry zone (REZ) of sensory nerves, in the head and neck, posterior mediastinum, retroperitoneum, and the *flexor surface of the extremities*. Intracranially, most common site is on the *superior vestibular nerve* where it originates in the internal auditory canal at the REZ (vestibular schwannoma). Second most common site is the trigeminal nerve (5%), and these

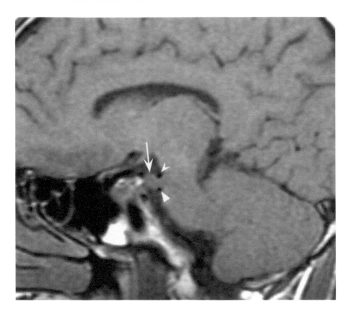

Fig. 3.19 Sagittal T1-weighted image demonstrates an ovoid, isointense mass (*arrow*) located between the PCA (*concave arrowhead*) and SCA (*straight arrowhead*). Note that it appears to be in contiguity with the ventral midbrain.

are located in the middle fossa (50%), both middle and posterior fossa (dumbbell, 25%), or posterior fossa (25%). Rarely, they are intraaxial in the brain or spinal cord when they form on perivascular nerves. Spinal schwan-

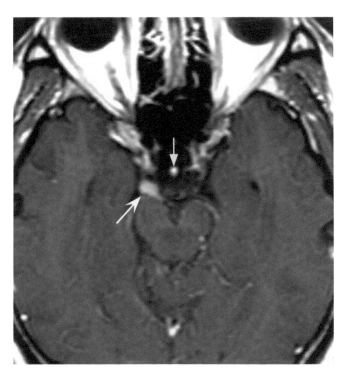

Fig. 3.20 Axial post-gadolinium T1-weighted image demonstrates intense enhancement of the mass (*concave arrow*). The mass follows the expected course of CN III within the right perimesencephalic cistern, consistent with a schwannoma of CN III. Note the normal enhancement of the pituitary stalk (*straight arrow*).

nomas form on sensory nerve roots, account for 30% of spinal tumors, and may be within the spinal canal or dumbbell-shaped with extension into neural foramina.

- *Imaging.* Extraaxial, intradural masses that are isointense to hypointense on T1-weighted MRI scan, hyperintense on T2WI, contrast-enhancing, and are rarely calcified. Forty percent are partly cystic (especially when large). If spinal, may extend through intervertebral foramen resulting in hourglass or dumbbell appearance.
- *Pathology.* Schwann cells are derived from neural crest cells (nonglial neuroectodermal tumor). Grossly, firm and *encapsulated.* Initially fusiform when intraneural but then enlarge and become eccentric with epineurium as a capsule. Contain no axons. Microscopically, have biphasic pattern of compact *Antoni A* (fusiform cells, reticulin, and collagen) and loose *Antoni B* (stellate round cells in stroma) areas. *Verocay bodies* (nuclear palisading around anuclear fibrillary material within Antoni A areas) may be seen. They are frequently *cystic or hemorrhagic.* They grow slowly and *almost never undergo malignant change.*
- *Treatment.* Surgery if indicated and if resectable. Radiosurgery may be useful in some cases.

Case 3.4

A 3-year-old female presents with diplopia and left ptosis after several episodes of pneumococcal meningitis (**Fig. 3.21**).

Diagnosis

Oculomotor neuritis secondary to bacterial meningitis

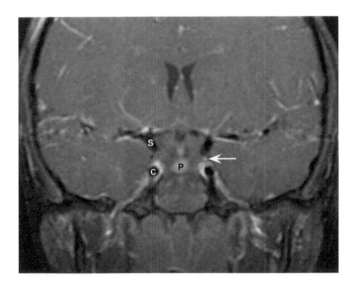

Fig. 3.21 Coronal post-gadolinium T1-weighted image with fat saturation at the level of the cavernous sinus and pituitary gland (P) demonstrates asymmetric enhancement (*arrow*) of the left CN III as it enters the superior aspect of the left cavernous sinus in this patient with oculomotor neuritis secondary to bacterial meningitis. Note the flow voids of the right cavernous carotid (C) and supraclinoid carotid (S) arteries.

Bacterial Meningitis

- *Epidemiology.* The three most common causes of meningitis are *Haemophilus influenzae*, *Streptococcus pneumoniae*, and *Neisseria meningitidis.* Incidence of *H. influenzae* meningitis dramatically reduced since introduction of Hib vaccination in the early 1990s. *Staphylococcus aureus* is associated with postoperative infections and *S. epidermidis* is the most common cause of ventriculoperitoneal shunt infections. *Listeria monocytogenes* may cause meningitis in the elderly and immunocompromised.
- *Clinical presentation.* Fever, meningismus, depressed mental status, occasionally focal neurologic deficits (due to infectious vasculitis and complicating parenchymal infarction, due to cranial neuritis, or due to complicating brain abscess).
- *Imaging.* Often normal, but may show communicating or noncommunicating hydrocephalus. Contrast studies may show leptomeningeal enhancement.
- *Pathology.* The subarachnoid space near the blood vessels fills first with neutrophils and fibrin, then macrophages, and then it eventually fibroses. Meningitis may be associated with arteritis, phlebitis, superior sagittal sinus thrombosis, and hydrocephalus.
- *Treatment.* Antibiotics ± steroids. Steroids can reduce the risk of deafness. Mortality and neurologic morbidity varies by age and infectious agent.

Case 3.5

A 42-year-old male presents with the "worst headache of his life" associated with meningismus, photophobia, and an enlarged right pupil (**Figs. 3.22, 3.23, 3.24**).

Diagnosis

Ruptured PcommA aneurysm with subarachnoid hemorrhage (SAH)

Cerebral Aneurysms

- *Epidemiology.* Most intracranial aneurysms are saccular and arise from the circle of Willis at the base of the brain. Ninety percent occur in the anterior circulation (PCommA 30%, anterior communicating artery [ACommA] 30%, middle cerebral artery [MCA] 20%, ICA 10%), 10% in the posterior circulation (basilar apex 5%, SCA, vertebrobasilar junction, posterior inferior cerebellar artery [PICA], and rarely anterior inferior cerebellar artery [AICA]. Rupture of cerebral aneurysms accounts for 85% of nontraumatic SAH. Risk of rupture is related to size and location. Risk factors for developing cerebral aneurysms include age, HTN, atherosclerosis, fibromuscular dysplasia, Marfan syndrome, Ehlers-Danlos syndrome, polycystic kidney disease, coarctation of the aorta, arteriovenous malformation (AVM), and family history of cerebral aneurysm.
- *Clinical presentation.* Most common nonhemorrhagic, neuroophthalmologic sign of aneurysm is CN III palsy

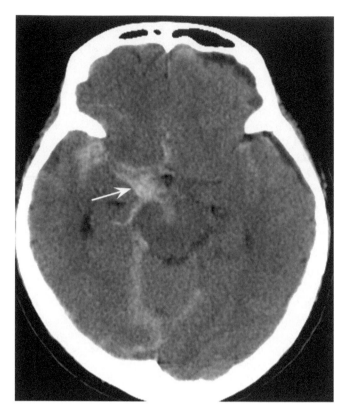

Fig. 3.22 Axial noncontrast CT scan demonstrates high-density material within the subarachnoid space, consistent with acute subarachnoid hemorrhage. The largest amount of blood is present in the right side of the suprasellar cistern (*arrow*), at the level of the right posterior communicating artery.

due to compression in subarachnoid space by PCommA aneurysm (see **Table 3.1**). The pupil is typically involved given the superficial location of pupillary fibers along the nerve bundle. Patients with complete CN III palsies may

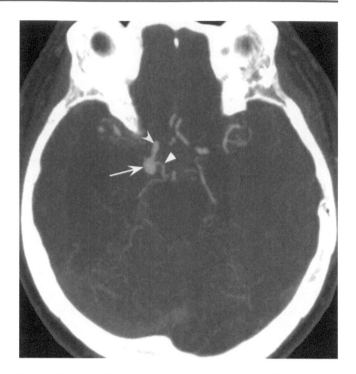

Fig. 3.23 Axial thin-slab reconstruction from a CT angiogram shows a saccular aneurysm (*arrow*) arising at the junction of the supraclinoid internal carotid artery (*concave arrowhead*) and posterior communicating artery (*straight arrowhead*).

not complain of diplopia if ptosis obscures the affected eye. Upon aneurysm rupture, severe headache ("worst headache of life"), meningismus, photosensitivity, depressed mental status, and/or focal neurologic findings may ensue. Important complications of aneurysmal SAH include *vasospasm* and *rehemorrhage*.

- *Imaging.* Noncontrast CT identifies acute SAH (~95%) in most cases, but lumbar puncture (LP) should be checked

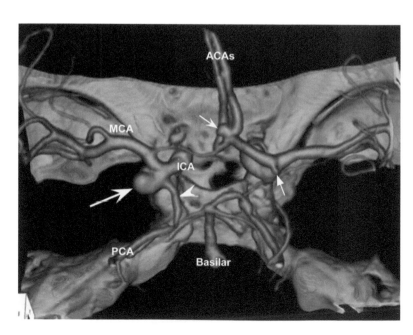

Fig. 3.24 Three-dimensional reconstruction of the CT angiographic data in the same patient as in **Fig. 3.23** shows the relationship of the aneurysm (*large arrow*) to the posterior communicating artery (*arrowhead*) and surrounding circle of Willis vessels in better detail. Note additional smaller aneurysms incidentally discovered at the anterior communicating artery (*small concave arrow*) and left carotid terminus (*small straight arrow*). (ACA, anterior cerebral artery; MCA, middle cerebral artery.)

for evidence of acute or subacute hemorrhage (xanthochromia) if clinical concern is high and CT is negative. If MRI is performed for headache, then fluid-attenuated inversion recovery (FLAIR) is the sequence most sensitive to SAH. CT angiography (CTA), MR angiography (MRA), and/or catheter angiography are all potentially useful to diagnose aneurysm, assess aneurysm anatomy (including relationship of aneurysm to parent vessel and perforators), and assess the presence or absence of vasospasm.

- *Pathology.* Pathologic examination reveals deterioration of internal elastic lamina (IEL) and muscularis at junction of vessel and aneurysm.
- *Treatment.* Treatment options include surgery (clipping, wrapping, or trapping) and endovascular coiling.

Case 3.6

A 25-year-old male is admitted with deteriorating mental status and a dilated left pupil following a high-speed motor vehicle accident (**Figs. 3.25, 3.26**).

Diagnosis

Left uncal herniation causing left CN III compression

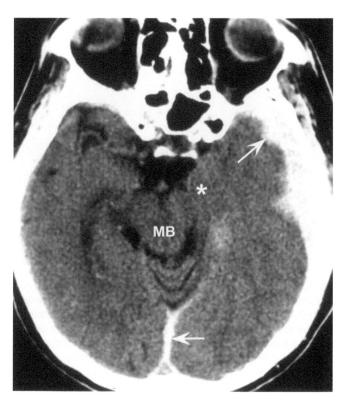

Fig. 3.25 Axial CT image at the level of the midbrain demonstrates mild left uncal herniation (*asterisk*), with mild rightward displacement of the midbrain (MB). Note acute subdural hematoma extending along the left middle cranial fossa and along the falx cerebri and tentorium cerebelli posteriorly (*arrows*). The subdural collection acts as a mass lesion, resulting in uncal herniation and the potential for brainstem and cranial nerve symptoms.

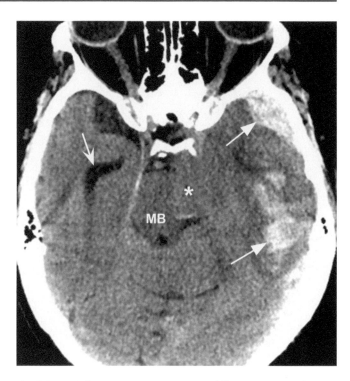

Fig. 3.26 Axial noncontrast CT image in a different patient with more severe left uncal herniation (*asterisk*) and therefore more severe compression of the midbrain (MB) and mass effect upon the expected course of CN III. Note the left temporal parenchymal hemorrhagic contusion and ipsilateral subdural hematoma (*straight arrows*). The right temporal horn (*concave arrow*) is dilated, consistent with trapping of the right lateral ventricle due to subfalcine herniation (not shown). This patient had extensive traumatic brain injury from a motor vehicle accident.

Case 3.7

A 44-year-old female presents with severe headache, dilated left pupil, and persistent diplopia (**Fig. 3.27**).

Diagnosis

Left extraaxial tumor (meningioma) with mass effect and uncal herniation

Clinical Pearls

- Dilated ("blown") pupil results from compression of the peripheral (pupillomotor) fibers of ipsilateral CN III by the uncus (medial temporal lobe).
- Treatment is based on individual lesions but may involve hyperosmotic therapy (mannitol) to reduce brain volume; steroid therapy for vasogenic (tumor-associated) edema, and/or surgical resection of the mass lesion. In cases of severe hemispheric brain swelling (e.g., following traumatic brain injury [TBI]), hemicraniectomy (bone removal) may occasionally be required to decompress the brainstem.
- Untreated, can lead to irreversible brainstem damage, coma, and death.

4 Trochlear Nerve

Functions

- General somatic efferent (GSE). Somatic motor innervation of the superior oblique (SO) muscle.

Anatomy

- The *trochlear nucleus* is in the inferior midbrain, inferior to the oculomotor nuclear complex, dorsal to the medial longitudinal fasciculus at the level of the inferior colliculus, ventrolateral to the cerebral aqueduct (**Fig. 4.1**).
- Trochlear nerve *fascicles* course posteroinferiorly around the cerebral aqueduct to *decussate in the superior medullary velum* of the midbrain and exit the contralateral side of the dorsal midbrain just below the inferior colliculus (**Fig. 4.2**). The *cisternal segment* runs anteriorly under the free edge of the tentorium, traversing the quadrigeminal, ambient (perimesencephalic), crural, and pontomesencephalic cisterns (**Fig. 4.3**). Cranial nerve (CN) IV then passes between the posterior cerebral artery (PCA) and the superior cerebellar artery (SCA) lateral to CN III and pierces the dura of the *cavernous sinus* along the lateral clivus below the petroclinoid ligament.

It travels in the lateral wall of the cavernous sinus below CN III and above CN V_1 (**Fig. 4.4**) and then enters the orbit through the superior orbital fissure (SOF) above the annulus of Zinn. It then crosses medially near the roof of the orbit over the levator palpebrae superioris (LPS) and superior rectus (SR) muscles to innervate the SO muscle.

- The tendon of the SO muscle passes through the trochlea (a "pulley" of variably calcified fibrocartilage) in the medial wall of the orbit and inserts on the sclera of the posterolateral globe. Therefore, contraction of the SO causes depression of the eye when the eye is adducted and inward rotation of the eye (intorsion) when the eye is abducted (**Fig. 4.5**).
- The trochlear nerve has several unique features among the CNs. It is the smallest CN (only ~2400 axons), the only CN to exit from the dorsum of the brainstem, the only CN in which all axons decussate, the only CN to decussate outside the CNS, and the CN with the longest intracranial course (~7.5 cm). *Note: because of the small size of CN IV, it is not visible on routine magnetic resonance imaging (MRI) sequences. It may be directly visualized with very high resolution MR imaging sequences or may be revealed in cases of nerve pathology (see below).*

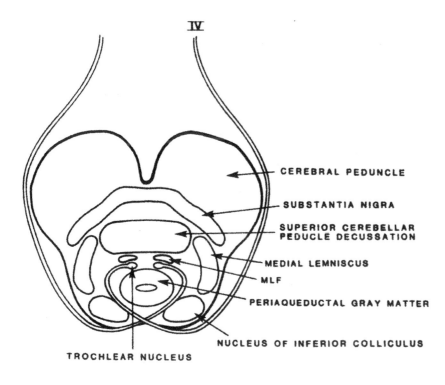

IV

CEREBRAL PEDUNCLE

SUBSTANTIA NIGRA

SUPERIOR CEREBELLAR PEDUCLE DECUSSATION

MEDIAL LEMNISCUS

MLF

PERIAQUEDUCTAL GRAY MATTER

NUCLEUS OF INFERIOR COLLICULUS

TROCHLEAR NUCLEUS

Fig. 4.1 Cross-section of midbrain at the level of the inferior colliculus demonstrating trochlear nucleus and course of CN IV (see text). (From Harnsberger HR. Handbook of Head and Neck Imaging [2nd ed.] St. Louis, MO: Mosby, 1995. Reprinted with permission.)

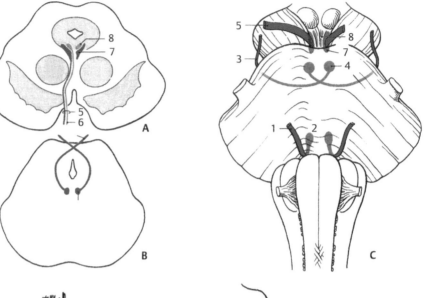

Fig. 4.2 Comparison of nuclear regions and exits of oculomotor, trochlear, and abducens nerves. **(A)** Midbrain at the level of the superior colliculus. **(B)** Midbrain at the level of the inferior colliculus. **(C)** Ventral view of brainstem. (1, abducens nerve; 2, abducens nucleus; 3, trochlear nerve; 4, trochlear nucleus; 5, oculomotor nerve; 6, visceromotor [parasympathetic] fibers; 7, oculomotor nucleus; 8, Edinger-Westphal nucleus.)

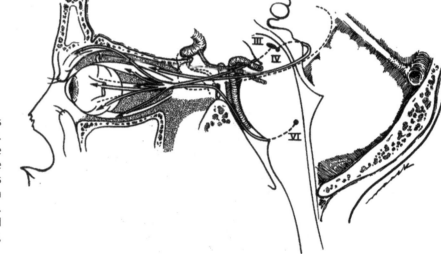

Fig. 4.3 Comparison of origins and courses of oculomotor, trochlear, and abducens nerves. The oculomotor and trochlear nerves originate in the midbrain, whereas the abducens nerve originates in the lower pons. All three nerves ultimately exit the cranial base into the eye via the superior orbital fissure (see text for details). (From Harnsberger HR. Handbook of Head and Neck Imaging [2nd ed.] St. Louis, MO: Mosby, 1995. Reprinted with permission.)

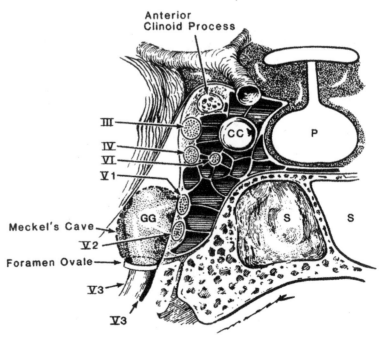

Fig. 4.4 Coronal view through the cavernous sinus demonstrates CN III, IV, VI, and V$_1$ and V$_2$ in the lateral wall of the cavernous sinus and CN VI within the cavernous sinus adjacent to the cavernous portion of the ICA. Note that CN V$_3$ does not enter the cavernous sinus but rather leaves the cranial base through the foramen ovale. (From Harnsberger HR. Handbook of Head and Neck Imaging [2nd ed.] St. Louis, MO: Mosby, 1995. Reprinted with permission.)

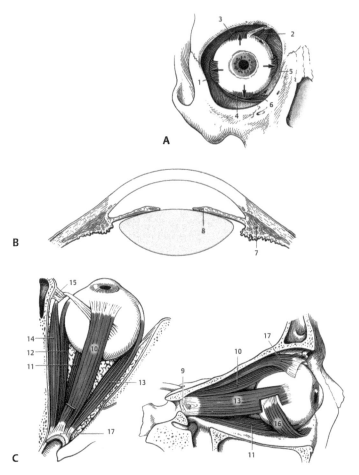

Fig. 4.5 Schematic of extraocular and intraocular muscles. **(A)** Anterior view. (1, LR muscle; 2, SO muscle; 3, SR muscle; 4, IR muscle; 5, MR muscle; 6, IO muscle.) **(B)** Intraocular muscles. (7, ciliary muscle; 8, sphincter pupillae muscle.) **(C)** Superior (left) and lateral (right) views. (9, common annular tendon [annulus of Zinn]; 10, SR muscle; 11, IR muscle; 12, MR muscle; 13, LR muscle; 14, SO muscle; 15, trochlea; 16, IO muscle; 17, LPS muscle.)

Trochlear Nerve Lesions

- The trochlear nerve is uncommonly affected in isolation.
- Trochlear palsy is the most common cause of vertical strabismus.
- A pure trochlear palsy is characterized by vertical or diagonal diplopia greatest on downward gaze directed to the opposite side. Excyclodeviation (outer rotation of globe) can be seen as well.
- Unilateral nuclear/fascicular lesion results in a contralateral SO palsy; lesions distal to the decussation result in an ipsilateral SO palsy.
- A patient with a unilateral SO palsy typically tilts his head to the side opposite the paretic muscle (*Biels-*

chowsky sign) to decrease diplopia, as contralateral head tilt counteracts excyclodeviation.
- Typically these patients have difficulty reading and going down stairs.
- Congenital trochlear palsies can be sporadic or familial (autosomal dominant). Longstanding head tilt observed in family photographs can aid in diagnosis.

Types

Brainstem Lesions (Nucleus or Fascicular Segment)

- Associated neurologic findings indicating dorsal midbrain injury can include internuclear ophthalmoplegia (due to medial longitudinal fasciculus [MLF] lesion), Horner syndrome (due to lesion of descending sympathetic fibers), and afferent pupillary defect (due to lesion of pretectal fibers) (see Appendix B).
- Specific causes of nuclear/fascicular lesions:
  ○ Trauma (trochlear nucleus may be involved by shear injury or contusion to the dorsolateral brainstem)
  ○ Ischemia (e.g., perforator infarct)
  ○ Tumor (e.g., brainstem glioma or metastasis)
  ○ Demyelinating disease (e.g., multiple sclerosis [MS]) (rare, perhaps because fascicular course of CN IV is so short)
  ○ Infectious/inflammatory

Lesions in the Subarachnoid Space (Cisternal Segment)

- Trauma (nerve avulsion or contusion, stretching or compression against tentorium)
- Ischemia (e.g., diabetic trochlear neuropathy)
- Increased intracranial pressure (ICP) (e.g., hydrocephalus)
- Vascular compression (e.g., SCA aneurysm in ambient cistern)
- Neoplasm (e.g., tentorial meningioma, CN IV schwannoma, perineural spread of tumor)
- Iatrogenic (injured during surgery under tentorial edge, radiation injury)
- Demyelinating disease (Miller-Fisher variant of Guillain-Barré syndrome, which includes ophthalmoplegia, ataxia, and areflexia)
- Inflammation/meningitis with secondary neuritis

Lesions in the Cavernous Sinus/Superior Orbital Fissure

- Neoplasm (e.g., meningioma, lymphoma, perineural spread of head and neck cancer)
- Vascular (carotid-cavernous fistula, giant ICA aneurysm). Most often affects CN VI first
- Inflammatory (e.g., sarcoidosis, Tolosa-Hunt syndrome)

- Infection (e.g., bacterial or fungal sphenoid sinusitis with extension to the cavernous sinus)
- Pituitary apoplexy (acute enlargement of the pituitary gland leads to acute cavernous sinus compression)
- Radiation injury (e.g., following radiosurgery for cavernous sinus meningiomas)

Lesions of the Orbit

- Lesions of the orbit do not typically lead to a palsy of CN IV.
- *Superior oblique myokymia* is a condition of intermittent vertical diplopia and oscillopsia caused by spontaneous firing of trochlear motor units. May be idiopathic or occur following recovery of a CN IV lesion, with posterior fossa lesions, or in MS.
- *Brown syndrome* (tenosynovitis of SO tendon, often occurring in association with rheumatologic disorders). May cause mechanical restriction of SO movement and may mimic a CN IV palsy.

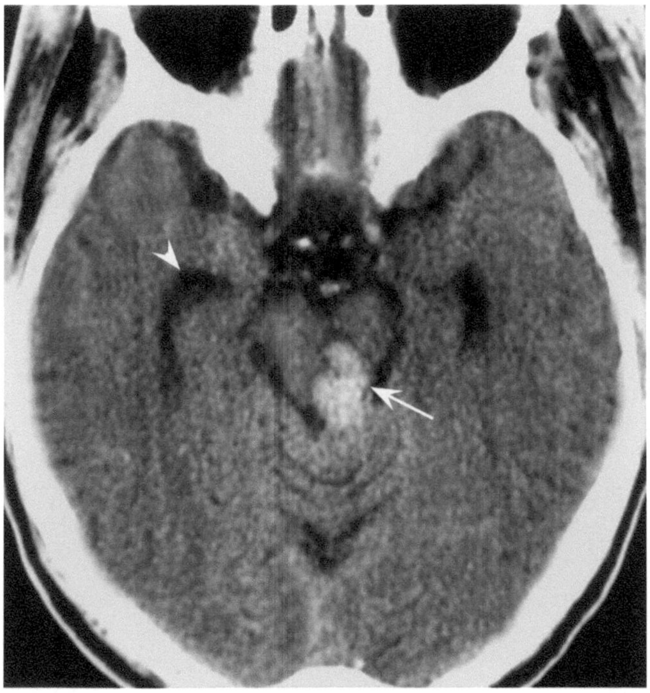

Treatment

- Correction of diplopia following CN IV injury may require prism therapy and/or strabismus surgery. Correction should not be undertaken until recovery is complete; in most cases the deficit stabilizes within ~6 months.

Trochlear Nerve: Pathologic Images

Case 4.1

A 21-year-old male status post–motor vehicle accident is found on examination to have left CN III and IV palsies (**Fig. 4.6**).

Diagnosis

Trauma (hemorrhagic brainstem contusion)

Case 4.2

An 18-year-old male status post–high-speed motorcycle accident presents with depressed mental status (Glasgow Coma Scale [GCS] 7). On examination he is found to have disconjugate gaze (**Fig. 4.7**).

Diagnosis

Trauma (hemorrhagic shear injury)

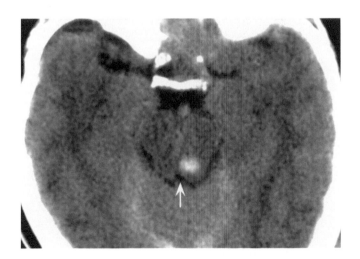

Fig. 4.6 Axial CT shows an acute hematoma (*arrow*) within the dorsolateral left midbrain, centered in the expected region of the CN III and IV nuclei. The hematoma involves the peripheral aspect of the brainstem, typical of contusion. Note the dilatation of the temporal horns (*arrowhead*) due to obstructive hydrocephalus related to mass effect upon the adjacent aqueduct of Sylvius (compressed and not visualized).

Fig. 4.7 Axial CT shows a small hemorrhage in the dorsal left midbrain at the level of the expected location of the CN IV nucleus, adjacent to the aqueduct of Sylvius (*arrow*). This lesion spares the periphery and is consistent with hemorrhagic shear injury of the dorsolateral brainstem. Also note increased density along the tentorium consistent with a tentorial subdural hematoma, as well as diffuse sulcal effacement due to posttraumatic cerebral swelling and small amounts of posttraumatic subarachnoid hemorrhage.

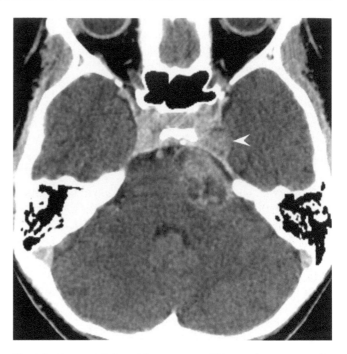

Fig. 4.9 A more inferior axial postcontrast CT image demonstrates the mass extending anteriorly into the left cavernous sinus (*arrowhead*).

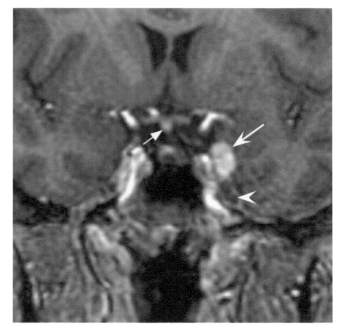

Fig. 4.10 A coronal postcontrast T1-weighted gradient-echo MRI scan at the level of the pituitary stalk (*straight arrow*) demonstrates the extension of the enhancing mass (*concave arrow*) into the superior aspect of the left cavernous sinus, above the level of Meckel's cave (*arrowhead*), along the course of CN IV.

Imaging Pearl

Shear injury involves the deep structures of the brain rather than the surface of the brain, and therefore does not typically extend to the surface of the brainstem. In cases of suspected shear injury (diffuse axonal injury), look for other sites of injury such as the supratentorial white matter and splenium of corpus callosum. Contusion, in contrast, involves the peripheral brainstem due to compression against the tentorium with resultant surface injury.

Case 4.3

A 17-year-old female presents with intermittent vertical diplopia. On examination she is found to have a left CN IV palsy (**Figs. 4.8, 4.9, 4.10**).

Diagnosis

CN IV schwannoma

Imaging Pearls

- Forty percent of schwannomas are cystic, especially when large.
- A schwannoma extending to the dorsal midbrain in the ambient cistern should be expected to arise from CN IV.

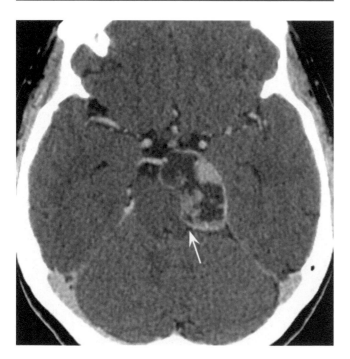

Fig. 4.8 Axial postcontrast CT image at the level of the lower midbrain shows a sharply circumscribed, heterogeneously enhancing extraaxial mass that displaces and compresses the adjacent brainstem. The mass extends posteriorly into the ambient cistern (*arrow*), compatible with a cystic schwannoma arising from CN IV.

Case 4.4

A 27-year-old female presents with right facial numbness (**Fig. 4.11**).

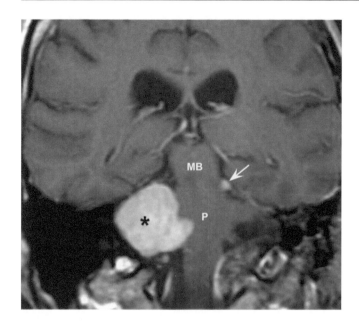

Fig. 4.11 Coronal postcontrast T1-weighted image shows a homogeneously enhancing mass (*asterisk*) lateral to the pons (P) in the right cerebellopontine angle that represents a large CN V schwannoma. Note the smaller enhancing mass (*arrow*) to the left of the inferior midbrain (MB) at the level of the pontomesencephalic junction, consistent with a CN IV schwannoma.

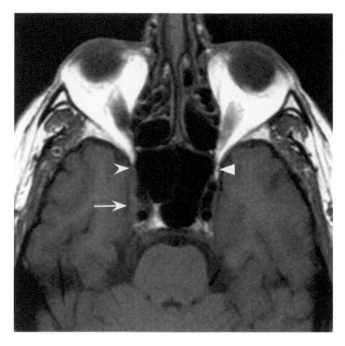

Fig. 4.12 Axial T1-weighted image shows asymmetric soft tissue along the lateral aspect of the right cavernous sinus (*arrow*). This effaces the normal fat at the right superior orbital fissure (*concave arrowhead*). Note bright signal of normal fat in the contralateral orbital fissure (*straight arrowhead*).

Diagnosis

Neurofibromatosis type 2 with multiple schwannomas, including a symptomatic right CN V schwannoma and an asymptomatic (incidental) left CN IV schwannoma (see Chapter 5, Case 5.6)

Case 4.5

A 62-year-old male presents with diplopia and retroorbital pain and is found to have a right CN IV palsy (**Figs. 4.12, 4.13, 4.14**).

Diagnosis

Tolosa-Hunt syndrome (see Chapter 3, Case 3.8)

Case 4.6

A 53-year-old female presents with headache, fever, proptosis, and vertical diplopia (**Figs. 4.15, 4.16, 4.17, 4.18**).

Diagnosis

Acute fungal sinusitis with CN IV palsy due to cavernous sinus involvement. Cultures revealed *Aspergillus fumigatus* and the patient was treated successfully with voriconazole.

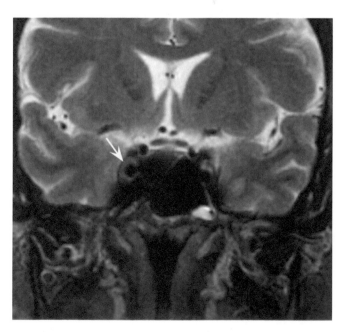

Fig. 4.13 Coronal fast spin echo T2-weighted image with fat saturation shows the subtle asymmetric soft tissue involving the right cavernous sinus (*arrow*). This tissue is intermediate in signal intensity on this T2-weighted image.

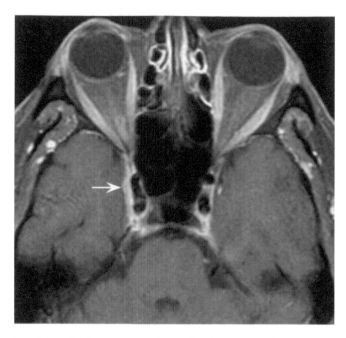

Fig. 4.14 Axial postcontrast T1-weighted image with fat saturation shows enhancement of the soft tissue (*arrow*) involving the lateral aspect of the right cavernous sinus and the superior orbital fissure.

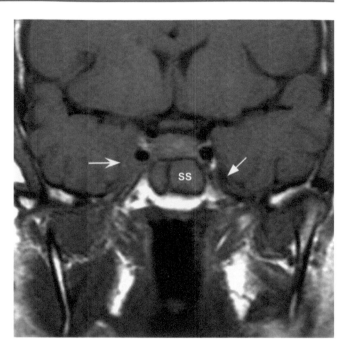

Fig. 4.15 Coronal precontrast T1-weighted image demonstrates soft tissue intensity material filling the sphenoid sinus (SS). Asymmetric soft tissue expands the right cavernous sinus (*concave arrow*) and extends into Meckel's cave. A normal Meckel's cave on the left (*straight arrow*) contains cerebrospinal fluid that is clearly not seen on the right.

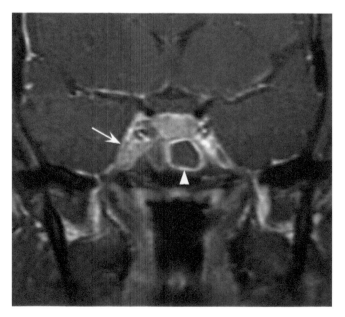

Fig. 4.16 Coronal postcontrast T1-weighted image shows peripheral enhancement of the mucosa of the sphenoid sinus (*arrowhead*), with nonenhancement of the secretions, consistent with inflammatory sinus disease. The soft tissue in the right cavernous sinus and Meckel's cave (*arrow*) shows slightly heterogeneous enhancement.

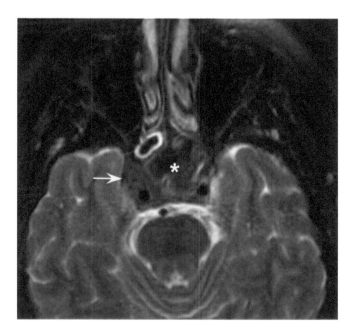

Fig. 4.17 Axial fast spin echo T2-weighted image (T2WI) with fat saturation demonstrates low signal intensity of the soft tissue within the right cavernous sinus (*arrow*). The material within the sphenoid sinus (*asterisk*) is also quite hypointense on T2WI. These findings are strongly suggestive of fungal sinusitis with cavernous sinus extension.

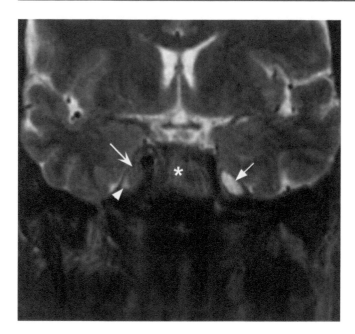

Fig. 4.18 Coronal fast spin echo T2-weighted image also shows the low signal intensity soft tissue within the sphenoid sinus (*asterisk*) and the right cavernous sinus (*concave arrow*) that effaces Meckel's cave. Note the tiny amount of residual cerebrospinal fluid (CSF) inferiorly (*arrowhead*) compared with the normal bright CSF signal within the contralateral Meckel's cave (*straight arrow*).

Fungal Sinusitis

- *Epidemiology.* Fungal infections of the paranasal sinuses are uncommon, and usually occur in those who are immunocompromised. The most common organisms responsible are *Aspergillus* and *Mucor* species.
- *Clinical presentation.* Noninvasive infections cause typical symptoms and signs of sinusitis (fever, sinus headache, tenderness, nasal drainage). Invasive infections can cause symptoms related to invasion of adjacent structures (skull base, central nervous system [CNS], orbit) such as cranial neuropathies, proptosis, and mental status changes.
- *Imaging.* Computed tomography (CT) is the imaging modality of choice for paranasal sinus disease although MRI adds considerably in the evaluation in complicated cases (such as the immunocompromised host with invasive sinus disease extending into the skull base or cavernous sinus). In the setting of invasive sinus disease, CT may show bony erosion, but MRI is often needed to evaluate extent of leptomeningeal and/or brain parenchymal involvement. Fungal sinus disease may be suspected when relatively high-density material is seen on CT, likely related to the presence of heavy metals such as *manganese and iron* within the inspissated secretions. On MRI, dark T2 signal (due to high protein and low water content) may be suggestive of fungal infection, though inspissated secretions can have a similar appearance. A potential pitfall is that, when dark enough, the signal void created by inspissated material may mimic normal aerated sinus.

- *Pathology.* Includes noninvasive and invasive forms, granulomatous fungal sinusitis, allergic fungal sinusitis, and sinus mycetoma. In acute invasive fungal sinusitis, there is hyphal invasion of the mucosa, submucosa, and blood vessels that may lead to vasculitis with thrombosis, hemorrhage, and tissue infarction.
- *Treatment.* Systemic antifungal therapy. Surgical debridement is used to restore sinus patency and for removal of sinus mycetoma ("fungus ball"). Surgical debridement is often used in cases of acute or chronic invasive fungal sinus disease as well, but it is generally not useful once infection has reached the skull base and adjacent soft tissues. Treatment of underlying immune deficiency, if present, is also useful.

Case 4.7

A 61-year-old male presents with vertical diplopia and left scalp numbness (**Figs. 4.19, 4.20, 4.21**).

Diagnosis

Mucocele of left anterior clinoid process with associated soft tissue inflammation

Mucocele

- *Clinical presentation.* Usually asymptomatic but can present with mass effect causing associated CN dysfunction and headache.

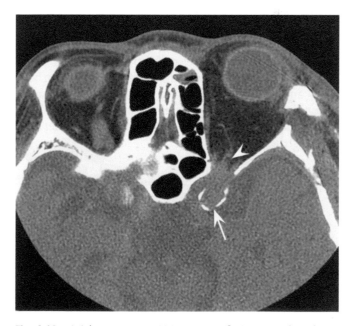

Fig. 4.19 Axial noncontrast CT image in soft tissue window shows expansion and opacification of the left anterior clinoid process (*arrow*). In addition, there is abnormal soft tissue infiltrating the fat of the left orbital apex (*arrowhead*).

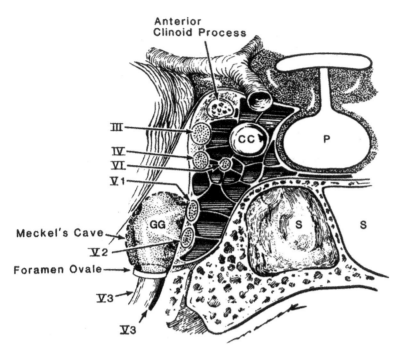

Fig. 5.2 Coronal view through the cavernous sinus demonstrates CN III, IV, V_1, and V_2 in the lateral wall of the cavernous sinus and CN VI within the cavernous sinus adjacent to the cavernous portion of the internal carotid artery. Note that CN V_3 does not enter the cavernous sinus but rather leaves the cranial base through the foramen ovale. (From Harnsberger HR. Handbook of Head and Neck Imaging [2nd ed.] St. Louis, MO: Mosby, 1995. Reprinted with permission.)

2. *Spinal trigeminal nucleus.* Extends from the principal sensory nucleus (in pons) caudally all the way to C-2 (cervical spinal cord), where it merges with the substantia gelatinosa (pain-related lamina in the spinal cord). The spinal trigeminal nucleus also gets input from CN VII, IX, and X. Fibers carrying pain and temperature (and crude touch as well) descend via the *spinal trigeminal tract,* synapse in the spinal trigeminal nucleus, then cross via the *ventral trigeminothalamic tract* to ascend to the VPM nucleus of the thalamus. There are also other pathways from the spinal trigeminal nucleus to intralaminar thalamic nuclei and the reticular formation that mediate affective and arousal components of facial pain.

3. *Mesencephalic nucleus of CN V.* Extends from principal sensory nucleus (in pons) cranially to superior colliculus (in midbrain). This nucleus contains the *primary sensory neurons* (i.e., there is no synapse in the trigeminal ganglion) involved in proprioception of head muscles (especially masticatory and extraocular muscles). This is the only case in which primary sensory neurons lie within the central nervous system (CNS) instead of in the peripheral ganglia.

• Information from the VPM nucleus of the thalamus travels to the ipsilateral somatosensory cortex (postcentral gyrus).

Ophthalmic Division (CN V_1) (Fig. 5.3)

• Purely sensory.
• From trigeminal ganglion courses in lateral wall of cavernous sinus inferior to CN IV (**Fig. 5.2**), enters orbit through superior orbital fissure (SOF)
• Structures in SOF: CNs III, IV, V_1 (nasociliary, frontal, and lacrimal branches), VI, sympathetic fibers from internal

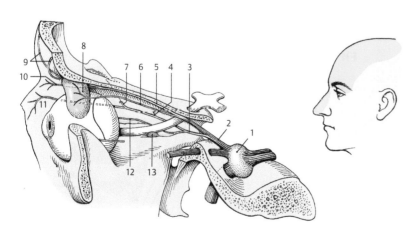

Fig. 5.3 Ophthalmic nerve (CN V_1). (1, gasserian [trigeminal, semilunar] ganglion; 2, ophthalmic nerve; 3, nasociliary nerve; 4, posterior ethmoidal nerve; 5, frontal nerve; 6, lacrimal nerve; 7, anterior ethmoidal nerve; 8, lacrimal gland; 9, supraorbital nerve; 10, supratrochlear nerve; 11, infratrochlear nerve; 12, long ciliary nerves; 13, ciliary ganglion.)

carotid artery (ICA) plexus, superior ophthalmic vein, orbital branch of middle meningeal artery, and recurrent meningeal branch of lacrimal artery

- Before leaving cavernous sinus, divides into
  1. *Tentorial (meningeal) branch.* Innervates dura of cavernous sinus, sphenoid wing, anterior fossa, petrous ridge, Meckel's cave, tentorium cerebelli, posterior falx cerebri, and dural venous sinuses. Note that this branch does *not* exit via the SOF.
  2. *Frontal nerve.* Enters orbit above annulus of Zinn, divides into *supraorbital nerve* (innervates frontal sinuses, forehead, scalp back to lambdoidal suture in midline) and *supratrochlear nerve* (medial conjunctiva, medial upper lid, forehead, side of nose).
  3. *Lacrimal nerve.* Enters orbit above annulus of Zinn. Innervates lateral conjunctiva and skin near lacrimal gland. Receives postganglionic parasympathetic fibers (from CN VII greater superficial petrosal nerve [GSPN]) for lacrimation from zygomatic nerve of CN V_2 (see below).
  4. *Nasociliary nerve.* Enters orbit through annulus of Zinn. Has several branches:
- *Infratrochlear nerve* innervates lacrimal sac, caruncle, conjunctiva, and skin of medial canthus.
- *Anterior and posterior ethmoidal nerves* innervate ethmoidal air cells.
- *Internal nasal nerve* innervates the anterior portion of the nasal septum.
- *External nasal nerve* innervates the skin of the dorsum and tip of the nose.
- *Long ciliary nerves* carry sensation from ciliary body, iris, and cornea. They also convey sympathetic fibers from the ICA to the *dilator pupillae* muscle.
- *Short ciliary nerves* carry sensation from the globe. They also convey postganglionic parasympathetic fibers (from CN III) from the ciliary ganglion to the *sphincter pupillae* and *ciliary muscles.*

Maxillary Division (CN V_2) (Fig. 5.4)

- Purely sensory.

- *Middle meningeal nerve* is given off from the maxillary nerve directly after its origin from the trigeminal ganglion. It accompanies the middle meningeal artery and innervates the dura of middle cranial fossa.
- From the trigeminal ganglion it courses in inferolateral wall of cavernous sinus inferior to CN V_1 (**Fig. 5.2**).
- Exits cranial vault via foramen rotundum to enter *pterygopalatine (sphenopalatine) fossa.*
- Contents of foramen rotundum: CN V_2, emissary veins, artery of foramen rotundum.
- In pterygopalatine fossa, branches into
  1. *Infraorbital nerve.* Enters orbit via inferior orbital fissure (IOF). Structures in IOF: infraorbital nerve, zygomatic nerve, infraorbital artery and vein, and inferior ophthalmic vein. Then infraorbital nerve travels under orbital periosteum; then enters and traverses the infraorbital canal and exits via the infraorbital foramen to innervate the midportion of the face. Along its course it gives off
     - *Posterior superior alveolar nerves.* To maxillary sinus, molar teeth of maxilla, and adjacent gums and cheek.
     - *Middle superior alveolar nerve.* To maxillary premolar teeth.
     - *Anterior superior alveolar nerves.* To the maxillary incisor and canine teeth.
     - *Inferior palpebral branches* to lower lid skin and conjunctiva, *external nasal branches* to side of nose, and *superior labial branches* to upper lip.
  2. *Zygomatic nerve.* It enters the orbit via the IOF, and gives off two branches:
     - *Zygomaticotemporal* nerve. Runs along lateral wall of the orbit and passes through the zygomaticotemporal foramen in the zygomatic bone to enter the temporal fossa and innervates the skin of the side of the forehead and the lateral angle of the orbit.
     - *Zygomaticofacial* nerve. Runs along inferolateral wall of the orbit and passes through the zygomaticofacial foramen in the zygomatic bone to reach the face and innervates the skin on the prominence of the cheek.
     - Postganglionic parasympathetic fibers originating from the GSPN of CN VII that have just synapsed

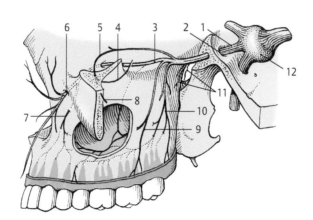
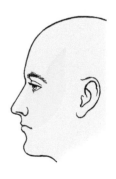

Fig. 5.4 Maxillary nerve (CN V_2). (1, maxillary nerve; 2, foramen rotundum; 3, infraorbital nerve; 4, zygomaticotemporal nerve; 5, zygomaticofacial nerve; 6, infraorbital foramen; 7, anterior superior alveolar nerves; 8, zygomatic nerve; 9, middle superior alveolar nerve; 10, posterior superior alveolar nerves; 11, ganglionic branches [fine filaments running to the pterygopalatine ganglion]; 12, gasserian [trigeminal, semilunar] ganglion.)

in the pterygopalatine ganglion join the zygomatic nerve and follow it into the IOF, travel with the zygomaticotemporal nerve, and then intraorbitally connect with fibers of the *lacrimal nerve* (of CN V$_1$), ultimately providing the lacrimal gland with secretomotor innervation.

3. *Other sensory fibers* pass through the pterygopalatine ganglion without synapsing and include the following:

   • *Orbital.* Several delicate filaments enter the IOF and innervate the orbital periosteum.

   • *Palatine.* The *greater palatine nerve* travels in the *greater palatine foramen* to the upper gingiva and hard palate. *Lesser palatine nerve* travels in the *lesser palatine foramen* to the soft palate, uvula, and tonsils. *Posterior inferior nasal nerves* arise from the greater palatine nerve, reach the nasal cavity via holes in the palatine bone, and innervate the inferior nasal concha.

   • *Posterior superior nasal.* These branches are distributed to the septum and lateral wall of the nasal fossa. They traverse the *sphenopalatine foramen* to reach the nasal cavity and the innervate superior and middle nasal conchae and posterior septum. One branch, larger than the others, is the *nasopalatine nerve*, which passes across the roof of the nasal cavity and descends to the roof of the mouth via the *incisive foramen*.

• *Pharyngeal.* This branch travels with the pharyngeal branch of the internal maxillary artery and innervates the mucous membrane of the nasopharynx.

Mandibular Division (CN V$_3$) (Fig. 5.5)

• Sensory and motor.
• Largest of the three divisions.
• In Meckel's cave, the sensory root of CN V$_3$ lies inferior to V$_1$ and V$_2$, and exits the skull via the foramen ovale. CN V$_3$ does *not* enter the cavernous sinus (**Fig. 5.2**). Contents of foramen ovale: CN V$_3$, lesser superficial petrosal nerve, emissary veins, and accessory meningeal artery. After CN V$_3$ exits foramen ovale, it joins the motor root to form the *mandibular nerve*. The mandibular nerve lies in the *infratemporal (zygomatic) fossa*, where it divides into

1. *Meningeal (recurrent) branch.* Reenters foramen spinosum along with the middle meningeal artery to innervate the dura of the middle cranial fossa and the mucous lining of the mastoid air cells.

2. *Medial pterygoid nerve.* Small branch to the deep surface of the medial pterygoid muscle.

3. *Masseteric nerve.* Passes laterally to cross mandibular notch to the deep surface of the masseter muscle.

4. *Deep temporal nerves.* Enter the deep surface of the temporalis muscle.

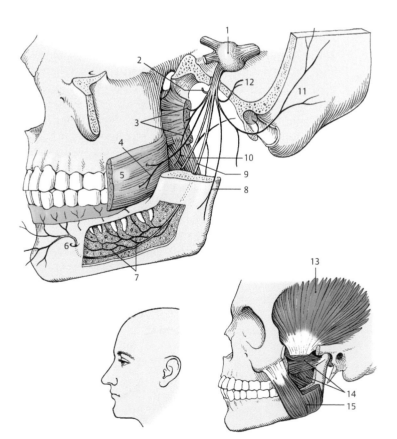

Fig. 5.5 Mandibular nerve (CN V$_3$). (1, gasserian [trigeminal, semilunar] ganglion; 2, deep temporal nerves; 3, pterygoid nerves; 4, buccal nerve; 5, buccinator muscle; 6, mental foramen; 7, inferior dental branches of inferior alveolar nerve; 8, masseteric nerve; 9, inferior alveolar nerve; 10, lingual nerve; 11, auriculotemporal nerve; 12, recurrent meningeal branch; 13, temporalis muscle; 14, pterygoid muscles; 15, masseter muscle.)

5. *Buccal nerve.* Innervates the skin over the buccinator muscle (note: motor innervation to the buccinator is provided by buccal branches of CN VII).
6. *Lateral pterygoid nerve.* Enters the deep surface of the lateral pterygoid muscle.
7. *Auriculotemporal nerve.* Runs posterior to the neck of the mandible, then turns upward with the superficial temporal artery under the parotid gland, then ascends over the zygomatic arch. Branches include
   - *Anterior auricular.* Innervate skin of the helix and tragus.
   - *Branches to the external acoustic meatus.* Innervate skin of the external acoustic meatus and tympanic membrane.
   - *Articular branches.* Innervate the temporomandibular joint.
   - *Superficial temporal branches.* Accompany the superficial temporal artery to the vertex of the skull and innervate the skin of temporal region.
   - Note that the auriculotemporal nerve conveys postganglionic parasympathetic fibers (from CN IX and the otic ganglion) to the parotid gland.
   - The auriculotemporal nerve also interacts with CN VII via communicating branches.
8. *Lingual nerve.* Innervates the mucous membrane of the mouth and gums and anterior two thirds of the tongue (*not* taste, which is supplied by CN VII). It is joined by the chorda tympani nerve (branch of CN VII), which transmits taste from anterior two thirds of the tongue and provides parasympathetic secretomotor innervation to the submandibular ganglion. Passes between the medial pterygoid and ramus of mandible and crosses obliquely to reach the tongue.
9. *Inferior alveolar nerve.* Largest branch of the mandibular nerve. It descends adjacent to the ramus of the mandible to the *mandibular foramen* to enter the mandibular canal and gives off
   - *Dental branches* innervating the mandibular molar and premolar teeth.
   - *Incisive branch* innervating the mandibular canine and incisor teeth.
   - *Mental nerve,* which emerges at the *mental foramen* and innervates skin of chin and lower lip.

Motor Portion (Portio Minor)

- Motor fibers receive supranuclear input from corticobulbar fibers that originate in the lower one third of the precentral gyrus and traverse the corona radiata, internal capsule, and cerebral peduncle, and then decussate in the pons and terminate in the motor nucleus in the midpons, medial to the principal sensory nucleus of CN V.
- Motor nucleus of CN V (**Fig. 5.1**) sends a motor root that leaves the pons, passes forward in the cerebellopontine angle cistern, and pierces dura beneath the attachment of the tentorium to the petrous temporal bone, enters

Meckel's cave, travels immediately beneath the trigeminal sensory ganglion and exits the skull via foramen ovale. The motor root and sensory root of CN V$_3$ then join to form the *mandibular nerve.*
- Motor component of the mandibular nerve gives branchial motor innervation to muscles of mastication:
  - *Masseter* (zygomatic arch to angle of mandible, closes mouth)
  - *Temporalis* (coronoid process of mandible to temporal bone up to superior temporal line, closes mouth)
  - *Medial pterygoid* (medial aspect of lateral pterygoid plate to angle of mandible, closes mouth)
  - *Lateral pterygoid* (lateral aspect of lateral pterygoid plate to top of mandible, opens mouth)
  - *Tensor tympani* (attached to malleus, involved in acoustic reflexes)
  - *Tensor veli palatini* (eustachian tube cartilage to pterygoid hamulus to soft palate, involved in equalizing pressure in the middle ear)
  - *Mylohyoid*
  - *Anterior belly of the digastric muscle*

Trigeminal Nerve: Normal Images (Figs. 5.6, 5.7, 5.8, 5.9, 5.10, 5.11)

Trigeminal Nerve Lesions

Evaluation

- *Sensory evaluation.* Somatic sensation (light touch, pain/temperature) tested on face and mucous membranes. Each of the three trigeminal divisions is tested and compared with the contralateral side. Lesions distal to the trigeminal ganglion result in sensory loss or paresthesias/dysesthesias confined to a single division. Lesions at or proximal to the ganglion result in sensory dysfunction over the whole ipsilateral face/forehead. The cutaneous area over the angle of the mandible is supplied by upper cervical roots (C-2/C-3) so a hemifacial sensory loss that spares the angle of the jaw makes anatomical sense. Dissociation of pain/temperature and light touch sensation on the face differentiates lesions affecting the spinal tract and nucleus of CN V from lesions affecting the principal sensory nucleus. It is important also to note that not all lesions result in complete sensory loss but rather may result in reduced sensation (hypesthesia), altered sensation (dysesthesia), abnormal sensation (paresthesia), or pain in the affected division.
- *Motor evaluation.* Test by having patient clench jaw (masseter, temporalis), open jaw, and move side to side against resistance (lateral pterygoids). Lesions of the motor nucleus or more distally result in lack of contraction of the ipsilateral masticatory muscles. When the mouth is opened, the jaw deviates to the paralyzed side (due to intact contralateral lateral pterygoid muscle). Other

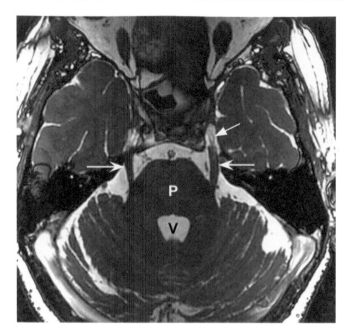

Fig. 5.6 Axial high-resolution FIESTA (fast imaging employing steady-state acquisition) image at the level of the fourth ventricle (V) demonstrates the normal CN V (*concave arrows*) exiting the mid-lateral pons (P) and dividing into smaller branches within Meckel cave (*straight arrow*).

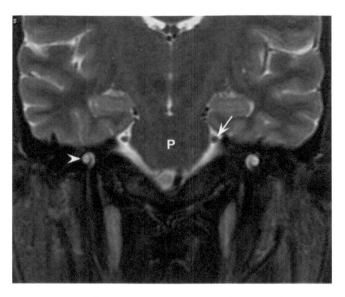

Fig. 5.7 Coronal T2-weighted image shows the cisternal segments of CN V (*arrow*) at the lateral aspect of the midpons (P). The more inferolateral cochlea (*arrowhead*) is well seen on this image.

muscles innervated by CN V (e.g., mylohyoid, anterior belly of the digastric, tensor tympani, tensor veli palatini) are difficult to test individually.

- *Reflex evaluation.*
  - *Corneal reflex.* Light touch to cornea leads to bilateral eyeblinks. Afferent arc is CN V_1 from upper cornea or CN V_2 from lower cornea to ipsilateral and contralateral CN VII motor nucleus. Efferent arc is CN VII to orbicularis oculi bilaterally for eyeblink.
  - *Jaw jerk reflex.* Tapping the lower jaw leads to contraction of the masseter and temporalis muscles. Afferent arc is proprioceptive sensory fibers to mesencephalic

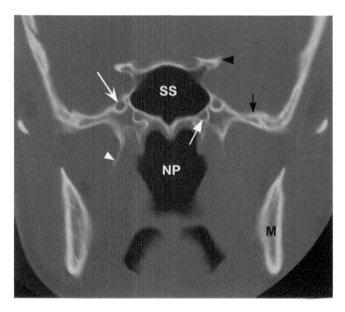

Fig. 5.8 Coronal CT image in bone window at the level of the midsphenoid sinus (SS) and nasopharynx (NP) shows the normal foramen rotundum (*white concave arrow*), the opening through which CN V_2 exits the skull base. Note that the vidian (pterygoid) canal (*white straight arrow*) is located inferior and medial to the foramen rotundum. The right lateral pterygoid plate (*white arrowhead*), left clinoid process (*black arrowhead*), left mandible (M) and greater wing of the left sphenoid bone (*black arrow*) are also indicated.

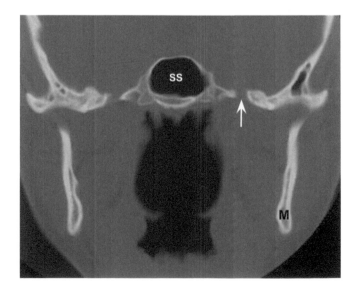

Fig. 5.9 A more posterior coronal CT image in bone window shows the normal foramen ovale (*arrow*), the opening through which CN V_3 exits the skull base.

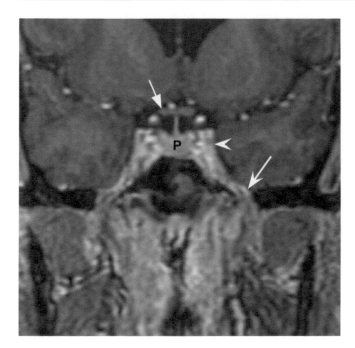

Fig. 5.10 Coronal postcontrast T1-weighted gradient-echo image in a different patient but at a similar plane as **Fig. 5.8** shows the normal appearance of foramen ovale (*concave arrow*) and the cavernous sinus (*arrowhead*). The foramen ovale can typically be identified on the same coronal image as the optic chiasm (*straight arrow*) and pituitary gland (P).

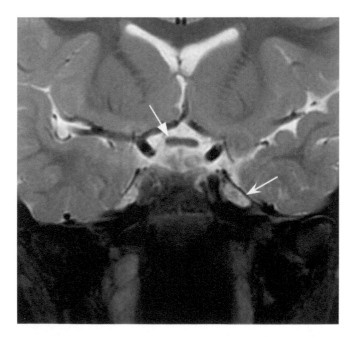

Fig. 5.11 Coronal T2-weighted image with fat saturation slightly more posteriorly shows the normal CSF-intensity signal within Meckel's cave (*concave arrow*). The optic chiasm (*straight arrow*) is also indicated.

nucleus of CN V. Efferent arc is motor nucleus of CN V to mandibular nerve to cause contraction of masseter and temporalis.

Types

Supranuclear Lesions

- Bilateral but predominantly contralateral control of muscles of mastication via corticobulbar fibers.
- Unilateral upper motor neuron lesions can interrupt the corticobulbar pathway from the motor cortex to pons. Because the jaw then deviates toward the paralyzed side (see above), it deviates away from the lesion.
- Bilateral upper motor neuron lesions lead to spastic masticatory paresis (pseudobulbar palsy).
- The sensory pathway may be interrupted anywhere from trigeminothalamic fibers to VPM thalamus to postcentral gyrus. For example, thalamic lesions can result in contralateral facial anesthesia.

Brainstem Lesions (Nucleus or Fascicular Portion)

- Motor and sensory nuclei may be affected by brainstem lesions. Like other brainstem lesions, the constellation of findings (e.g., long tract signs and other CN involvement) helps pinpoint the location of the lesion.
- Dorsal midpontine lesions affect motor nucleus. Findings include ipsilateral paresis/atrophy/fasciculations of masticatory muscles. Suggested also by involvement of corticospinal tract (contralateral hemiplegia), principal sensory nucleus of CN V (ipsilateral hemianesthesia of the face), spinothalamic tract (contralateral hemisensory loss of limbs and trunk), medial longitudinal fasciculus internuclear ophthalmoplegia (INO), descending sympathetic fibers (Horner syndrome) (see Appendix A).
- Lesions affecting lateral medulla or upper cervical cord affect the spinal tract and nucleus of CN V and cause ipsilateral facial pain/temperature loss, often along with involvement of the spinothalamic tract (leading to contralateral trunk and extremity pain/temperature loss) (e.g., as part of Wallenberg syndrome) (see Appendix A).
- Lower medullary or upper cervical spinal cord nuclear lesions can result in an *"onion-skin"* pattern of sensory loss over lateral forehead, cheek, and jaw. This reflects the somatotopic organization of the spinal nucleus of CN V (perioral area—rostral; lateral face—caudal).
- Specific lesions:
  - Tumors
  - Cavernous vascular malformations
  - Demyelinating disease
  - Inflammatory disease
  - Ischemia/infarction
  - Syringobulbia. Cranial extension of *syringomyelia* (dilatation of central canal) from the upper cervical cord into the medulla may affect spinal nucleus of CN V.

Lesions in the Subarachnoid Space

- Lesions affecting the preganglionic trigeminal nerve typically cause ipsilateral motor (masticatory) paresis and/or ipsilateral facial pain/sensory loss with a depressed corneal reflex.
- Concurrent involvement of adjacent CNs (VII and VIII) suggests a cerebellopontine angle lesion
- Specific lesions:
  - Cerebellopontine angle tumors (e.g., vestibular schwannoma, meningioma, epidermoid cyst)
  - Infectious/inflammatory disease (e.g., viral neuritis, meningitis, arachnoiditis, sarcoidosis, syphilis, tuberculosis [TB])
  - Trauma
  - Neurovascular compression (e.g., *trigeminal neuralgia* is a syndrome of severe lancinating facial pain often due to irritation/compression of the trigeminal nerve at the root entry zone by vascular branches).
  - Perineural spread of tumor

Lesions at the Petrous Apex and Meckel's Cave

- May affect the main trunk of the trigeminal nerve and/or the trigeminal ganglion, leading to severe hemifacial pain or numbness (or may involve only select divisions of the trigeminal nerve).
- Specific lesions:
  - Infectious lesions (e.g., petrous apicitis, skull base osteomyelitis) (see *Gradenigo syndrome* below)
  - Neoplasms (e.g., meningiomas, schwannomas, perineural spread of head and neck cancer, chordomas, chondrosarcomas, nasopharyngeal carcinomas, metastases)
  - Inflammatory lesions (e.g., cholesterol granuloma, cholesteatoma, mucocele)
  - Trauma (skull base fracture)
- *Raeder paratrigeminal syndrome.* Unilateral oculosympathetic paresis (Horner syndrome) and ipsilateral trigeminal involvement. The Horner syndrome is postganglionic (ptosis, miosis without anhidrosis), and trigeminal involvement consists of ipsilateral head, facial, or retroorbital pain. Classically described as due to lesions in the middle cranial fossa near the trigeminal ganglion (hence "paratrigeminal") and the petrous portion of the internal carotid artery, at the petrous apex. Postganglionic Horner syndrome would result from involvement of sympathetic fibers in the internal carotid plexus. Lesions that can cause this syndrome include parasellar mass lesions, aneurysm, trauma, and infection. Involvement of other CNs (III, IV, VI) would suggest cavernous sinus syndrome instead.
- *Gradenigo syndrome.* Gradenigo syndrome is caused by inflammation of the petrous apex (petrous apicitis) which leads to injury to the trigeminal (CN V) and abducens (CN VI) nerves with facial pain/numbness and ipsilateral lateral rectus palsy. The clinical "Gradenigo triad" includes retroorbital pain, abducens nerve palsy, and otorrhea. This is usually due to otitis media and/or mastoiditis complicated by infection of petrous apex air cells and sometimes skull base osteomyelitis. See Case 6.8, Chapter 6.
- *Herpes zoster.* Caused by varicella-zoster virus (VSV, member of herpesvirus family). After varicella (chickenpox), the virus remains latent in sensory ganglia, including the trigeminal ganglion. Upon reactivation, it multiplies and spreads distally causing pain and skin eruptions (vesicles). Any division of CN V can be involved, but by far it most commonly involves CN V_1 (called *herpes zoster ophthalmicus*). Involvement of cornea and conjunctiva can lead to permanent visual loss. Treatment is with acyclovir and its derivatives.

Lesions at the Cavernous Sinus/Superior Orbital Fissure

- *Cavernous sinus syndrome.* Dysfunction of CN III, IV, VI, V_1, V_2 due to cavernous sinus lesion and leading to unilateral ophthalmoplegia with pain/sensory loss in CN V_1 and V_2 distribution, ± oculosympathetic paresis (Horner syndrome). Often only one or a few CNs are affected by lesions of the cavernous sinus, with the full-blown syndrome being rare.
- *Superior orbital fissure syndrome.* Dysfunction of CN III, IV, VI, V_1 leading to ophthalmoplegia and pain/sensory loss in CN V_1 distribution ± oculosympathetic paresis, as well as possible exophthalmos (due to blockage of superior ophthalmic vein).
- The presence or absence of CN V_2 involvement can help differentiate between these two syndromes and help to localize the lesion.
- Specific lesions:
  - Neoplasm (e.g., meningioma, lymphoma, metastatic disease)
  - Vascular (carotid-cavernous fistula, giant ICA aneurysm)
  - Inflammatory (e.g., sarcoidosis, Tolosa-Hunt syndrome)
  - Infection (e.g., bacterial or fungal sphenoid sinusitis with extension to the cavernous sinus)
  - Pituitary apoplexy (acute enlargement of the pituitary gland with secondary acute cavernous sinus compression)
  - Radiation injury (e.g., following radiosurgery for cavernous sinus meningiomas)

Distal Trigeminal Lesions

- Distal trigeminal branches may be involved by local trauma, inflammation (e.g., viral neuritis) or tumor (e.g., lymphoma, squamous cell carcinoma, adenoid cystic carcinoma, melanoma).
- Trauma to distal trigeminal branches:
  - CN V_1. Supraorbital and supratrochlear nerves are most frequently injured after frontal head trauma. Na-

sociliary nerve is often damaged after frontoethmoid injury.

- CN V$_2$. Infraorbital nerve is often injured during orbital floor "blow-out" fractures. Greater and lesser palatine nerves can be injured with fractures of the hard palate.
- CN V$_3$. The inferior alveolar nerves can be injured by mandibular fractures.

- *Numb cheek syndrome.* Secondary to lesions in infraorbital foramen causing numbness of cheek and upper lip (infraorbital nerve).
- *Numb chin syndrome.* Isolated mental neuropathy leads to pain, swelling, and jaw numbness. Can be caused by perineural spread of head and neck cancer arising from the skin of the chin or lower buccal or gingival mucosa, lymphoproliferative neoplasms, or metastases to the mandible.

Trigeminal Nerve: Pathologic Images

Case 5.1

A 26-year-old female presents with stabbing left facial pain (**Figs. 5.12, 5.13**).

Diagnosis

Trigeminal neuralgia due to multiple sclerosis

Case 5.2

A 78-year-old female presents with intractable lancinating left facial pain (**Figs. 5.14, 5.15**).

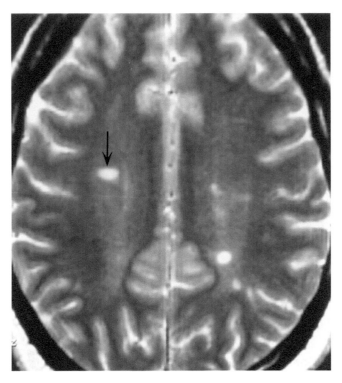

Fig. 5.13 Axial T2-weighted image at the level of the centrum semiovale (above the lateral ventricles) shows additional hyperintense lesions within the periventricular white matter. Note a horizontally aligned lesion (*arrow*), which is typical of the periventricular demyelinating plaques of multiple sclerosis.

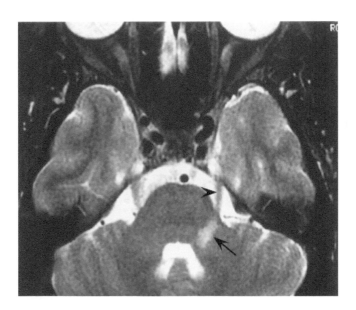

Fig. 5.12 Axial T2-weighted image at the level of the pons and fourth ventricle shows a hyperintense lesion (*arrow*) within the left middle cerebellar peduncle, at the level of the exiting left CN V (*arrowhead*).

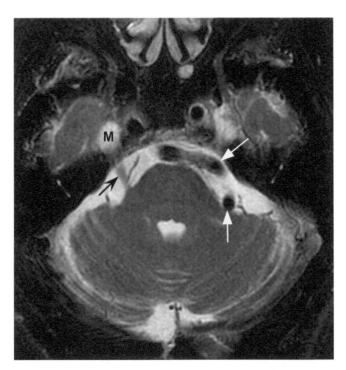

Fig. 5.14 Axial T2-weighted image demonstrates dilatation and marked tortuosity of the basilar artery (*white straight arrows*), at the level of the expected location of the cisternal segment of the left CN V. Note the normal right CN V (*black arrow*) as it exits the pons and heads toward Meckel cave (M).

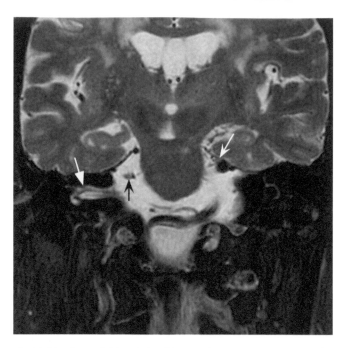

Fig. 5.15 Coronal T2-weighted image demonstrates superior displacement of a small left CN V (*white concave arrow*) by the tortuous basilar artery as compared with the normal position of the right CN V (*black arrow*), just above the right internal auditory canal (*white straight arrow*). Neurovascular compression of the trigeminal nerve.

Diagnosis

Trigeminal neuralgia due to neurovascular compression

Trigeminal Neuralgia (Also Called Tic Douloureux)
- *Epidemiology.* Uncommon. Female:male ratio 3:2.
- *Clinical presentation.* Lancinating (stabbing or shock-like), paroxysmal, intense, usually unilateral facial pain. Most commonly affects *CN V_2 > V_3 > V_1 distributions*, and it is typically associated with only minimal sensory deficit. The pain episodes are typically sudden in onset, last for a few seconds, and may occur frequently over several weeks. Often incited by touch or other stimuli to trigger zones on the face (e.g., shaving, face washing, chewing).
- *Pathology.* Most commonly due to irritation/compression of root entry zone (REZ) by vascular structures, either venous or arterial. May also be due to demyelinating plaques, brainstem neoplasms, or perineural spread of tumor.
- *Imaging.* Imaging may demonstrate a tortuous vessel or vascular loop in the region of the CN V REZ, or may be normal. Dedicated skull base magnetic resonance imaging (MRI) with thin cuts and/or MR angiography is usually necessary to identify these small compressive vascular structures. Other vascular pathologies such as dural arteriovenous fistulae may occasionally be demonstrated. Demyelinating plaques or compressive or infiltrative neoplastic lesions may also be identified.

- *Treatment.* Medical treatment is with *carbamazepine* (Tegretol), phenytoin (Dilantin), baclofen, clonazepam, and/or amitriptyline (Elavil). *Opiates offer little relief.* If no relief occurs with carbamazepine, the diagnosis should be questioned, and imaging can be useful to assess for more unusual causes of trigeminal neuralgia such as neoplasm or demyelination. Surgical options include peripheral nerve injections or peripheral neurectomy, percutaneous radiofrequency (RF) or glycerol rhizotomies, percutaneous balloon gangliolysis, open retrogasserian rhizotomy, microvascular decompression, and stereotactic radiosurgery. Percutaneous procedures have high initial success rates but may be associated with paresthesias/dysesthesias and occasionally anesthesia dolorosa and neuroparalytic keratitis. Open retrosigmoid craniotomy for microvascular decompression, although most invasive, is highly effective, and no sensory impairment occurs with this option.

Case 5.3

A 47-year-old female with known right frontal lobe glioblastoma multiforme (GBM) presents with new right facial numbness (**Figs. 5.16, 5.17, 5.18**).

Diagnosis

Multifocal GBM, affecting trigeminal nuclei and extending into cisternal segment of trigeminal nerve

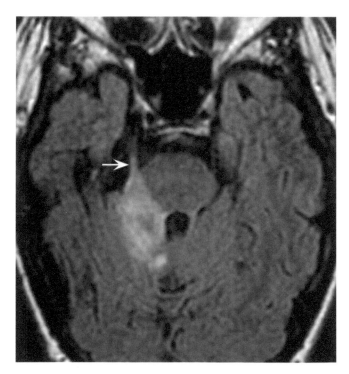

Fig. 5.16 Axial FLAIR image shows a hyperintense expansile lesion with ill-defined margins, especially posterolaterally, involving the right pons, middle cerebellar peduncle, and cerebellum. The lesion infiltrates anteriorly into the exiting right CN V (*arrow*).

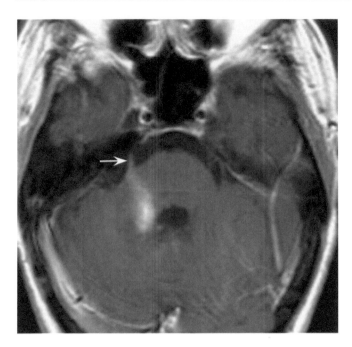

Fig. 5.17 Axial postcontrast T1-weighted image shows irregular enhancement within this mass and along the right CN V (*arrow*).

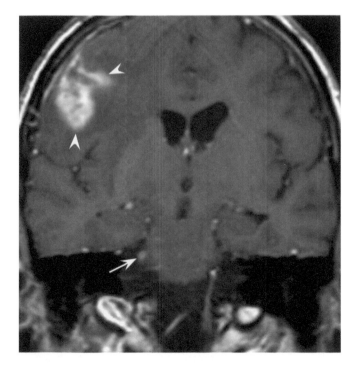

Fig. 5.18 Coronal postcontrast T1-weighted image shows enhancement of the cisternal segment of the right trigeminal nerve (*arrow*). Note also the heterogeneously enhancing mass (*arrowheads*) within the right frontal lobe. Multifocal glioblastoma multiforme with involvement of the cisternal segment of CN V.

Glioblastoma Multiforme

- *Epidemiology.* GBM is the most frequent primary brain tumor, accounting for ~12 to 15% of all intracranial neoplasms and 50 to 60% of all astrocytic tumors. Incidence is ~2 to 3 new cases per 100,000 people per year. Predominantly affects adults (peak incidence age 45–70).
- *Clinical presentation.* Usually present with headaches, progressive neurologic deficits, altered mental status, signs/symptoms of increased intracranial pressure, and/ or seizures. Presentation with CN deficits is rare (as in this case).
- *Pathology.* GBMs may be classified as primary (developing de novo) or secondary (developing from a lower-grade glioma), which appear to represent distinct genotypic alterations leading to the identical phenotypic end point. They are highly malignant and invasive. Distinguishing characteristics include hypercellularity, nuclear atypia/ pleomorphism, necrosis, and microvascular proliferation (Grade IV, World Health Organization [WHO] classification). Multifocal GBMs constitute an uncommon but increasingly recognized subgroup associated with an even poorer prognosis than solitary lesions.
- *Imaging.* MRI may reveal a heterogeneous rim-enhancing mass on T1-weighted images with central necrosis or an ill-defined infiltrative mass. Intense enhancement with gadolinium is common but not invariable. Peritumoral edema appears hyperintense on T2 and hypointense on T1. These tumors tend to spread along white matter tracts such as the corpus callosum ("butterfly" glioma) or internal capsule. Multifocal GBMs may appear as anatomically separate and distant lesions.
- *Treatment.* Surgical resection for accessible solitary lesions + XRT ± chemotherapy. Biopsy + XRT for unresectable and/or multiple lesions. Prognosis is affected by histologic grade, age, preoperative neurologic status, extent of resection, addition of radiation therapy, and multiplicity of lesions. Steroids are useful in treating vasogenic edema, and anticonvulsants are used following documented seizures.

Case 5.4

A 34-year-old male presents with acute left perioral numbness (**Fig. 5.19**).

Diagnosis

Cranial neuritis affecting the left CN V (presumably postviral)

Case 5.5

A 20-year-old male presents with progressive right facial numbness. On examination, he has weakness of the right masticatory muscles, and the jaw deviates to the right (**Figs. 5.20, 5.21**).

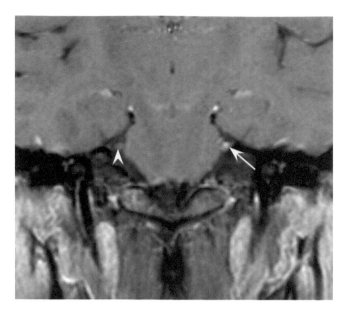

Fig. 5.19 Coronal postcontrast T1-weighted image shows enhancement of the left CN V (*arrow*) when compared with the normal contralateral right CN V (*arrowhead*). Viral neuritis.

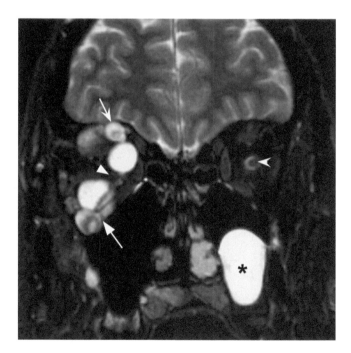

Fig. 5.20 Coronal fast spin echo T2-weighted image with fat saturation shows multiple lobulated, predominantly hyperintense, right intraorbital and infraorbital masses along the first division (CN V₁, *concave arrow*) and second division (CN V₂, *straight arrow*) of the trigeminal nerve. Several of these lesions have the "target" morphology typical of neurofibromas, with concentric rings of T2 hyperintensity alternating with areas of intermediate signal intensity. A normal left optic nerve-sheath complex (*concave arrowhead*) is clearly identified. The right optic nerve sheath complex (*straight arrowhead*) can be faintly seen despite being severely displaced and compressed by the multiple intraorbital neurofibromas. The hyperintense mass within the left maxillary sinus (*asterisk*) represents an incidental mucosal retention cyst or polyp.

Diagnosis
Multiple neurofibromas in a patient with neurofibromatosis type 1 (NF-1) with involvement of right CNs V₁ to V₃

German Neurofibromatosis Type 1 (von Recklinghausen Neurofibromatosis, Peripheral Form)
- *Epidemiology*. Occurs in 1 in 3000 births. Autosomal dominant transmission, chromosome 17 (neurofibromin gene). Fifty percent occur by spontaneous mutation without family history.
- *Clinical presentation*. Inclusion criteria are at least two of the following: six *café-au-lait spots*, two neurofibromas, *one plexiform neurofibroma*, axillary or inguinal freckling, an osseous lesion (*sphenoid dysplasia* or thinning of long bones or cortex), an *optic glioma*, two Lisch nodules (pigmented iris hamartomas, appear as translucent yellow/brown elevations, only seen with NF-1), and a relative with NF-1.
- *Imaging*. May show multiple intra- or extracranial masses that are hyperintense on T2, isointense to hypointense on T1 and show mild to intense contrast enhancement. Fusiform enlargement of optic nerves, optic tracts, and/or optic chiasm in cases of optic pathway glioma. Nonenhancing foci of T2 hyperintensity within the deep gray nuclei and white matter are thought to represent areas of myelin vacuolization. Parenchymal tumors (usually astrocytomas) show T2 hyperintensity and variable enhancement and have predilection for thalami and basal ganglia. Brainstem gliomas (BSG) in setting of NF-1

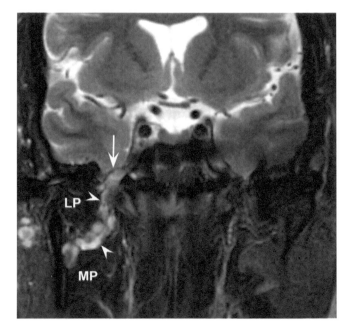

Fig. 5.21 More posteriorly, there is multilobulated enlargement of CN V₃ (*arrowheads*) as it exits through the foramen ovale (*arrow*) and passes between the medial (MP) and lateral (LP) pterygoid muscles. Multiple neurofibromas involving CN V₁, V₂, and V₃ in a patient with neurofibromatosis type 1.

have a more indolent course and better prognosis than isolated BSGs. Sphenoid wing dysplasia may be present and is usually associated with plexiform neurofibroma and buphthalmos (enlarged eye resulting from increased intraocular pressure). Spinal neurofibromas develop on the posterior nerve roots and may be completely intradural or "dumbbell" (intra- and extradural), ± widening of the neural foramina with bony remodeling of adjacent pedicle.

- *Pathology.* Neurofibromas contain Schwann cells, fibroblasts, collagen, and reticulin. They are fusiform, *unencapsulated*, infiltrate nerves (contain axons), and *rarely have cystic, fatty, or hemorrhagic changes.* Most are solitary cutaneous nodules coming from small terminal nerves. Approximately 5% undergo malignant change.
- *Associated tumors.* Optic gliomas, ependymomas, rare unilateral vestibular neuromas and meningiomas, *astrocytomas, pheochromocytoma, and malignant peripheral nerve sheath tumor.*
- *Other associated conditions. Scoliosis,* widened spinal canal, *posterior vertebral body scalloping* (due to dural ectasia), meningocele, renal artery stenosis, aqueductal stenosis, retinal phakomas, *moyamoya-type arterial occlusions,* aneurysms, arteriovenous malformations (AVMs), mental retardation (5%), and learning disability (40%).
- *Treatment.* Surgery for removal or debulking of symptomatic lesions. Gross total removal can cause deficit as neurofibromas infiltrate into nerves.

Case 5.6

A 24-year-old male with a known genetic syndrome develops bilateral facial numbness and paresthesiae (**Figs. 5.22, 5.23, 5.24**).

Diagnosis

NF-2 with multiple schwannomas

Neurofibromatosis Type 2 (Central Form)
- *Epidemiology.* Occurs in 1 in 30,000 births. Autosomal dominant transmission, chromosome 22 (schwannomin gene). Later onset than NF-1.
- *Clinical presentation.* Related to location of tumors (e.g., progressive hearing loss related to vestibular schwannomas). *Paucity* of cutaneous lesions.
- *Imaging. Schwannomas:* round to ovoid extraaxial masses that have iso- to hypointense T1 signal and iso- to hyperintense T2 signal as compared with brain parenchyma (may be indistinguishable from neurofibromas, though neurofibromas may have central T2 hypointensity in some cases, a so-called "target" appearance). Moderate, homogeneous enhancement is typical, unless the lesion is hemorrhagic or cystic. *Bilateral enhancing cerebellopontine angle (CPA) tumors* (bilateral vestibular schwannomas) are pathognomonic. *Meningiomas:* dural-based

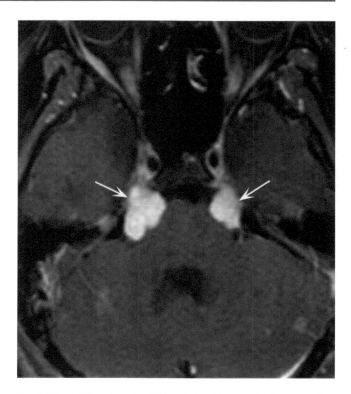

Fig. 5.22 Axial postcontrast T1-weighted image with fat saturation demonstrate enlarged enhancing masses (*concave arrows*) along both CNs V.

extraaxial masses, often associated with a dural "tail." Typically isodense to brain on computed tomography (CT) and isointense to gray matter on MRI. Usually intense and homogeneous enhancement. May be calcified. *Spinal tumors* (usually schwannomas) may occur in as many as 90% of patients with NF-2 and are most

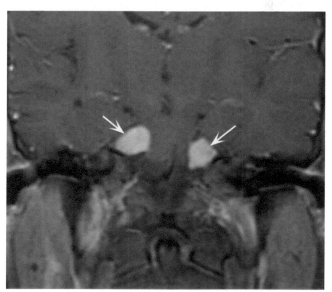

Fig. 5.23 Coronal postcontrast T1-weighted image with fat saturation in the same patient shows the bilateral enhancing masses (*concave arrows*) adjacent to the pons along the course of the trigeminal nerve.

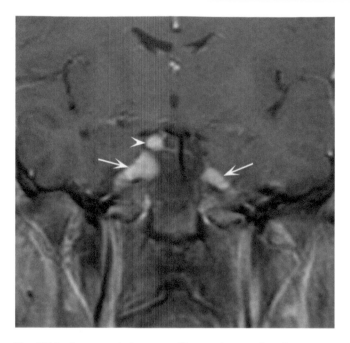

Fig. 5.24 A more anterior coronal image shows enhancing masses along bilateral CN V (*arrows*) and the right CN III (*arrowhead*), consistent with multiple CN schwannomas in this patient with neurofibromatosis type 2.

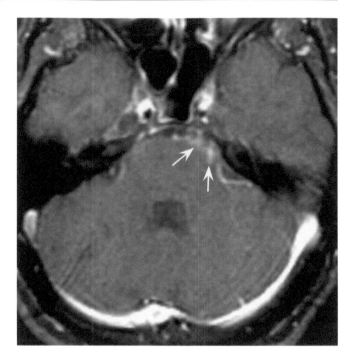

Fig. 5.25 Axial post-contrast T1-weighted image with fat saturation at the level of the pons demonstrates abnormal enhancement (*arrows*) involving the left prepontine cistern and the surface of the pons more diffusely. Enhancement is most intense at the root entry zone of the left CN V.

sensitively detected on fat-saturated postcontrast MRI. Imaging of brain or spine should include the lower CNs because patients may also have had tumors of cranial nerves X and XII. Two to 10% of all patients with vestibular schwannomas have NF-2. Hemorrhage into a vestibular schwannoma may result in sudden hearing loss or acute hydrocephalus.

- *Associated lesions.* Other associated tumors include *meningiomas, spinal ependymomas* (spinal astrocytomas are more common in NF-1), and *nerve root schwannomas.* There are rare café-au-lait spots, cutaneous neurofibromas (more likely to be schwannomas), and plexiform neurofibromas. There are no *Lisch nodules.*
- *Pathology.* Pathology for schwannomas is previously described (Chapter 3).
- *Treatment.* Surgery or radiosurgery for vestibular schwannomas; other lesion-specific therapies.

Case 5.7

A 40-year-old male with acquired immune deficiency syndrome (AIDS) presents with altered mental status, left facial numbness, and intermittent diplopia (**Figs. 5.25, 5.26, 5.27, 5.28**).

Diagnosis

Fungal encephalitis, ventriculitis, and meningitis at autopsy (*Pseudallescheria boydii* infection, a saprophytic fungus)

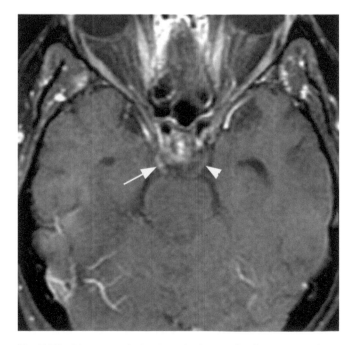

Fig. 5.26 More superiorly, there is abnormal enhancement along the right CN III (*arrow*) compared with the left (*arrowhead*).

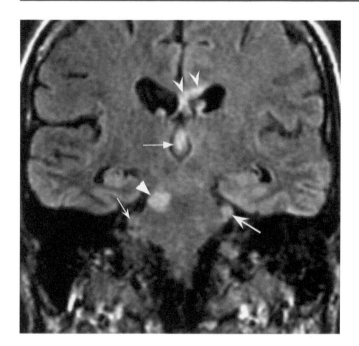

Fig. 5.27 Coronal FLAIR image at the level of the ventral pons shows abnormal enlargement and hyperintensity of the left CN V (*large concave arrow*) as well as more subtle hyperintensity of the right CN V (*small concave arrow*). Parenchymal hyperintensity is seen within the right brainstem (*straight arrowhead*) at the pontomesencephalic junction. Also note the abnormal hyperintensity (*concave arrowheads*) along the septum pellucidum and ependymal surface of the left lateral ventricle. Focal bright signal within the third ventricle (*small straight arrow*) is a common CSF flow related artifact but may mimic an intraventricular lesion.

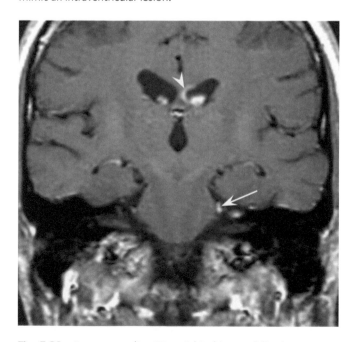

Fig. 5.28 A corresponding T1-weighted image following contrast but without fat saturation shows abnormal enhancement along the left CN V (*arrow*), as well as the ependymal surface (*arrowhead*) of the left frontal horn, compatible with an infectious/inflammatory ventriculitis or neoplastic involvement by lymphoma. A diagnosis of fungal meningitis was made by CSF analysis.

Clinical Pearl

Fungal meningitis is most often seen in the setting of immunodeficiency (e.g., AIDS, posttransplantation, cancer chemotherapy), with the notable exception of *Coccidioidomyces,* which frequently affect immune competent hosts in the southwestern and western United States. *Basilar meningitis* (with cranial neuropathies, hydrocephalus, and arteritis causing strokes) is characteristic. CSF reveals increased lymphocytes and decreased glucose. The most common fungal organisms isolated are *Cryptococcus, Coccidioidomyces, Aspergillus,* and *Mucor,* but many species may be isolated. *Aspergillus* and *Mucor* are particularly associated with rapid clinical deterioration.

Imaging Pearl

CT imaging is often normal in the setting of meningitis, though hydrocephalus (check for mild dilatation of the temporal horns) may be the first imaging clue. Fluid-attenuated inversion recovery (FLAIR) images are very sensitive to alterations in CSF composition, and the presence of elevated protein and/or cells will result in high signal intensity in sulci on FLAIR images. As with CT, hydrocephalus may also be seen on MRI in the setting of meningitis. CN involvement is best evaluated by fat-saturated postcontrast MRI, with thin cuts through the skull base. CN and leptomeningeal enhancement may be seen with fungal meningitis. Parenchymal infarcts and/or edema may be seen due to inflammation and occlusion of small perforating vessels at the base of the brain, or in the setting of infection with angioinvasive organisms (e.g. *Aspergillus*) leading to large vessel occlusions. If ventriculitis is suspected, subtle edema and/or enhancement may be seen along the ependymal surface, or there may be debris within the ventricles. Remember: normal imaging never rules out infection!

Case 5.8

A 51-year-old male presents with left CN V$_2$ numbness and decreased vision (**Figs. 5.29, 5.30, 5.31, 5.32, 5.33, 5.34**).

Diagnosis

Nasopharyngeal carcinoma with both perineural spread of tumor and direct extension of tumor to the skull base

Nasopharyngeal Carcinoma

- *Epidemiology.* Endemic in China, Southeast Asia, and portions of Africa. Male:female ratio 2:1. Bimodal age distribution with peaks in adolescence and at 50 to 60 years.
- *Clinical presentation.* Nasopharyngeal carcinoma can lead to nasal obstruction, changes in hearing (blockage of eustachian tube and serous otitis media), epistaxis, and

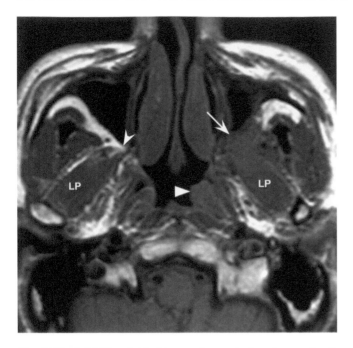

Fig. 5.29 Axial T1-weighted image demonstrates abnormal soft tissue infiltrating the left pterygopalatine fossa (*arrow*) and involving the adjacent lateral pterygoid muscle (LP). Note normal fat signal within the right pterygopalatine fossa (*concave arrowhead*). Also present is a soft tissue mass in the left nasopharynx (*straight arrowhead*).

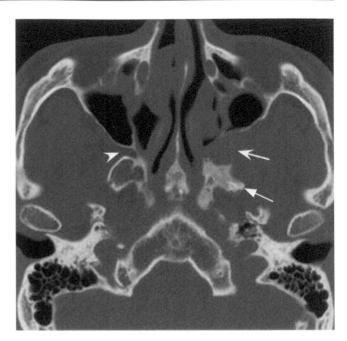

Fig. 5.30 Axial CT (bone window) in the same patient as in **Fig. 5.28** shows marked widening of the left pterygopalatine fossa (*concave arrow*) compared with the normal right side (*arrowhead*). There is bony sclerosis of the left pterygoid process of the sphenoid bone (*straight arrow*).

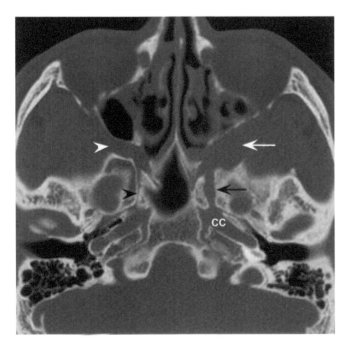

Fig. 5.31 A more superior axial CT image in bone window again shows asymmetric enlargement and remodeling of the left pterygopalatine fossa (*white arrow*) compared with the normal right side (*white arrowhead*), as well as widening of the left vidian canal (*black arrow*) compared with the normal right vidian canal (*black arrowhead*), consistent with tumor spread along the vidian nerve toward the carotid canal (CC).

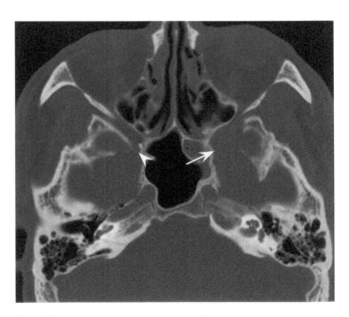

Fig. 5.32 More superiorly, an axial CT image in bone window shows erosion of the greater wing of the sphenoid bone and marked widening of the left foramen rotundum (*arrow*). Note the normal right foramen rotundum (*arrowhead*).

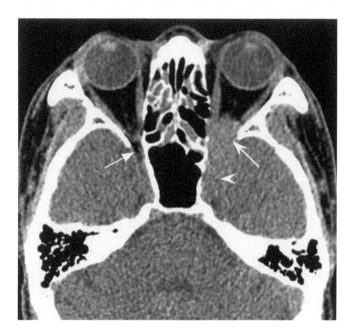

Fig. 5.33 Somewhat more superiorly, an axial CT image in soft tissue window demonstrates a soft tissue mass extending from the level of the cavernous sinus (*arrowhead*) through a markedly widened superior orbital fissure (*concave arrow*) into the orbital apex. Low-density fat is seen in the normal contralateral right superior orbital fissure (*straight arrow*).

CN palsies (from extension into skull base via floor of the middle fossa or perineural extension). Other associated findings are headache and cervical lymphadenopathy.
- *Imaging.* Soft tissue mass usually centered near the fossa of Rosenmüller (lateral nasopharyngeal recess), typically

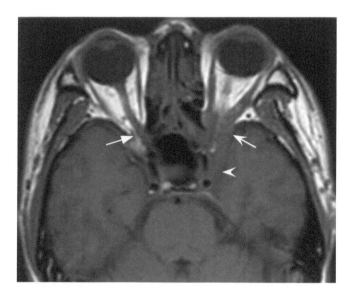

Fig. 5.34 An axial T1-weighted image in the same patient as in **Figs. 5.29, 5.30, 5.31, 5.32, 5.33** shows the abnormal infiltrative soft tissue extending from the left cavernous sinus (*arrowhead*) into the left orbit (*concave arrow*). On the right, normal fat is seen in the posterior orbit, adjacent to the optic nerve (*straight arrow*). Nasopharyngeal carcinoma with extensive, direct skull base and orbital extension, as well as perineural extension.

with intermediate T2 signal and homogenous enhancement. Signal characteristics may mimic lymphoma. Patient demographics and lesion location and morphology usually help to differentiate from other malignancies, but final diagnosis requires tissue confirmation. Obstruction of the eustachian tube results in ipsilateral mastoid effusion. Intracranial extension may result from direct skull base invasion, typically through the foramen lacerum to the middle cranial fossa, or via perineural spread along the adjacent CNs.
- *Pathology.* Arises from the epithelium of the nasopharynx. Epstein-Barr virus (EBV) is associated etiologic agent in endemic cases. WHO has classified three categories of nasopharyngeal carcinoma: WHO-1 is the most differentiated and is also known as keratinizing squamous cell carcinoma. WHO-2 is referred to as nonkeratinizing, and it is the least common. WHO-3 is also called undifferentiated carcinoma, represents the EBV-associated endemic form, and is the most common.
- *Treatment.* Biopsy for diagnosis. Radiation therapy is the mainstay of treatment, with chemotherapy used in advanced cases.

Case 5.9

A 17-year-old male with known acute lymphocytic leukemia (ALL) presents with right facial numbness and intermittent diplopia (**Figs. 5.35, 5.36**).

Diagnosis

CNS spread of tumor in a patient with ALL involving cavernous sinus, Meckel's cave, and multiple CNs

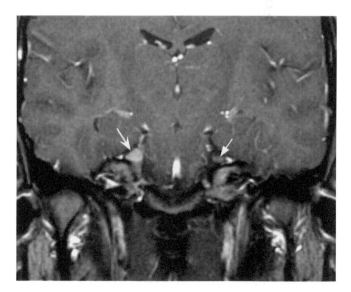

Fig. 5.35 Coronal postcontrast T1-weighted image with fat saturation at the level of the ventral pons shows clear-cut enlargement and enhancement of CN V on the right (*concave arrow*). CN V on the left (*straight arrow*) is not enlarged but may show subtle abnormal enhancement.

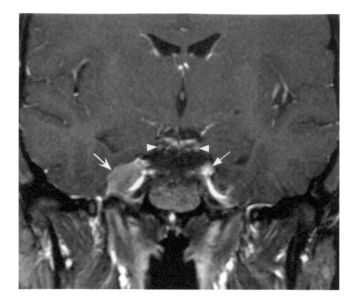

Fig. 5.36 A more anterior coronal postcontrast T1-weighted image with fat saturation demonstrates a large soft tissue mass in Meckel's cave on the right (*concave arrow*). In addition, due to the leptomeningeal involvement by leukemic cells, both oculomotor nerves (*arrowheads*) are seen to be slightly enlarged and abnormally enhancing, with the left being greater than the right. Pathologic enhancement is also seen on the left (*straight arrow*) at the level where CN VI is crossing the anteromedial petrous ridge on its way to the cavernous sinus. Leukemic leptomeningitis.

Clinical Pearl

Leptomeningeal spread of tumor occurs in ~20% of patients with cancer. It is most commonly found in adults with breast carcinoma, lung carcinoma, or melanoma, and in children with hematologic malignancies (as in this case) or primitive neuroectodermal tumors (PNET). The leptomeninges enclose the subarachnoid space and extend along the CNs, allowing access by tumor cells within the CSF. Patients present with symptoms caused by irritation/compression of CNs in the subarachnoid space, direct invasion into the brain and/or spinal cord, and/or hydrocephalus. Definitive diagnosis is obtained by CSF cytology or in some cases by leptomeningeal biopsy. Therapy is lesion-specific, potentially including intrathecal chemotherapy and/or radiation therapy.

Imaging Pearl

Contrast-enhanced imaging studies demonstrate focal or diffuse leptomeningeal enhancement (*zuckerguss*, German for sugar icing). This enhancement may be very subtle and in some cases diagnosis can be improved with double- or triple-dose of a gadolinium-based agent or FLAIR or post-gadolinium FLAIR imaging. The involved CNs may demonstrate enhancement, enlargement, or both. This finding may also be quite subtle and often requires thin-section, fat-saturated post-gadolinium imaging to confirm the diagnosis.

Case 5.10

A 66-year-old male presents with right forehead pain and paresthesias (**Figs. 5.37, 5.38, 5.39, 5.40**).

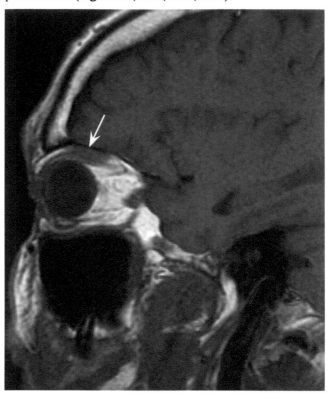

Fig. 5.37 Sagittal T1-weighted image demonstrates focal soft tissue thickening (*arrow*) within the superior aspect of the right orbit, above the superior rectus/levator palpebrae superioris muscle complex.

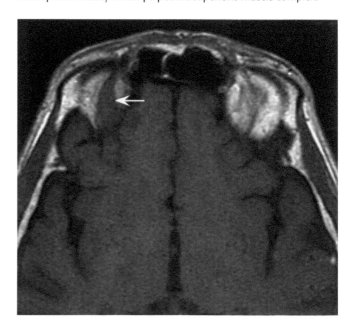

Fig. 5.38 Axial T1-weighted image in the same patient shows asymmetric soft tissue (*arrow*) within the superior aspect of the right orbit, above the superior rectus/levator palpebrae superioris muscle complex and along the expected course of CN V_1.

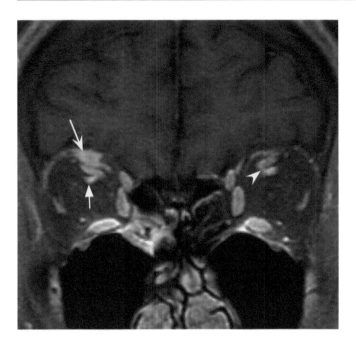

Fig. 5.39 Coronal postcontrast T1-weighted image with fat saturation in the same patient shows an enhancing soft tissue mass (*concave arrow*) above the superior rectus/levator palpebrae superioris complex musculature (*arrowhead*) and superior ophthalmic vein (*straight arrow*).

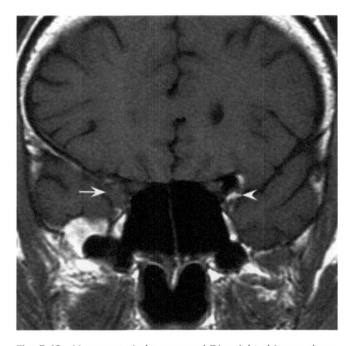

Fig. 5.40 More posteriorly, a coronal T1-weighted image shows soft tissue within the right superior orbital fissure (SOF) (*arrow*), effacing the fat that is typically present in the SOF. Compare the normal, bright fat signal in the SOF on the contralateral side (*arrowhead*). Perineural spread of squamous cell carcinoma was confirmed with tissue sampling.

Diagnosis

Perineural spread of tumor (squamous cell carcinoma) involving the intraorbital portion of CN V$_1$

Clinical Pearl

Perineural spread of tumor refers to extension of tumor along a nerve, usually a named branch of a CN. It most commonly occurs with malignant tumors such as squamous cell carcinoma, adenoid cystic carcinoma, or melanoma arising from various sites in the head and neck. Because of their extensive distal ramification and wide distribution with resultant proximity to most head and neck tumors, CNs V and VII are most commonly involved by perineural spread, and indeed tumors can spread perineurally from one nerve to the other. The two most common CN V to CN VII connections are via the auriculotemporal nerve and the greater superficial petrosal nerve. Clinical findings include CN dysfunction, pain or dysesthesias, or muscle denervation atrophy in advanced cases.

Imaging Pearl

CT is often unremarkable although it may show bony remodeling or expansion of the CN foramina within the skull base. MR is the imaging modality of choice and typically demonstrates enhancement and/or enlargement of the CNs. Noncontrast T1-weighted images may show replacement of normal fat planes with soft tissue along the course of the nerve. Skull base invasion may also result in the replacement of normal fatty marrow by tumor. It is important to image the entire course of the involved CN as well as its associated target organs (e.g., perineural spread along CN VII requires imaging of the parotid gland). In cases of spread along motor nerves (such as CN V$_3$, VII, and X), denervation changes may be seen in innervated muscle groups.

Case 5.11

A 45-year-old male presents with right brow numbness and paresthesias (**Figs. 5.41, 5.42**).

Diagnosis

CN V$_1$ schwannoma

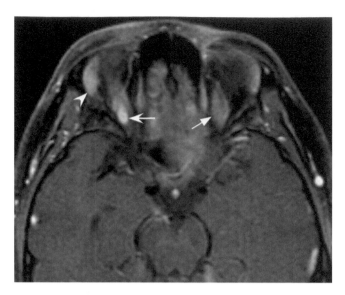

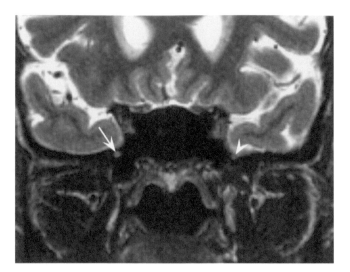

Fig. 5.41 Axial postcontrast T1-weighted image with fat saturation demonstrates a small, focal, rounded enhancing mass (*concave arrow*) just superior to the superior rectus (SR) muscle (*straight arrow* is on contralateral SR muscle). An enhancing structure (*concave arrowhead*) in the superolateral aspect of the orbit represents the normal lacrimal gland.

Fig. 5.43 Coronal T2-weighted image shows subtle enlargement and high signal intensity of the right CN V_2 (*arrow*) within the foramen rotundum. Note the normal signal of the left CN V_2 (*arrowhead*).

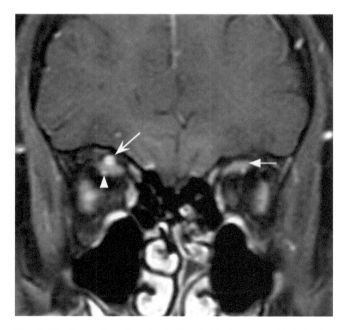

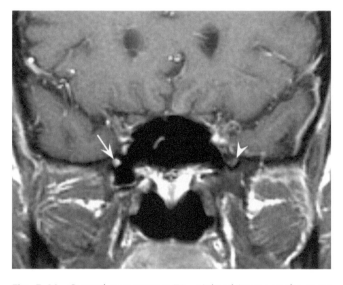

Fig. 5.42 Coronal postcontrast T1-weighted image with fat saturation shows the small, rounded enhancing mass (*concave arrow*) along the expected course of the right CN V_1 (frontal branch) just superior to the superior rectus muscle (*straight arrow*). Note the tiny focus of enhancement (*straight arrowhead*) inferior to the muscle that represents the superior ophthalmic vein. Schwannoma arising from CN V_1.

Fig. 5.44 Coronal postcontrast T1-weighted image at the same level shows abnormal enhancement of the right CN V_2 (*arrow*) compared with the normal signal of the left CN V_2 (*arrowhead*). The patient's imaging and clinical findings resolved after a course of steroids and acyclovir. Viral neuritis.

Diagnosis

CN V_2 neuritis

Case 5.12

A 55-year-old female presents with right cheek numbness (**Figs. 5.43, 5.44**).

Case 5.13

A 74-year-old with prior history of squamous cell carcinoma presents with right lateral nose and cheek numbness (**Figs. 5.45, 5.46, 5.47**).

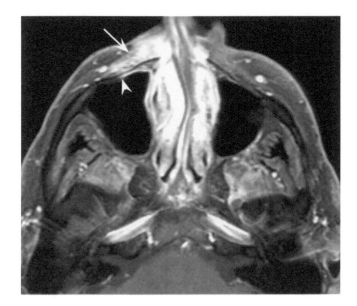

Fig. 5.45 Axial postcontrast T1-weighted image with fat saturation demonstrates an abnormal, ill-defined enhancing mass (*arrow*) in the right premaxillary soft tissues, extending to the expected location of the infraorbital foramen (*arrowhead*).

Diagnosis

Perineural spread of recurrent tumor (squamous cell carcinoma) involving right infraorbital nerve (of CN V$_2$)

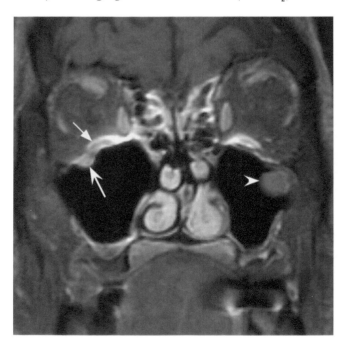

Fig. 5.47 Coronal postcontrast T1-weighted image with fat saturation at the same level shows focal asymmetric enhancement of the right infraorbital nerve (*concave arrow*) within the infraorbital foramen, beneath the normal inferior rectus muscle (*straight arrow*). A small mucosal polyp or retention cyst (*arrowhead*) within the left maxillary sinus does not enhance and should not be confused with an enlarged infraorbital nerve. Perineural spread of recurrent squamous cell carcinoma along CN V$_2$.

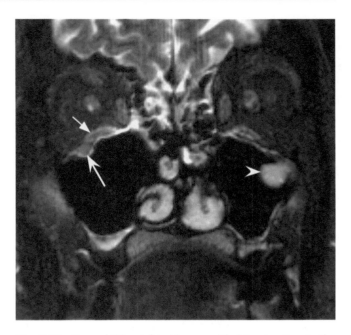

Fig. 5.46 Coronal T2-weighted image with fat saturation in the same patient shows asymmetric enlargement of the right infraorbital nerve (branch of CN V$_2$, *concave arrow*) within the infraorbital canal, beneath the normal inferior rectus muscle (*straight arrow*). A small mucosal polyp or retention cyst (*arrowhead*) within the left maxillary sinus is incidentally noted.

Case 5.14

A 59-year-old male presents with left jaw numbness (**Figs. 5.48, 5.49**).

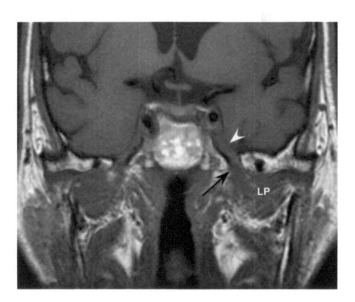

Fig. 5.48 Coronal T1-weighted image demonstrates asymmetric widening of the left foramen ovale (*arrow*) and asymmetric thickening of CN V$_3$ as it heads toward the lateral pterygoid muscle (LP). Soft tissue fullness is also seen in the region of Meckel's cave (*arrowhead*). Also note that the muscles of mastication are decreased in size on the left as compared with the right.

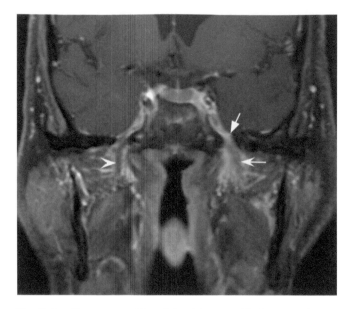

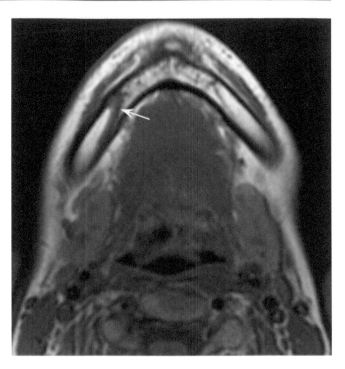

Fig. 5.49 Postcontrast T1-weighted image with fat saturation at the same level shows asymmetric enhancement along the course of CN V₃ (*concave arrow*) and at the level of foramen ovale (*straight arrow*). Note the normal appearance of the right CN V₃ nerve (*concave arrowhead*) and its surrounding vascular plexus. Perineural spread of squamous cell carcinoma proximally along CN V₃ and through the foramen ovale.

Fig. 5.50 Axial T1-weighted image demonstrates increased soft tissue within the right inferior alveolar canal (*arrow*) along the course of the inferior alveolar nerve.

Diagnosis

Melanoma with perineural spread along left CN V₃

Case 5.15

A 35-year-old male presents with right lower mouth and chin numbness (**Figs. 5.50, 5.51**).

Diagnosis

Gingivobuccal sulcus squamous carcinoma with perineural spread along the right inferior alveolar nerve

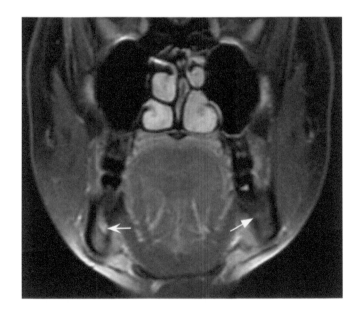

Fig. 5.51 Coronal postcontrast T1-weighted image with fat saturation in the same patient shows an enlarged and enhancing right inferior alveolar nerve (*concave arrow*) compared with the normal-sized contralateral nerve (*straight arrow* on left inferior alveolar canal). Perineural spread of tumor was confirmed at the time of segmental mandibular resection.

6 Abducens Nerve

Functions

- General somatic efferent (GSE). Somatic motor innervation to the lateral rectus (LR) muscle.

Anatomy

- The *abducens nucleus* is in the dorsal pontine tegmentum at the level of the lower pons, just ventral to the fourth ventricle (separated from floor of the fourth ventricle by genu of facial nerve) (**Figs. 6.1, 7.1**).

- *Fascicles* course ventrally through the pons and through the medial lemniscus (ML) medial to facial nerve fascicles to emerge at the pontomedullary junction just lateral to the pyramid (**Fig. 6.2**). The *cisternal segment* ascends in the prepontine cistern through the subarachnoid space of the posterior fossa and traverses *Dorello's canal*, extending over the petrous apex and beneath Grüber's (petroclinoid) ligament to enter the cavernous sinus. The petroclinoid ligament is a fibrous band connecting the lateral margin of the dorsum sellae to the upper border of the petrous part of the temporal bone. *Dorello's canal* is a fibroosseous channel bounded by the

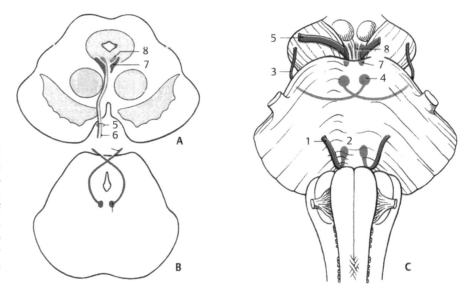

Fig. 6.1 Comparison of nuclear regions and exits of oculomotor, trochlear, and abducens nerves. (**A**) Midbrain at the level of the superior colliculus. (**B**) Midbrain at the level of the inferior colliculus. (**C**) Ventral view of brainstem. (1, abducens nerve; 2, abducens nucleus; 3, trochlear nerve; 4, trochlear nucleus; 5, oculomotor nerve; 6, visceromotor [parasympathetic] fibers; 7, oculomotor nucleus; 8, Edinger-Westphal nucleus.)

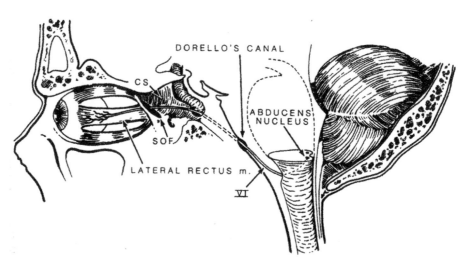

Fig. 6.2 Sagittal view of the abducens nerve from nuclear origin in the lower pontine tegmentum to its end point in the lateral rectus muscle (see text). (From Harnsberger HR. Handbook of Head and Neck Imaging [2nd ed.] St. Louis, MO: Mosby, 1995. Reprinted with permission.)

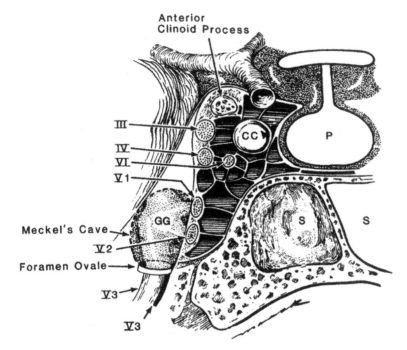

Fig. 6.3 Coronal view through the cavernous sinus demonstrates CN III, IV, V$_1$ and V$_2$ in the lateral wall of the cavernous sinus and CN VI within the cavernous sinus adjacent to the cavernous portion of the ICA. Note that CN V$_3$ does not enter cavernous sinus but rather leaves cranial base through the foramen ovale. (From Harnsberger HR. Handbook of Head and Neck Imaging [2nd ed.] St. Louis, MO: Mosby, 1995. Reprinted with permission.)

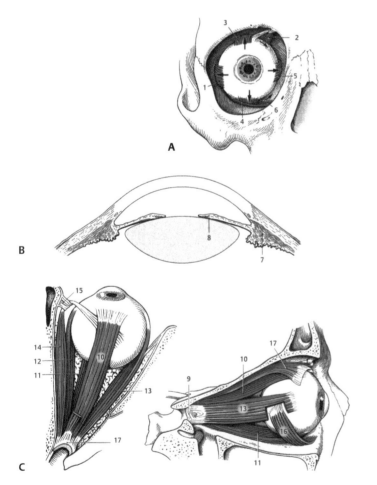

Fig. 6.4 Schematic of extraocular and intraocular muscles. **(A)** Anterior view. (1, LR muscle; 2, SO muscle; 3, SR muscle; 4, IR muscle; 5, MR muscle; 6, IO muscle.) **(B)** Intraocular muscles. (7, ciliary muscle; 8, sphincter pupillae muscle.) **(C)** Superior (left) and lateral (right) views. (9, common annular tendon [annulus of Zinn]; 10, SR muscle; 11, IR muscle; 12, MR muscle; 13, LR muscle; 14, SO muscle; 15, trochlea; 16, IO muscle; 17, LPS muscle.)

apex of the petrous bone inferolaterally, the petroclinoid ligament superiorly and the dorsum sella medially. Once in the cavernous sinus, cranial nerve (CN) VI travels just lateral to the internal carotid artery (ICA) and medial to CN V$_1$ (**Fig. 6.3**), then enters the orbit at the medial end of the superior orbital fissure (SOF), traverses the annulus of Zinn (tendinous ring), and innervates the LR muscle. Note that unlike the other CNs (III, IV, V$_1$, V$_2$) which lie between the two leaves of dura that make up the lateral wall of the cavernous sinus, CN VI actually lies *within* the cavernous sinus adjacent to the ICA (**Fig. 6.3**).

• LR muscle functions to abduct the eye (**Fig. 6.4**).

Abducens Nerve: Normal Images (Figs. 6.5, 6.6, 6.7)

Abducens Nerve Lesions

• Lesions of the abducens nerve cause impaired ipsilateral lateral gaze. Therefore, patients with unilateral abducens palsy complain of horizontal diplopia, worst in the direction of the paretic LR muscle.

• Unlike a peripheral CN VI lesion, a nuclear CN VI lesion impairs ipsilateral gaze of *both* eyes. This is due to the fact that the abducens nuclear complex contains interneurons projecting via the medial longitudinal fasciculus (MLF) to the contralateral oculomotor nucleus (innervating the contralateral MR muscle). Therefore, a right-sided lesion of the abducens *nucleus* impairs rightward gaze of *both* eyes, whereas a right-sided lesion of the abducens *nerve* impairs rightward gaze of the *right* eye only (and hence horizontal diplopia with image separation worst on far rightward gaze). This is the only cra-

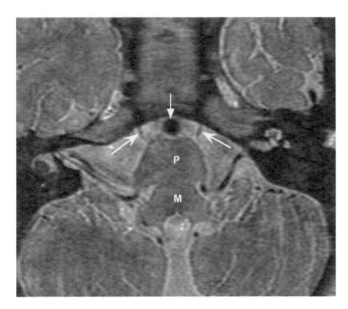

Fig. 6.5 Axial T2-weighted image shows bilateral CN VI (*concave arrows*) exiting the ventral aspect of the pontomedullary junction and ascending in the prepontine cistern lateral to the basilar artery (*straight arrow*). Here we see the upper medulla (M) but also the belly of the pons (P) given the angle of slice acquisition.

nial nerve in which lesion of the root fibers and nucleus do not produce the same effect.

- Rare congenital lesions of CN VI include *Möbius syndrome* (a genetic disorder caused by absence or underdevelopment of CNs VI and VII, characterized by horizontal gaze palsy associated with facial diplegia) and *Duane retrac-*

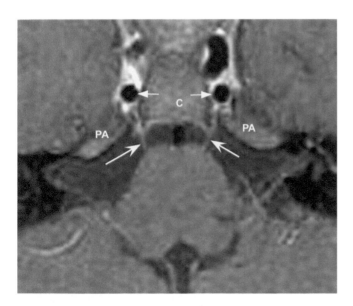

Fig. 6.7 Axial postcontrast T1-weighted image shows faint normal enhancement of CN VI. On this image, the nerves (*concave arrows*) are seen extending over the medial aspect of the petrous apices (PA) as they head for Dorello's canal. Note the cavernous carotid artery flow voids (*straight arrows*) within the cavernous sinus lateral to the clivus (C).

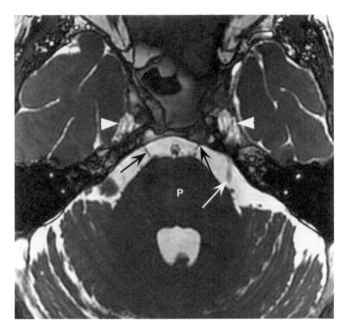

Fig. 6.6 Axial fast imaging employing steady-state acquisition (FIESTA) sequence shows in fine detail the cisternal segments of CN VI (*black arrows*) at the level of the mid pons (P) and fourth ventricle, as CN VI courses toward Dorello's canal. The left CN V (*white arrow*) is faintly seen. Note the normal CSF within Meckel's cave bilaterally (*arrowheads*).

tion syndrome (congenital unilateral horizontal abduction deficit due to absence of the abducens nerve on one side, characterized by gaze palsy with globe retraction).

Types

Brainstem Lesions (Abducens Nuclear Lesions)

- Produce a conjugate (both eyes involved) horizontal gaze palsy toward the side of the lesion
- Often associated with other neurologic signs of injury to the pons (usually ipsilateral peripheral CN VII palsy)

Fascicular Lesions

- Result in an ipsilateral abduction deficit
- Also associated with damage to nearby pontine structures (anterior paramedian pontine lesions)
- Paramedian pontine lesions (including nuclear and fascicular lesions) may be caused by
  ○ ischemia,
  ○ inflammation,
  ○ demyelination (e.g., multiple sclerosis [MS]),
  ○ compressive mass lesion (tumor, abscess, cavernous vascular malformation).
- *Millard-Gubler syndrome.* Unilateral lesion of ventrocaudal pons affecting corticospinal tract, CN VI fascicles and CN VII with contralateral hemiplegia, ipsilateral LR paresis, and facial paresis

Lesions of the Cisternal Segment (in Prepontine Cistern)

- Result in isolated abduction deficits
- Associated with contralateral hemiparesis if corticospinal tract involved by extrinsic compression
- Causes include the following:
  - Ischemia (e.g., ischemic abducens neuropathy from diabetes)
  - Neoplasm (e.g., cerebellopontine angle tumors, clival meningioma, clival chordoma, chondrosarcoma, schwannoma, nasopharyngeal carcinoma)
  - Vascular (e.g., dolichoectatic basilar arteries, aneurysms)
  - Trauma (nerve stretching and/or compression)
  - Inflammation (e.g., meningitis with secondary neuritis)
  - Demyelinating disease (Miller-Fisher variant of Guillain-Barré syndrome includes ophthalmoplegia, ataxia, and areflexia)
  - Changes in intracranial pressure (ICP). CN VI palsies are noted both with increased ICP but also with decreased ICP (e.g., from intracranial hypotension related to a dural cerebrospinal fluid [CSF] leak). Therefore an ipsilateral CN VI palsy often turns out to be a "false localizing sign" in the absence of localizing pathology.
  - Radiation injury

Lesions at the Petrous Apex and Dorello's Canal

- Concomitant involvement of CN V is frequent.
- Causes include the following:
  - Infectious lesions.
    - Skull base osteomyelitis.
    - Petrous apicitis.
    - *Gradenigo syndrome.* Inflammation of the petrous apex (petrous apicitis) leads to damage to the trigeminal (CN V) and abducens (CN VI) nerves with facial pain/numbness and ipsilateral lateral rectus palsy.
  - Trauma (e.g., skull base fracture involving clivus and petrous apex).
  - Neoplasms (e.g., meningiomas, schwannomas, chordomas, chondrosarcomas, nasopharyngeal carcinomas, metastases).
  - Inflammatory lesions (e.g., cholesterol granuloma, cholesteatoma, mucocele).
  - Intrapetrous carotid artery aneurysms are rare but may cause CN VI palsy.

Lesions in the Cavernous Sinus/Superior Orbital Fissure

- Concomitant Horner syndrome suggests cavernous lesion (because sympathetic fibers travel with the cavernous portion of the ICA).
- Neoplasm (e.g., meningioma, lymphoma, metastasis).
- Vascular (carotid-cavernous fistula, giant ICA aneurysm).
- Inflammatory (e.g., sarcoidosis, Tolosa-Hunt syndrome).
- Infection (e.g., bacterial or fungal sphenoid sinusitis with extension to the cavernous sinus).
- Pituitary apoplexy (acute enlargement of the pituitary gland leads to acute cavernous sinus compression).
- Radiation injury (e.g., following radiosurgery for cavernous sinus meningiomas).

Lesions of the Orbit

- Lesions of the orbit do not typically lead to a palsy of CN VI.
- Other conditions of the orbit may present with an isolated abduction deficit (e.g., thyroid orbitopathy, myasthenia gravis). In thyroid orbitopathy, inflammatory infiltration and interstitial edema result in increased fatty mass and muscle enlargement, leading to mechanical restriction of the globe. In myasthenia gravis, weakness of extraocular muscles may present as diplopia, often accompanied by ptosis due to weakness of the levator palpebrae superioris (LPS) muscle; indeed in ~20% of patients weakness remains confined to the extraocular and eyelid muscles (*ocular myasthenia*).

Treatment

- Correction of diplopia following CN VI injury may require prism therapy and/or strabismus surgery. Correction should not be undertaken until recovery is complete. Occasionally, botulinum toxin is injected into the contralateral medial rectus muscle to minimize diplopia.

Abducens Nerve: Pathologic Images

Case 6.1

A 28-year-old female presents with horizontal diplopia and is found to have a left CN VI palsy (**Figs. 6.8, 6.9, 6.10, 6.11**).

Diagnosis

MS affecting left CN VI nucleus/fascicles

Multiple Sclerosis
- *Epidemiology.* Affects ~400,000 people in the United States. Peak age 20 to 40 years, with female predominance (2:1). The highest incidence is in Northern Europe. Risk is related to one's geographic location before age 15 years. Etiology is unknown, but influences are considered to be geographic origin (distance from the equator), family history, and an infectious process (possibly viral) that triggers autoimmunity to myelin.
- *Clinical presentation.* Neurologic deficits including visual (*optic neuritis* 25%), autonomic, and sensorimotor (50%).

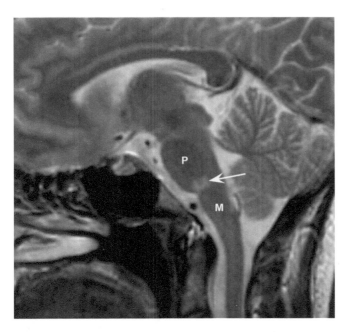

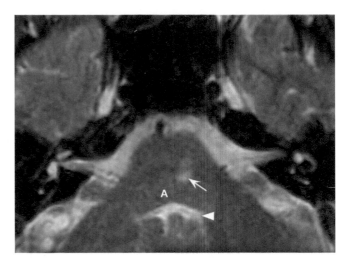

Fig. 6.9 Axial T2-weighted image shows the hyperintense lesion (*arrow*) near the expected location of the CN VI fascicles as they exit ventrally from the abducens nucleus within the dorsal pontomedullary junction at the level of the mid fourth ventricle (*arrowhead*). Note the approximate location of the abducens nucleus on the right (A).

Fig. 6.8 Sagittal T2-weighted image demonstrates a hyperintense lesion (*arrow*) within the inferior pons (P) at the level of the pontomedullary junction (M, medulla).

Fifty percent of patients who have optic neuritis will eventually be diagnosed with MS. *Bilateral internuclear ophthalmoplegia* (INO) is characteristic of MS. Trigeminal neuralgia may also occur. Lhermitte sign (electrical shock or tingling up and down the spine) is common but not specific to demyelinating diseases. MS is usually *relapsing/remitting* (Charcot type), but 10% of cases are progressive. Diagnosis is aided by magnetic resonance imaging (MRI), the presence of CSF oligoclonal bands, and abnormal sensory evoked potentials (e.g., visual or auditory).

• *Imaging.* Typically shows periventricular white matter low attenuation (computed tomography, CT) or T2-hyperintense (MRI) foci (a nonspecific finding that may

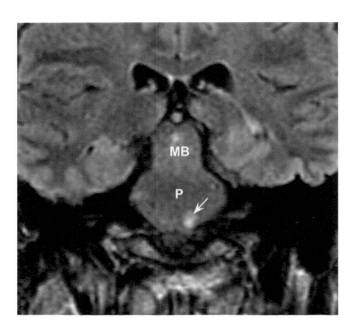

Fig. 6.10 Coronal FLAIR image at the level of the midbrain (MB) demonstrates the hyperintense lesion (*arrow*) at the inferior aspect of the pons (P).

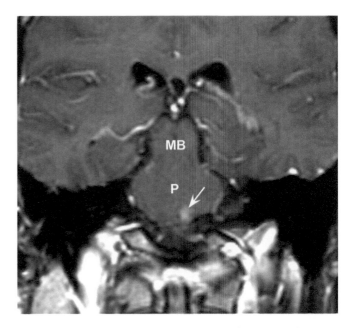

Fig. 6.11 Coronal postcontrast T1-weighted image at the same level shows focal enhancement of the lesion (*arrow*). This is most consistent with an active inflammatory/demyelinating process in this young woman, but in the absence of a known diagnosis, infectious, vascular, and neoplastic possibilities would also have to be considered. (MB, midbrain; P, pons.)

mimic to some extent the small vessel ischemic changes commonly seen in diabetic, hypertensive, or elderly patients). On T2 or fluid-attenuated inversion recovery (FLAIR) sequences, focal hyperintense lesions are present in nearly all definite MS cases. MS often involves the brainstem and cerebellar white matter tracts as well. More specific findings include perivenular lesions (*Dawson's fingers*) within deep white matter perpendicular to the lateral ventricles and/or involvement of the undersurface of the corpus callosum. Callosal thinning and white matter volume loss are nonspecific and indicate long-standing disease. Contrast enhancement suggests active plaques.

- *Pathology.* Immune-mediated CNS demyelination. Gross pathologic examination reveals plaques that are gelatinous, firm, ovoid, *perpendicular to the ventricles*, and in the superolateral *periventricular white matter*, corpus callosum, subcortical white matter, optic nerves/chiasm/tracts, brainstem, and spinal cord. Microscopic examination of an *active plaque* demonstrates decreased myelin, macrophages, destruction of and/or proliferation of oligodendrocytes, perivascular inflammatory infiltrate (T > B cells), reactive astrocytosis, and edema. Relative axonal sparing is seen early in the disease but chronic progressive disease is associated with axonal loss leading to permanent disability.

- *Treatment.* Immune modulation with high-dose steroids followed by slow taper. Steroids reduce duration and severity of exacerbations but do not change frequency or outcome. β-interferons have been shown to reduce the number and severity of exacerbations in relapsing-remitting MS. Copolymer 1 (or Copaxone, glatiramer acetate), a synthetic form of myelin basic protein, is also approved for the treatment of relapsing-remitting MS. An immunosuppressant treatment, mitoxantrone (Novantrone), is approved for the treatment of advanced or chronic MS.

Case 6.2

An 8-year-old female presents with nausea, ataxia, and inability to look to the left. No other cranial abnormalities are found on physical examination (**Fig. 6.12, 6.13, 6.14**).

Diagnosis

Brainstem abscess

Brainstem Abscess

- *Epidemiology.* Rare (<1% of intracranial abscesses). Pons is the most common site, followed by the midbrain and the medulla.
- *Clinical presentation.* Occasional fever and headache, followed by CN deficits and long-tract signs, nausea/vomiting, and cerebellar dysfunction.

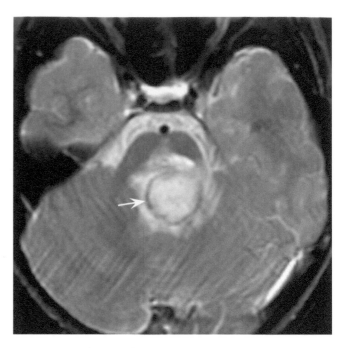

Fig. 6.12 Axial T2-weighted image shows a dorsal pontine mass with central hyperintensity, a peripheral hypointense rim (*arrow*), and surrounding high signal intensity consistent with vasogenic edema. This appearance is nonspecific but typical of a pyogenic abscess.

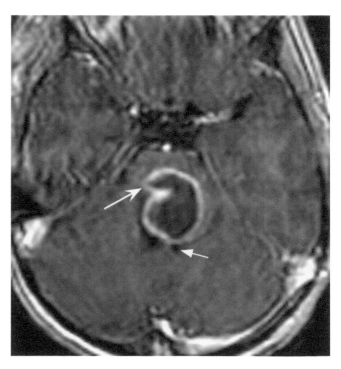

Fig. 6.13 Axial postcontrast image demonstrates a rim-enhancing mass centered within the dorsal pons which compresses the fourth ventricle (*straight arrow*). Note the partially septated component (*concave arrow*) or so called developing daughter lesion that is often seen with abscess.

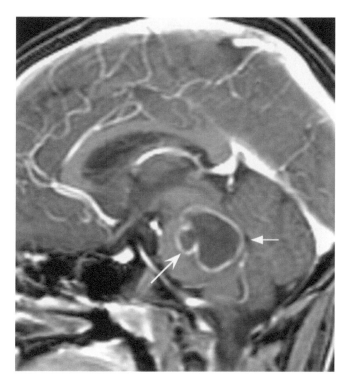

Fig. 6.14 Sagittal postcontrast image confirms location within the dorsal pons (*straight arrow*) and shows more clearly the developing daughter lesion anteriorly (*concave arrow*). Brainstem abscess.

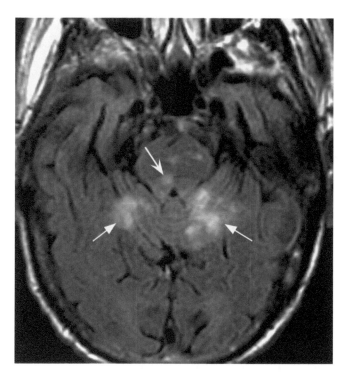

Fig. 6.15 Axial FLAIR image demonstrates patchy hyperintense signal within the superior cerebellar hemispheres bilaterally (*straight arrows*), as well as scattered hyperintense foci within the pons. A small focus of T2 hyperintensity is seen in the expected location of the right medial longitudinal fasciculus (MLF) (*concave arrow*).

- *Imaging.* CT: central hypodensity with a thin, smooth enhancing wall. MRI: central T1 hypointensity and T2 hyperintensity with peripheral ring enhancement following gadolinium administration. A peripheral rim of dark T2 signal is suggestive of abscess. Markedly reduced diffusion within the central region of a peripherally enhancing mass lesion is characteristic of pyogenic abscess, but this appearance may be seen on occasion with primary or metastatic brain tumors. Nonpyogenic parenchymal infectious cysts or abscesses (e.g., neurocysticercosis, tuberculosis) will generally not show reduced diffusion.
- *Pathology. Staphylococcus, Streptococcus,* and anaerobic species are the most common organisms isolated, especially in immunocompetent hosts.
- *Treatment.* Medical therapy (antibiotics), stereotactic aspiration, and/or open microsurgical exploration and drainage. Six to 8 weeks of parenteral antibiotics based on microbiologic diagnosis, if possible. Morbidity is high.

Case 6.3

An 86-year-old male with a history of hypertension and hypercholesterolemia presents with acute ataxia, somnolence, slurred speech and diplopia on left lateral gaze. On examination he is found to have internuclear ophthalmoplegia (INO), with impaired adduction of the right eye (**Figs. 6.15, 6.16**).

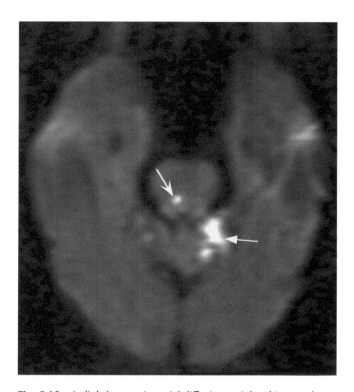

Fig. 6.16 A slightly superior axial diffusion-weighted image shows marked hyperintensity consistent with areas of acute tissue injury in the superior cerebellum (*straight arrow*) and right dorsal pons (*concave arrow*). Posterior circulation ischemia/infarction.

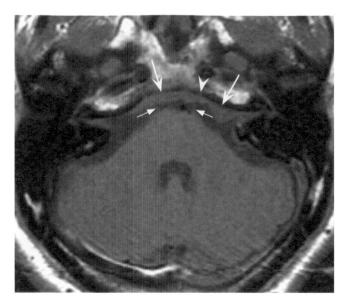

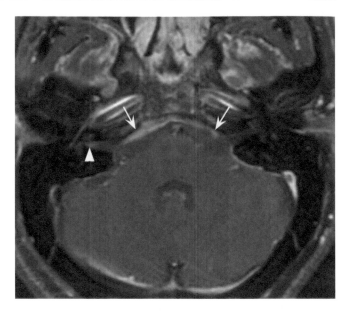

Fig. 6.17 Axial T1-weighted image demonstrates isointense soft tissue (*concave arrows*) dorsal to the clivus at the level of the mid pons, consistent with thickening of the dura. Note the tiny defect (*arrowhead*) in the cortical bone in the expected region of Dorello's canal. Also, the bilateral CN VI (*straight arrows*) can be faintly seen as they course toward the abnormally thickened dura on their way to the petrous apices.

Fig. 6.18 Axial postcontrast T1-weighted image shows diffuse enhancement of the retroclival soft tissue (*arrows*) as well as mild linear dural enhancement along the posterior petrous faces bilaterally. In addition, there is faint enhancement within the apex of the right internal auditory canal (*arrowhead*), consistent with involvement of dura within the internal auditory canal (IAC). The differential diagnosis includes neoplasm, infection, sarcoidosis, and idiopathic pachymeningitis.

Diagnosis

Bilateral cerebellar infarcts and right MLF lesion/right INO secondary to posterior circulation ischemia and infarction

Clinical Pearls

- INO is due to a lesion in the MLF and is characterized by adduction paresis on the side of the MLF lesion.
- INO may be unilateral or bilateral. Unilateral INO may result from brainstem infarction; other causes include Wernicke encephalopathy, trauma, encephalitis, neurosyphilis, and neoplasm. Bilateral INO is characteristic of MS but may also be seen with ischemic lesions.
- If a lesion damages the abducens nucleus in addition to the MLF, then *one-and-a-half syndrome* occurs: loss of conjugate gaze toward the side of the lesion (one) and adduction paresis on the side of the lesion (half).

Case 6.4

A 60-year-old male presents with diplopia and on examination is found to have a right abducens palsy (**Figs. 6.17, 6.18**).

Diagnosis

Idiopathic pachymeningitis

Clinical Pearl

- Differential diagnosis of pachymeningitis includes sarcoidosis, lymphoma, infection, neoplasm, and idiopathic pachymeningitis. Treatment with steroids in this case led to clinical improvement although a definitive diagnosis was never made.

Case 6.5

A 15-year-old male presents with diplopia and is found on examination to have a right CN VI palsy (**Figs. 6.19, 6.20, 6.21, 6.22, 6.23**).

Diagnosis

Clival chordoma presenting with palsy of CN VI

Clival Chordoma
- *Epidemiology.* Rare intracranial tumor. Usually presents in the third to fifth decade. Thirty-five percent of all chordomas occur in the *clivus* and 50% in the *sacrum,* with the remainder arising in the vertebral column or unusual sites (paranasal sinus, soft tissues of head and neck).
- *Clinical presentation.* Generally slow-growing but locally aggressive, destroying surrounding bone and infiltrating

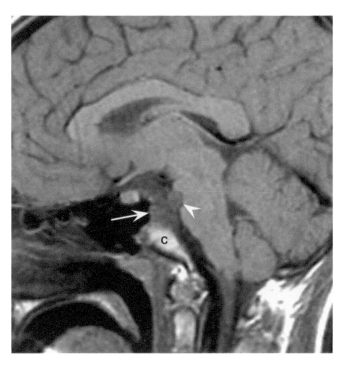

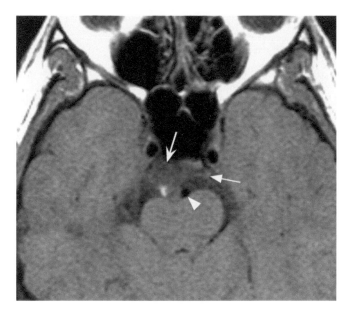

Fig. 6.19 The sagittal T1-weighted image demonstrates a mildly hypointense lesion (*white arrow*) replacing the fatty marrow of the upper aspect of the clivus (C) and dorsum sella with posterior extension to efface the prepontine cistern and focally deform the ventral pons (*arrowhead*).

Fig. 6.20 The axial T1-weighted image shows the right paracentral lesion (*concave arrow*) involving the dorsum sella, deforming the pons and displacing the basilar artery (*arrowhead*) to the left. The left CN VI (*straight arrow*) can be faintly seen. The right CN VI cannot be seen but would be expected to be ascending in the right side of the prepontine cistern and is presumably compressed by this mass.

adjacent soft tissues, making it very difficult to resect completely. Presenting findings include headache, double vision (CN VI palsy most common), and progressive

cranial neuropathies such as hoarseness/dysphagia, facial numbness/pain, hearing loss/vertigo, or brainstem signs. Metastases occur in ~40% of patients, but generally late in the course of the disease.

- *Imaging.* Destructive midline mass centered on the clivus. CT: lytic bone destruction, mixed density due to

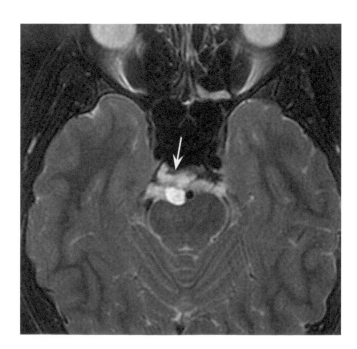

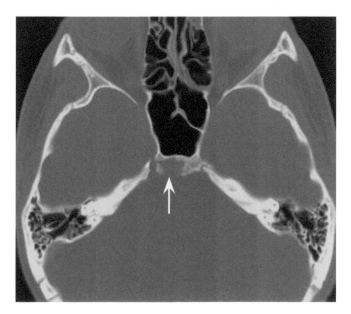

Fig. 6.21 Axial T2-weighted image with fat saturation shows that the prepontine mass (*arrow*) is lobulated and hyperintense.

Fig. 6.22 Axial CT image confirms a lytic lesion (*arrow*) involving the clivus.

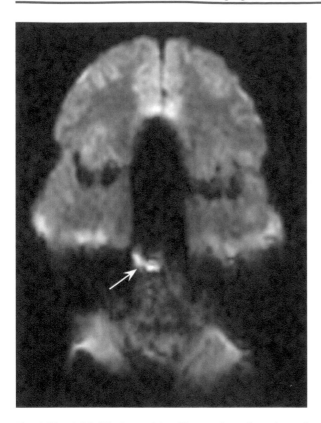

Fig. 6.23 Axial diffusion-weighted image shows hyperintensity (*arrow*) consistent with reduced diffusion. Although reduced diffusion in an extra-axial mass is typical of an epidermoid, other lesions may also have reduced diffusion. At surgery, this lesion was confirmed to represent a chordoma arising from the posterosuperior aspect of the clivus.

mucoid component. The calcification described in 30 to 70% of patients represents fragments of clival bone within the mass in most cases rather than actual tumor matrix calcification. MRI: usually hypo- or isointense to soft tissue on T1-weighted images, with *hyperintense* T2 signal. Enhancement is variable and heterogeneous. May extend into cavernous sinus, sella, petrous apex, sphenoid sinus, and/or nasopharynx and displace or compress basilar artery and brainstem posteriorly. Imaging differential includes chondrosarcoma, though these tend to arise more laterally.

- *Pathology.* Derived from *notochord remnants* (as is the nucleus pulposus) at the extremes of the axial skeleton. Lobulated, gray, soft, with sheets or cords of large vacuolated cells (*physalipherous* or bubble-bearing cells) in mucin-rich stroma. Immunohistochemistry is similar to the notochord with characteristics of both mesenchyme and epithelium and is critical for distinguishing chordomas from chondrosarcomas.
- *Treatment.* Slow-growing but difficult to cure, and many will eventually metastasize. Also may recur along the surgical track. Surgical resection followed by radiation therapy is used most commonly.

Case 6.6

A 50-year-old female with a remote history of left sphenoid sinus surgery presents 20 years later with intermittent horizontal diplopia. On examination, she is found to have bilateral CN VI palsies (**Figs. 6.24, 6.25, 6.26, 6.27**).

Diagnosis

Cholesterol granuloma affecting bilateral CN VI

Cholesterol Granuloma
- *Epidemiology.* Most common pathologic entity of the petrous apex.
- *Clinical presentation.* Presents with local mass effect causing headache and cranial neuropathies (e.g., CN VI palsy, hearing loss, vertigo, tinnitus, facial numbness).
- *Imaging.* CT demonstrates a sharply marginated expansile lesion of the petrous apex. MRI: high T1 and T2 signal (related to blood products, cholesterol crystals). Typically nonenhancing, though a thin rim of enhancing tissue may be observed around the periphery of the lesion. Differential diagnosis includes trapped fluid/petrous apex effusion (no bony abnormalities, low T1 signal), congenital or acquired cholesteatoma (usually not bright on T1-weighted image, shows reduced diffusion), mucocele (can have similar imaging characteristics, but usually not

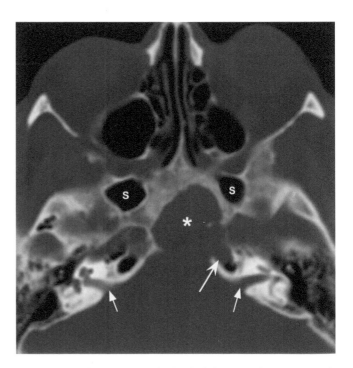

Fig. 6.24 Axial CT image at the level of the internal auditory canals (*straight arrows*) shows smoothly marginated erosive change in the clivus (*asterisk*). Partial aeration of the uninvolved right petrous apex is present, but on the left, there is erosion and mild expansion of the petrous apex (*concave arrow*), and this communicates with the erosive process of the clivus. Some aeration of the lateral sphenoid recesses (S) is present.

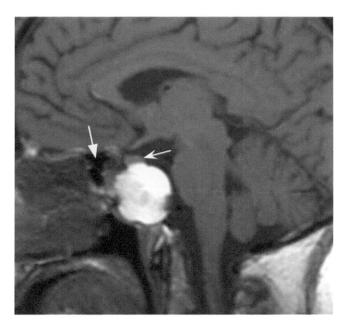

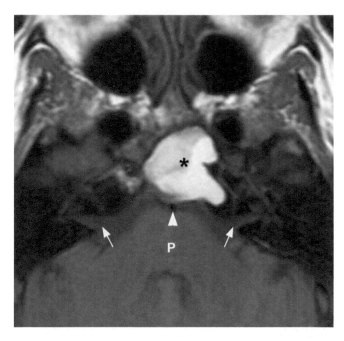

Fig. 6.25 Sagittal T1-weighted image demonstrates that the clival lesion is intrinsically bright. Note the upward displacement of the normal-appearing pituitary gland (*concave arrow*) and the small sphenoid sinus (*straight arrow*).

Fig. 6.26 Axial T1-weighted image at the level of the pons (P) and internal auditory canals (*straight arrows*) shows mild signal heterogeneity within the left petrous apex and clivus lesion (*asterisk*). There is slight protrusion into the prepontine cistern, with posterior displacement of the basilar artery (*arrowhead*). The bright signal is consistent with hemorrhagic and/or highly proteinaceous content.

so bright on T1-weighted images) and petrous apicitis (rim enhancing, low T1 signal).

- *Pathology.* May occur in any area of pneumatized temporal bone, but typically at petrous apex. May also involve middle ear and mastoid or may extend into clivus and cer-

ebellopontine angle. When the pneumatized cavity becomes obstructed, usually due to mucosal inflammatory disease, the subsequent decrease in air pressure causes fluid accumulation and intralesional bleeding. Hemoglobin breakdown promotes cholesterol crystal formation and a granulomatous "foreign-body" reaction.

- *Treatment.* Open surgical drainage to reduce local mass effect and establish a permanent drainage pathway.

Case 6.7

A 49-year-old male presents with diplopia and left ptosis and is found to have left CN III and CN VI palsies (**Figs. 6.28, 6.29**).

Diagnosis

Giant aneurysm of the cavernous segment of the left ICA

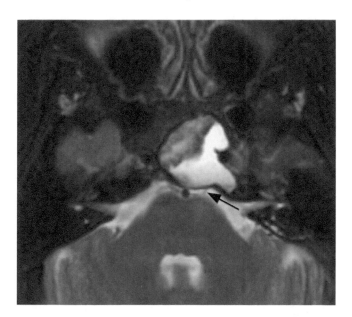

Fig. 6.27 Axial T2-weighted image with fat saturation shows the mass to be heterogeneous, consistent with variable protein content of the secretions and probably areas of prior hemorrhage as well. Note the course of the left CN VI (*arrow*) as it approaches the expected location of Dorello's canal. The imaging appearance is most consistent with a cholesterol granuloma of the petrous apex, longstanding, with remodeling of the clivus. This was confirmed at subsequent drainage.

> **Imaging Pearl**
>
> CT may reveal linear calcification along the peripheral rim of an aneurysm, while postcontrast CT or CTA will typically show dense enhancement. A partially thrombosed aneurysm, however, will have heterogeneous enhancement, and a completely thrombosed aneurysm will not enhance. Flow within an aneurysm will result in signal void and/or pulsation artifact on spin-echo MRI, and high signal intensity on flow-sensitive sequences.

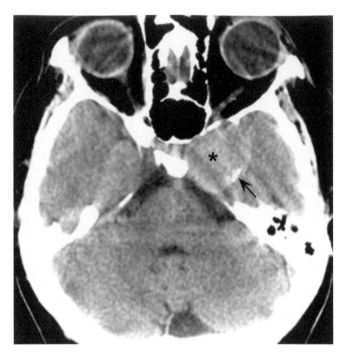

Fig. 6.28 Axial noncontrast CT demonstrates a rounded, intermediate density mass (*asterisk*) arising from the left cavernous sinus. Note the focus of high density (*arrow*) along the peripheral margin of the lesion, consistent with calcification of the wall of this giant aneurysm.

Case 6.8

A 45-year-old female with recent history of mastoiditis and mastoidectomy presents with fever, headache, left CN VI palsy and left forehead numbness (CN V₁ distribution) (**Figs. 6.30, 6.31, 6.32, 6.33**).

Diagnosis

Gradenigo syndrome

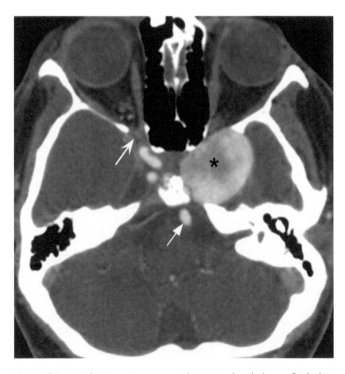

Fig. 6.29 Axial CT angiogram at the same level shows fairly homogeneous intense enhancement of this mass (*asterisk*) to almost the same degree as the adjacent carotid and basilar (*straight arrow*) arteries. There is bony remodeling of the left superior orbital fissure when compared with the normal right side (*concave arrow*). These imaging findings are diagnostic of a giant aneurysm of the cavernous internal carotid artery.

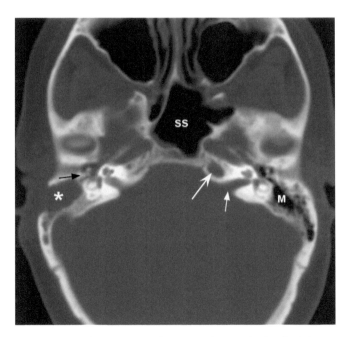

Fig. 6.30 Axial CT image in bone window at the level of the internal auditory canals (*straight arrow*) shows a bony defect in the right mastoid (*) compatible with prior mastoidectomy. Soft tissue within the right mastoid and surrounding the ossicles (*black arrow*) is nonspecific but is suggestive of either residual cholesteatoma or otitis media. A rounded area of soft tissue density is seen in the left petrous apex (*concave arrow*). Normal aeration is seen in the left mastoid air cells (M) and middle ear cavity. Minimal mucosal thickening is seen in the sphenoid sinus (SS).

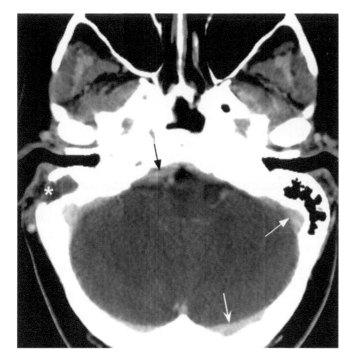

Fig. 6.31 Just below the level shown in Figure 6.30, an axial post-contrast CT image in soft tissue window shows the right mastoid bony defect (*asterisk*) and abnormal thickening and enhancement of the dura in the retroclival region (*black arrow*). Normal vascular enhancement is seen in the left transverse sinus (*white concave arrow*) and sigmoid sinus (*white straight arrow*). The venous sinuses on the right are patent as well.

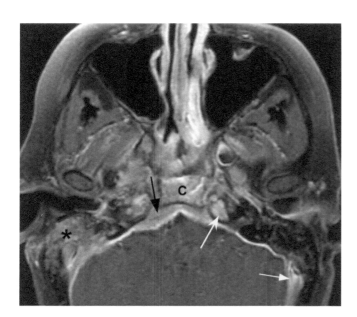

Fig. 6.32 Axial postcontrast T1-weighted image with fat saturation at a similar level as in **Fig. 6.31** demonstrates abnormal dural thickening and enhancement (*black arrow*) posterior to the clivus (C) that extends to the heterogeneously enhancing right mastoid (*asterisk*). Enhancement of the clivus suggests osteomyelitis. High T1 signal is seen in the left petrous apex, likely representing enhancement although precontrast T1 images would be needed to confirm this. The right petrous apex is also mildly enhancing. Normal enhancement is again seen at the left sigmoid sinus (*straight white arrow*).

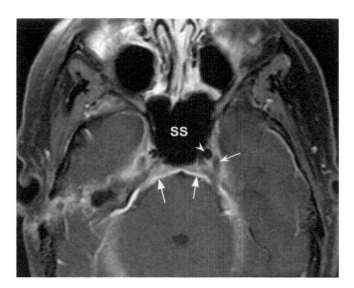

Fig. 6.33 More superiorly, an axial postcontrast T1-weighted image with fat saturation shows abnormal retroclival dural enhancement (*straight arrows*) encasing the left trigeminal nerve (*concave arrow*) as it enters Meckel's cave. The left cavernous carotid artery flow void is normal. Diagnosis: Gradenigo syndrome with petrous apicitis, as well as retroclival phlegmon, clival osteomyelitis, and infectious pachymeningitis.

Clinical Pearl

- Gradenigo syndrome is caused by inflammation of the petrous apex (petrous apicitis) that leads to injury to the trigeminal (CN V) and abducens (CN VI) nerves with facial pain/numbness and ipsilateral LR palsy. The clinical "Gradenigo triad" includes retroorbital pain, abducens nerve palsy, and otorrhea. It typically occurs as a complication of otitis media and mastoiditis. Treatment involves intravenous antibiotics. Failure to respond to antibiotics and/or worsening CN involvement necessitates open surgical drainage.

Imaging Pearls

- CT may demonstrate destruction of bony septa within an opacified petrous apex. Gradenigo syndrome typically occurs in the setting of a pneumatized but then inflamed petrous apex, and the contralateral petrous apex will often show normal pneumatization in these cases. Middle ear and mastoid are often involved. MRI shows enhancement around fluid within the petrous apex. Adjacent meninges may be thickened and enhancing.
- Petrous apex imaging differential will include the following:
  1. *Petrous apicitis* (T1 hypointense, T2 hyperintense, rim-enhancing) (Case 6.8)
  2. *Cholesterol granuloma* (T1 and T2 hyperintense, no enhancement, expansile) (Case 6.6)
  3. *Cholesteatoma* (T1 hypointense, T2 hyperintense, no enhancement, expansile, reduced diffusion)
  4. *Chondrosarcoma* (T1 hypointense, T2 hyperintense, intense enhancement, variable calcification on CT)
  5. *Mucocele* (variable T1 and T2 depending on protein + water content, expansile) (Chapter 4, Case 4.7)

Anatomy of Peripheral Course of Facial Nerve

- After emerging from the ventrolateral pons, the motor division and nervus intermedius traverse the cerebellopontine angle cistern with CN VIII and then enter the

IAC in the petrous temporal bone, along with the labyrinthine artery and vein (**Fig. 7.3**). Four intratemporal segments of the nerve are described (**Fig. 7.4**):

○ *Meatal (intracanalicular) segment.* Within the IAC, the motor division of CN VII is located anterosuperior, the cochlear nerve anteroinferior, the superior vestibu-

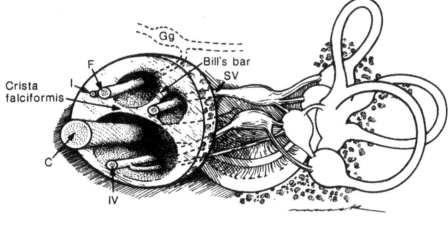

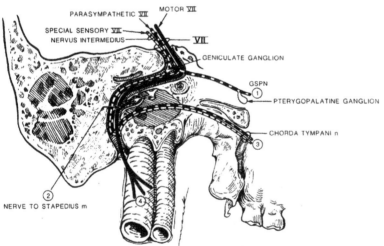

Fig. 7.3 Internal auditory canal. The facial nerve (F) and nervus intermedius (I) are found in the anterior-superior quadrant, the cochlear nerve (C) in the anterior-inferior quadrant, the superior vestibular nerve (SV) in the posterior-superior quadrant, and the inferior vestibular nerve (IV) in the posterior-inferior quadrant. The *crista falciformis* (falciform crest) is a horizontal bony strut separating the superior and inferior halves of the fundus of the IAC. *Bill's bar* is a surgical landmark separating CN VII from the superior vestibular nerve. (Gg, geniculate ganglion.) (From Harnsberger HR. Handbook of Head and Neck Imaging [2nd ed.]. St. Louis, MO: Mosby, 1995. Reprinted with permission.)

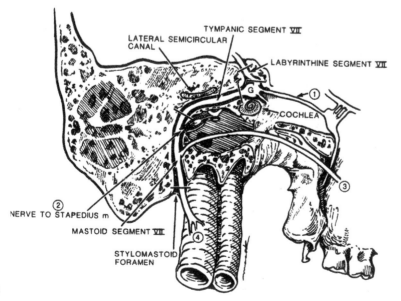

Fig. 7.4 Detailed course of the facial nerve through the temporal bone. **(A)** The parasympathetic portion (*dashed line*) branches at the anterior genu to supply the lacrimal gland via the GSPN (1) before continuing as part of the chorda tympani nerve to supply secretomotor function to the submandibular and sublingual glands. Special sensory fibers (*dotted line*) comprise the majority of the chorda tympani nerve (conveying taste) (3), with cell bodies in the geniculate ganglion. The branchial motor portion (*solid line*) gives off the nerve to the stapedius muscle (2) before continuing to innervate the muscles of facial expression (4). **(B)** Segments of the facial nerve within the temporal bone in order: meatal or intracanalicular (not shown), labyrinthine, tympanic (also called horizontal segment), and mastoid (also called vertical segment). (From Harnsberger HR. Handbook of Head and Neck Imaging [2nd ed.]. St. Louis, MO: Mosby, 1995. Reprinted with permission.)

lar nerve posterosuperior, and the inferior vestibular nerve posteroinferior. The nervus intermedius travels between CN VII and CN VIII at the porus acusticus and then joins CN VII to travel in the anterosuperior quadrant (superior to the crista falciformis and anterior to the Bill bar) (**Fig. 7.3**).

○ *Labyrinthine segment.* The bony fallopian canal courses anterolaterally from the fundus of the IAC and carries the labyrinthine segment of CN VII to the geniculate ganglion. The GSPN arises from the apex of the geniculate ganglion.

○ *Horizontal (tympanic) segment.* From the geniculate ganglion, CN VII travels posteriorly and horizontally just inferior to the lateral semicircular canal. No branches arise from this segment of the facial nerve.

○ *Mastoid (vertical) segment.* At the posterior aspect of the middle ear, CN VII turns inferiorly to form the mastoid segment. Three branches arise from this segment of CN VII: the *nerve to the stapedius muscle*, the *chorda tympani nerve* (see above), and the *sensory auricular branch* (innervates external auditory meatus and the auricle and retroauricular area). CN VII then exits the bony facial canal at the level of the *stylomastoid foramen* and immediately gives off the *posterior auricular nerve* (to occipitalis, posterior auricular, and oblique auricular muscles), the *digastric branch* (to the posterior belly of the digastric muscle), and the *stylohyoid branch* (to the stylohyoid muscle).

○ CN VII then enters the parotid gland and divides into temporofacial and cervicofacial branches. These then divide into temporal, zygomatic, buccal, marginal mandibular, and cervical branches (TEN ZEBRAS BIT MY CLOCK), which innervate the many muscles of facial expression (listed at beginning of chapter).

○ The distribution and functions of CN VII are summarized in **Fig. 7.5**.

Greater Superficial Petrosal Nerve

• GVE (parasympathetic).

• GSPN arises from the geniculate ganglion, courses anteromedially, and exits the petrous temporal bone via the greater petrosal foramen (facial hiatus) to the middle fossa.

• GSPN passes deep to the trigeminal (gasserian) ganglion in Meckel's cave and down the foramen lacerum to the pterygoid canal (vidian canal), where it joins with the *deep petrosal nerve* (sympathetic fibers from ICA plexus; cell bodies in superior cervical ganglion) to form the *nerve of the pterygoid canal (vidian nerve)*.

Nerve of the Pterygoid Canal (Vidian Nerve)

• GVE (parasympathetic) + sympathetic.

• Traverses pterygoid (vidian) canal to the pterygopalatine fossa, where the *parasympathetics* synapse in the pterygopalatine (sphenopalatine) ganglion.

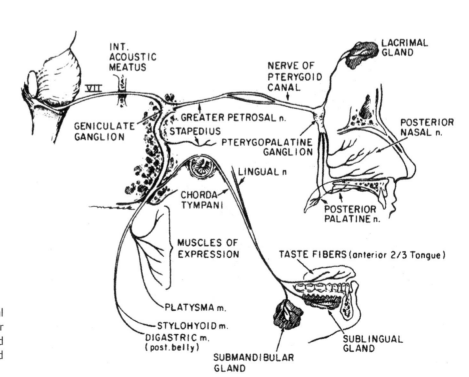

Fig. 7.5 Schematic of functions of the facial nerve. See text for details. (From Harnsberger HR. Handbook of Head and Neck Imaging [2nd ed.]. St. Louis, MO: Mosby, 1995. Reprinted with permission.)

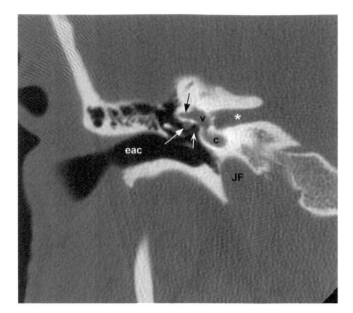

Fig. 7.11 A coronal CT image in bone window demonstrates normal temporal bone anatomy at the level of the internal auditory canal (*). The horizontal or tympanic segment of the facial nerve canal (*white straight arrow*) is seen immediately beneath the horizontal semicircular canal (*black arrow*) and superolateral to the stapes (faintly seen, *white concave arrow*) within the oval window. Normal inner ear anatomy includes the vestibule (v) and cochlea (c). Normal jugular foramen (JF) and external auditory canal (eac) are also shown.

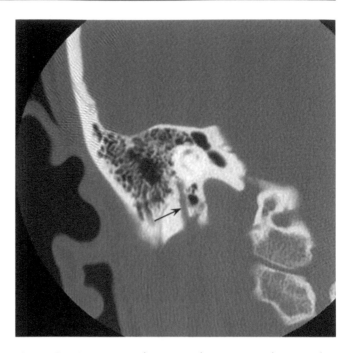

Fig. 7.12 More posteriorly, a coronal CT image in bone window shows the normal descending (vertical) mastoid segment of the facial nerve canal (*arrow*) extending inferiorly to the stylomastoid foramen.

Normal MRIs

• (**Figs. 7.14, 7.15, 7.16, 7.17 and 7.18**)

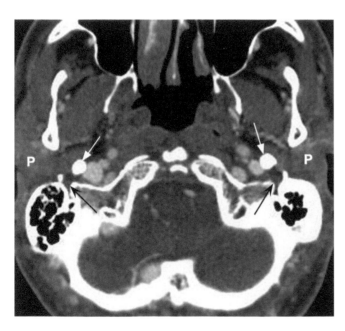

Fig. 7.13 An axial postcontrast CT in soft tissue window through the lower skull base shows the normal stylomastoid foramina bilaterally (*black arrows*), posterolateral to large styloid processes (*white arrows*). Normal parotid glands (P).

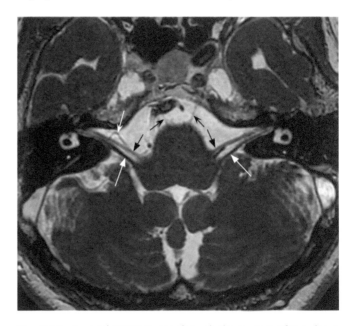

Fig. 7.14 An axial FIESTA image through the posterior fossa shows normal CN VII and CN VIII exiting the lateral aspect of the pontomedullary junction (*black straight arrows*: CN VII; *white straight arrows*: CN VIII, vestibular division) and coursing into the internal auditory canal. Bilateral VI nerves (*small black arrows*) exit the ventral pontomedullary junction and traverse the prepontine cistern. Note the small flow void on the right (*white concave arrow*) that typically represents a loop of AICA and is commonly seen in asymptomatic patients.

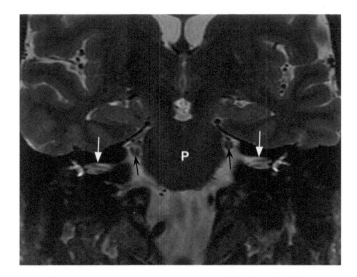

Fig. 7.15 A thin-section coronal T2-weighted image with fat saturation shows normal IACs (*white arrows*), with CN VII and VIII coursing through them. The IACs lie inferior to the cisternal segments of the trigeminal nerves (*black arrows*), at the level of the midpons (P).

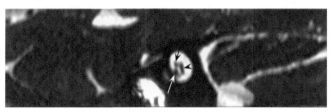

Fig. 7.16 An oblique parasagittal high-resolution FIESTA image through the internal auditory canal shows the normal positions of CNs VII and VIII. CN VII (*black cconcave arrow*) is located anterosuperiorly and is slightly smaller in size than the anteroinferiorly located cochlear nerve (*white arrow*). Posteriorly, the vestibular component of CN VIII (*black arrowhead*) is starting to divide into superior and inferior divisions.

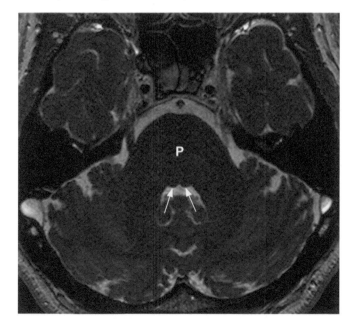

Fig. 7.17 An axial FIESTA image through the posterior fossa at the level of the midpons (P) shows normal facial colliculi bilaterally (*arrows*). The facial colliculus is a small bulge of the dorsal pons into the fourth ventricle at the site where the facial nerve loops around the abducens nucleus.

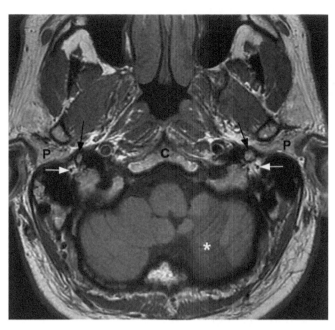

Fig. 7.18 An axial T1-weighted image through the lower skull base demonstrates normal bilateral stylomastoid foramina filled with fat. The centrally located dot of dark signal (*white arrows*) is the normal CN VII traversing the foramen prior to entering the parotid glands. Normal parotid tissue (P) is noted anterolaterally. Dark signal lateral to the foramina represents air within the inferior mastoid air cells. Anteromedial to the foramina, the normal styloid processes (*black arrows*) are seen: a rim of dark signal represents cortical bone and the central hyperintensity represents fatty marrow. A remote left inferior cerebellar infarct (*asterisk*) is present. (C, clivus.)

Facial Nerve Lesions

Types

Supranuclear Lesions

- Lead to contralateral paresis/palsy of lower portion of face ("central CN VII" lesion).
- Upper part of the face is spared due to bilateral supranuclear innervation.

Nuclear and Fascicular Lesions

- Lead to ipsilateral paresis/palsy of entire face ("peripheral CN VII" lesion).
- Lesion within pons may affect nearby structures, for example, CN V, CN VI, paramedian pontine reticular formation (PPRF), corticospinal tract (CST), spinothalamic tract (STT).
- *Millard-Gubler syndrome*. Lesion in ventral pons affecting CN VI, CN VII, CST. CN VII involvement is due to involvement of the fascicles of CN VII, not the more dorsally lo-

cated CN VII motor nucleus. Characterized by ipsilateral peripheral CN VII paralysis, ipsilateral abducens palsy, contralateral hemiplegia.

- *Foville syndrome.* Lesion in pons affecting CN VII, CN VI, PPRF, CST. Characterized by ipsilateral peripheral CN VII paralysis, ipsilateral conjugate gaze paralysis, contralateral hemiplegia.
- See Appendix A (The Brainstem) for a review of anatomical details.

Cerebellopontine Angle Lesions

- In the cerebellopontine angle (CPA) cistern, CN VII travels with nervus intermedius and near CN VIII. Masses of the CPA cistern (e.g., acoustic neuroma, meningioma) result variably in ipsilateral peripheral CN VII paralysis, loss of taste over anterior two thirds of tongue, hyperacusis, ipsilateral tinnitus, hearing loss, and/or vertigo. CPA masses affect CN VIII function far more commonly than CN VII function.
- Lesions in CPA may displace or compress pons, cerebellum, or other CNs (e.g., CN V, CN VI).
- *Hemifacial spasm.* Usually due to neurovascular compression of the motor root of CN VII in the CPA (see Case 7.8).
- *Geniculate neuralgia* (also called nervus intermedius neuralgia or Hunt neuralgia). Neuralgia affecting the sensory root of CN VII (nervus intermedius), causing paroxysmal otalgia similar to the ear form of glossopharyngeal neuralgia (see Chapter 9). Attributed to vascular—usually anterior inferior cerebellar artery (AICA)—compression of nervus intermedius. Treatment is with carbamazepine, microvascular decompression, or sectioning of the nervus intermedius and/or geniculate ganglion.

More Peripheral Lesions

- Most common causes of unilateral complete facial paralysis are Bell's palsy, trauma, and Ramsay Hunt syndrome (herpes zoster oticus).
- *Bell's palsy* (idiopathic facial palsy). Unilateral CN VII dysfunction with sudden onset (see case discussion below).
- *Ramsay Hunt syndrome* (herpes zoster oticus) (see Case 7.6).
- *Posttraumatic facial palsy.* The facial nerve is the most commonly injured motor CN (see Case 7.13).
- *Möbius syndrome.* Congenital bilateral CN VI and CN VII palsies due to neural underdevelopment.
- Additional causes of peripheral facial palsy include
  - Malignancy (e.g., parotid, temporal bone).
  - Infectious/inflammatory (e.g., varicella-zoster virus [VZV], Lyme disease, syphilis, acquired immunodeficiency syndrome [AIDS], mononucleosis, Guillian-Barré syndrome [Miller-Fisher variant]).
  - Iatrogenic (e.g., parotid surgery, temporal bone surgery).

- Granulomatous and connective tissue diseases (e.g., sarcoidosis, Wegener granulomatosis).
- Facial nerve dysfunction is most commonly described using the House-Brackmann classification scheme (**Table 7.2**).

Table 7.2 House-Brackmann Classification of Facial Nerve Dysfunction

Grade	Definition
I	Normal facial function
II	Slight weakness noticeable on close inspection Forehead—moderate-to-good function Eye—complete closure with minimal effort Mouth—slight asymmetry
III	Obvious weakness, but not disfiguring Forehead—slight-to-moderate movement Eye—complete closure with effort Mouth—slightly weak with maximum effort
IV	Obvious weakness and/or disfiguring asymmetry Forehead—no motion Eye—incomplete closure Mouth—asymmetric with maximum effort
V	Only barely perceptible motion Forehead—no motion Eye—incomplete closure Mouth—slight movement
VI	No movement (complete facial paralysis)

Facial Nerve: Pathologic Images

Congenital Anomalies Affecting the Course of the Facial Nerve

- Congenital anomalies of the temporal bone and inner ear often alter the bony anatomy of the facial nerve canal; this may have major implications for treatment planning (i.e., surgery).
- A situation where the facial nerve has an abnormal intratemporal course is exemplified by external auditory canal (EAC) atresia.
- (**Figs. 7.19, 7.20**).

Clinical Pearl

- EAC atresia is associated with auricle deformity and microtia and leads to conductive hearing loss. Bilateral involvement is usually syndromic.

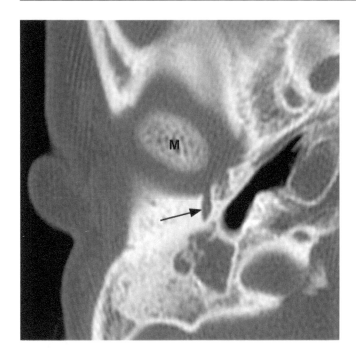

Fig. 7.19 An axial CT image in bone window through the skull base and inferior right temporal bone in a patient with external auditory canal atresia demonstrates an aberrant course of the right facial nerve canal (*arrow*). CN VII exits into the glenoid fossa of the temporomandibular joint instead of normally into the stylomastoid foramen. (M, condylar head of the mandible.) Also note the presence of microtia, with a small deformed right pinna.

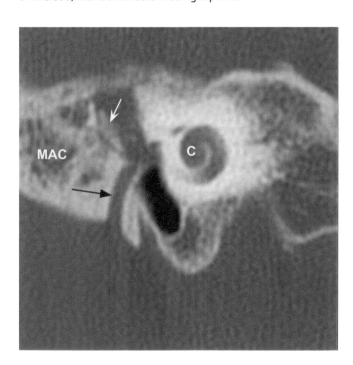

Fig. 7.20 A coronal CT image in bone window through the right temporal bone in the same patient also demonstrates the aberrant and abnormally short right facial nerve canal (*black arrow*). The ossicles (*white arrow*) are dysplastic and laterally positioned within an abnormally small and opacified middle ear cavity. The mastoid air cells (MAC) are also underdeveloped in this patient with external auditory canal atresia. (C, cochlea.)

Imaging Pearls

- Bony or membranous stenosis or atresia of the EAC is associated with underdeveloped mastoid air cells, a small tympanic cavity, and ossicular malformations. It may also be associated with congenital cholesteatoma. The inner ear is typically normal. It is important to assess the facial nerve canal in all cases. Aberrant course of the tympanic and mastoid segments is common and can result in operative injury during reconstructive surgery. The tympanic segment is often dehiscent and the mastoid segment is usually displaced anteriorly. CN VII often exits anteriorly into the glenoid fossa (temporomandibular joint; TMJ), or lateral to the styloid process.
- Oval window (OW) atresia or hypoplasia is another situation where the facial nerve canal may be aberrant and CN VII can be injured if the surgeon does not appreciate the abnormal course and position of the nerve.
- (**Figs. 7.21, 7.22**).

Clinical Pearl

- OW atresia is an uncommon embryological defect characterized by severe conductive hearing loss from birth or early childhood without associated external ear anomalies or any history of otomastoiditis or trauma.

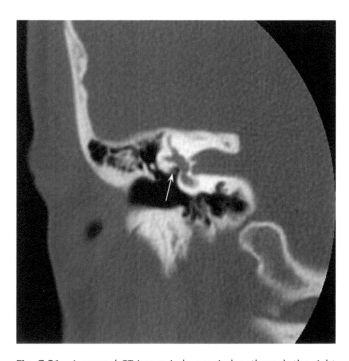

Fig. 7.21 A coronal CT image in bone window through the right temporal bone demonstrates hypoplasia of the oval window and absence of the stapes. The tympanic segment of CN VII (*arrow*) has an abnormal position and partially overlies the hypoplastic oval window. Its bony covering also appears dehiscent.

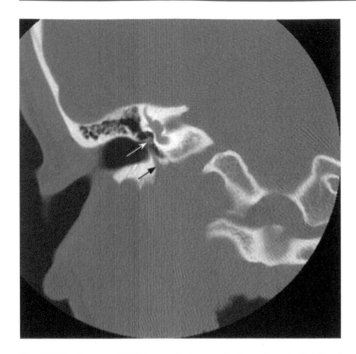

Fig. 7.22 A coronal CT image in bone window at a similar level in a different patient demonstrates complete bony atresia of the oval window and an even more abnormal position of the tympanic segment of CN VII (*white arrow*). Aberrant course of the descending mastoid segment of the facial nerve canal is also noted (*black arrow*).

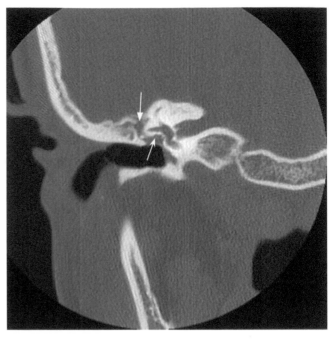

Fig. 7.23 A coronal CT image in bone window through the right temporal bone demonstrates abnormal soft tissue in the middle ear cavity medial to a retracted tympanic membrane. Soft tissue fills the oval window, and the bony wall of the tympanic segment of CN VII (*concave arrow*) is dehiscent. The mastoid (*straight arrow*) is underdeveloped and opacified in this patient with a known cholesteatoma and facial nerve palsy. The ossicles are not well visualized due to either erosion or prior surgical removal.

Imaging Pearl

- Thin-section temporal bone CT in the coronal plane best demonstrates OW hypoplasia or atresia. The EAC is typically normal. OW atresia is associated with anomalies of the stapes and incus. It is also frequently associated with anomalous development of the horizontal facial nerve canal, making surgical treatment difficult if not absolutely contraindicated.

Acquired Lesions That May Affect the Bony Facial Nerve Canal

- Cholesteatoma is an important cause of hearing loss in adults and children. Cholesteatomas may be congenital or acquired, with acquired cholesteatoma being far more common. Cholesteatomas frequently erode into and involve the facial nerve canal, hence the facial nerve canal must be traced carefully in all cases (**Fig. 7.23**).

Clinical Pearl

- Cholesteatoma is associated with conductive hearing loss and occurs most commonly in the setting of chronic otitis media. Cholesteatomas are usually located within the middle ear in association with a retracted or perforated tympanic membrane. The cholesteatoma mass consists of exfoliated keratin with underlying squamous epithelium.

Imaging Pearl

- Temporal bone CT best shows a non-specific soft tissue mass with variable bone erosion that most commonly involves the ossicles, the tympanic segment of the facial nerve canal, and/or the lateral semicircular canal. MRI shows a T2-hyperintense and T1-hypointense nonenhancing mass with high signal on diffusion-weighted imaging. Though CT is the study of choice to assess middle ear and mastoid extent of cholesteatoma, MR is indicated for assessment of intracranial extension and intracranial complications.

Clinical Cases

Case 7.1

An 11-year-old male presents with right CN VI and CN VII palsies (**Figs. 7.24, 7.25**).

Diagnosis

• Pilocytic astrocytoma

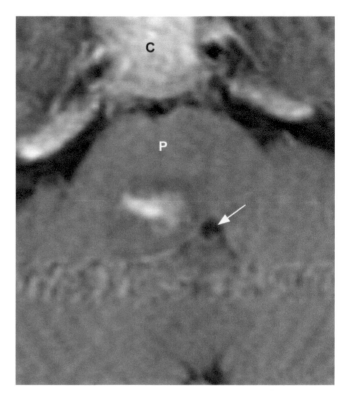

Fig. 7.25 An axial post-contrast T1-weighted Image through the same level shows moderate central enhancement of the mass. Again demonstrated is mass effect upon the fourth ventricle (*arrow*), which is significantly compressed and shifted slightly to the left. This lesion is consistent with a pilocytic astrocytoma of the brainstem. (C, clivus; P, pons.)

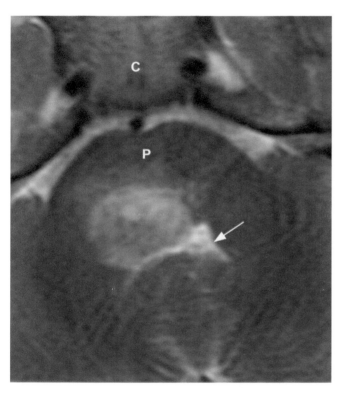

Fig. 7.24 An axial T2-weighted image through the pons at the level of the upper clivus (C) demonstrates a slightly heterogeneous but mostly hyperintense intraaxial mass within the central and dorsal aspect of the pons (P) resulting in mass effect upon the fourth ventricle (*arrow*). The lesion is centered at the level of the nuclei and proximal tracts of CN VI and CN VII.

Imaging Pearl

• Pilocytic astrocytomas are World Health Organization (WHO) Grade 1 brain tumors that are most commonly diagnosed in the first decade of life. They most frequently arise in the cerebellum, but they also occur in the brainstem, the cerebral hemispheres, and the hypothalamic-chiasmal region. They tend to be well-circumscribed and T2-hyperintense with little or no surrounding edema. They are often associated with cysts, particularly when they occur in the cerebellum. Enhancement is variable and may be nodular, diffuse and homogeneous, or multifocal. The prognosis is excellent when gross total surgical removal can be accomplished.

Case 7.2

An 8-year-old male presents with right facial numbness and weakness as well as left body weakness and numbness (**Figs. 7.26, 7.27**).

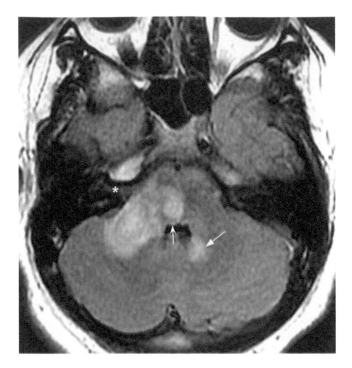

Fig. 7.26 An axial fluid-attenuated inversion recovery (FLAIR) image through the pons at the level of the right internal auditory canal (*asterisk*) demonstrates an area of abnormal high signal intensity and swelling centered within the right middle cerebellar peduncle, extending into the right side of the pons. Abnormal signal involves the region of the right facial colliculus (*concave arrow*) at the ventral aspect of the fourth ventricle, and also the expected path of CN VII as its fibers travel to its root exit zone. An additional hyperintense lesion (*straight arrow*) is noted within the left deep cerebellum, adjacent to the posterolateral aspect of the fourth ventricle.

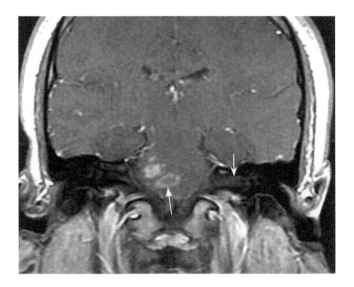

Fig. 7.27 A coronal postcontrast T1-weighted image in the same patient at the level of the pons and left internal auditory canal (*concave arrow*) demonstrates areas of irregular ring enhancement (*straight arrow*) within the central and right pons. Clinical, CSF, and imaging findings were consistent with ADEM.

Diagnosis

- Acute disseminated encephalomyelitis (ADEM) (see Chapter 2, Case 2.2, for further discussion).

Case 7.3

A 41-year-old female presents with recurrent episodes of right facial weakness and diplopia which have now become persistent (**Figs. 7.28, 7.29**).

Diagnosis

- Brainstem cavernous malformation (see Chapter 12, Case 12.1, for further discussion).

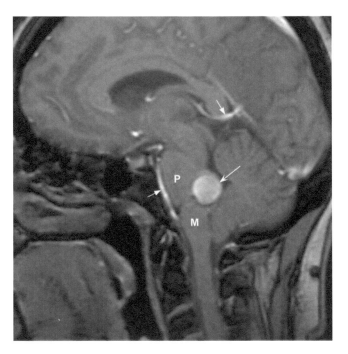

Fig. 7.28 A sagittal, precontrast, T1-weighted gradient-echo sequence through the midline demonstrates a round hyperintense intraaxial mass centered within the dorsal brainstem at the pontomedullary junction. The mass (*white concave arrow*) protrudes into and partially effaces the fourth ventricle. The intrinsic high T1 signal within the mass is consistent with hemorrhage. The bright signal within the intracranial vessels (*small straight arrows: upper arrow* on internal cerebral vein, *lower arrow* on basilar artery) and the low signal intensity within bone marrow is expected for this sequence. (M, medulla; P, pons.)

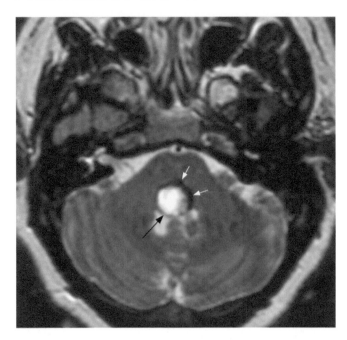

Fig. 7.29 An axial T2-weighted image in the same patient through the midpons level demonstrates a round intra-axial centrally hyperintense mass (*black arrow*) within the dorsal pons. A peripheral rim of low signal (*white arrows*) is due to hemosiderin. The T1 and T2 signal characteristics are consistent with both subacute and chronic blood products secondary to repeated hemorrhages into a cavernous malformation, and subsequent surgical removal confirmed the diagnosis of cavernous malformation.

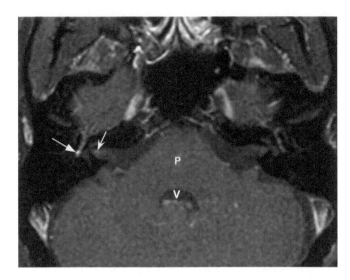

Fig. 7.30 An axial postcontrast T1-weighted image with fat saturation through the pons (P), fourth ventricle (v), and bilateral internal auditory canals demonstrates asymmetric increased enhancement within the tympanic (horizontal) segment of the right CN VII (*straight arrow*). In addition, there is faint enhancement of CN VII within the fundus of the right internal auditory canal (*concave arrow*).

Case 7.4

A 53-year-old male presents with acute onset of right CN VII palsy (**Figs. 7.30, 7.31,** and **7.32; Figs. 7.33, 7.34,** and **7.35** are from a different patient with the same diagnosis).

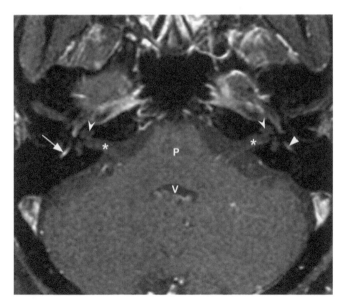

Fig. 7.31 More inferiorly in the same patient, an axial postcontrast T1-weighted image with fat saturation through the internal auditory canals (*asterisk*) demonstrates asymmetric increased enhancement of the tympanic segment (*straight arrow*) of the right facial nerve. Mild enhancement of the facial nerve as seen on the left (*straight arrowhead*) is a normal finding. Cochleae (*concave arrowheads*), pons (P), and fourth ventricle (V) are shown.

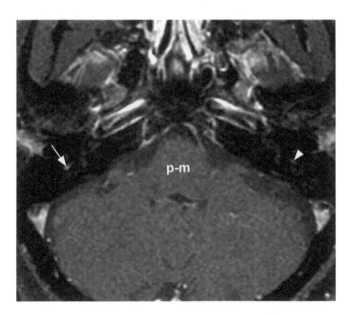

Fig. 7.32 More inferiorly in the same patient, an axial postcontrast T1-weighted image with fat saturation through the pontomedullary junction (p-m) shows asymmetric abnormal enhancement of the descending mastoid segment of the right facial nerve (*arrow*) when compared with the normal left side (*arrowhead*).

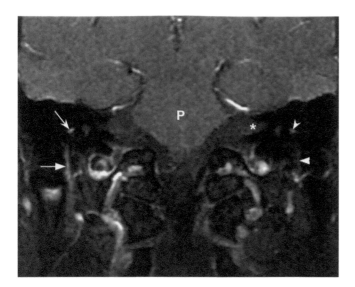

Fig. 7.33 A coronal postcontrast T1-weighted image with fat saturation in the same patient through the pons (P) and left internal auditory canal (*asterisk*) demonstrates asymmetric abnormal enhancement of the descending mastoid (vertical) segment (*straight arrow*) and tympanic (horizontal) segment (*concave arrow*) of the right CN VII. The descending mastoid segment (*straight arrowhead*) and tympanic segment (*concave arrowhead*) of the left CN VII are normal.

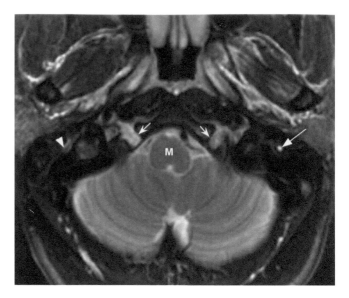

Fig. 7.34 An axial T2-weighted image with fat saturation through the lower skull base and medulla (M) in a different patient with Bell's palsy demonstrates abnormal hyperintensity in the descending mastoid segment of the left CN VII (*straight arrow*) as it enters the left stylomastoid foramen. Normal signal is noted within CN VII in the right stylomastoid foramen (*arrowhead*). Hypoglossal canals (*concave arrows*) are indicated.

Diagnosis

- Bell's palsy

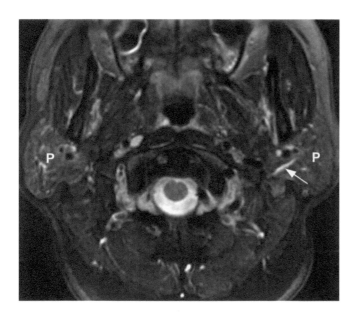

Fig. 7.35 More inferiorly, an axial T2-weighted image with fat saturation at the level of the parotid glands (P) in the same patient shows abnormal enlargement and hyperintensity of the left facial nerve (*arrow*) as it courses through the parotid gland. On postcontrast images (not shown), there was abnormal enhancement as well.

Clinical Pearl

- *Bell's palsy* (idiopathic facial palsy) is characterized by sudden onset of unilateral peripheral (lower motor neuron) CN VII dysfunction. Herpes simplex virus is considered by many to be the causative agent. Weakness typically peaks in 2 to 5 days. Bell's palsy may be associated with dysgeusia (impaired taste), impaired salivation and lacrimation, and hyperacusis. Treatment is with systemic corticosteroids, often with the addition of acyclovir; prevention of corneal damage (due to impaired eye closure and also to decreased lacrimation) is also important. Approximately 80 to 85% of patients recover completely within 2 to 4 months. "Atypical" Bell's palsy (~15% of cases) is characterized by slow onset and/or resolution, recurrence, the presence of other CN palsies, and/or an atypical degree of pain. Though typical Bell's palsy does not require MR imaging, MR imaging is generally suggested for atypical cases.

- Imaging is not generally required unless the CN VII palsy is atypical or recurrent. When imaging is done in "typical" Bell's palsy, the post-gadolinium images typically show increased enhancement involving one or more segments of the facial nerve without irregularity or nodularity. T2 hyperintensity of the nerve may also be seen. Thick, irregular, and/or nodular enhancement is atypical for Bell's palsy and raises the concern for an underlying neoplastic etiology (e.g., perineural spread of tumor). The parotid gland should be fully included in the imaging volume and carefully inspected for a mass lesion in a patient with atypical Bell palsy.

Case 7.5

A 52-year-old male presents with acute onset of bilateral CN VII weakness (**Figs. 7.36, 7.37**).

Diagnosis

- Bilateral Bell's palsy

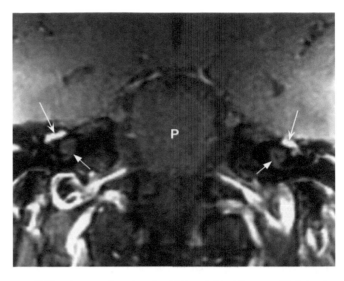

Fig. 7.37 A coronal postcontrast T1-weighted image with fat saturation through the skull base at the level of the pons (P) and cochleae (*straight white arrows*) shows marked enhancement of the bilateral geniculate ganglia of the facial nerves (*concave white arrows*) in this patient with bilateral Bell's palsy.

- Bilateral Bell's palsy is uncommon. Whereas Bell's palsy has an annual incidence of 20–30/100,000, bilateral cases account for only 0.3–2%. Bilateral Bell's palsy is more common in human immunodeficiency virus (HIV)+ patients, and also has a higher association with systemic causes (e.g., Miller-Fisher syndrome, syphilis, sarcoidosis, Lyme disease).

Case 7.6

A 45-year-old HIV+ male presents with acute right-sided peripheral facial palsy, otalgia, hearing loss, and vertigo. Examination reveals several vesicular lesions of the soft palate and EAC (**Figs. 7.38, 7.39**).

Diagnosis

- Ramsay Hunt syndrome (herpes zoster oticus)

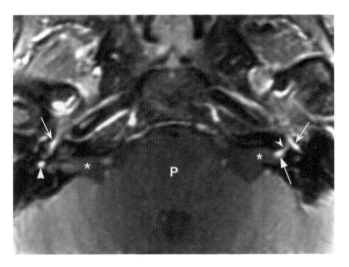

Fig. 7.36 An axial postcontrast T1-weighted image with fat saturation through the level of the internal auditory canals (*asterisk*) and pons (P) demonstrates abnormal enhancement along the bilateral CNs VII, including the intracanalicular segment at the fundus of the internal auditory canal (*straight arrow* on left), left labyrinthine segment (*concave arrowhead*), bilateral horizontal (tympanic) segments (*concave arrows*), and right posterior genu (*straight arrowhead*).

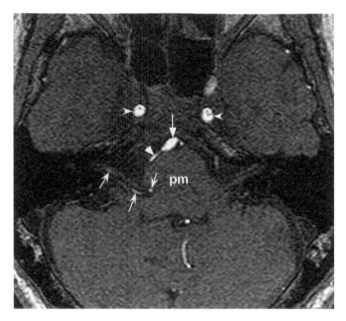

Fig. 7.44 An axial source image from a three dimensional time-of-flight intracranial MR angiogram confirms a vascular loop (*concave arrows*) traversing the right pontomedullary angle and subsequently continuing into the right internal auditory canal. This vessel is a tortuous right AICA, seen arising (*straight arrowhead*) from the basilar artery (*straight arrow*). Although the AICA may also be tortuous in asymptomatic patients, neurovascular compression is likely the cause of hemifacial spasm in this patient. Internal carotid arteries, cavernous segments (*concave arrowheads*) are shown.

Clinical Pearl

- *Hemifacial spasm* is characterized by adult-onset (40–60 years of age, female predominance) painless, irregular clonic contractions on one side of the face; it may also involve the stapedius (clicking). Spasms start near the eye (orbicularis oculi) and move caudally. Hemifacial spasm is thought to be caused by compression of the motor root of CN VII with segmental demyelination leading to ephaptic (nonsynaptic contact site) transmission. It is usually associated with neurovascular compression in the CPA (most commonly the AICA, although other blood vessels also are implicated: posterior inferior cerebellar artery (PICA), vertebral artery (VA), ectatic basilar artery [BA]), but it may be due to other vascular and nonvascular lesions (tumors, vascular malformations, aneurysms) compressing the facial nerve. Medical treatment is with carbamazepine or botulinum toxin injections. In many cases surgical microvascular decompression is used to separate the vascular compressive lesion from the underlying nerves and is highly effective.

Imaging Pearl

- MRI is the study of choice for imaging evaluation of hemifacial spasm. High-resolution heavily T2-weighted sequences or MR angiography with attention to the posterior fossa are most helpful for identifying the offending vessel. The vessel should be seen to contact the nerve root at its exit zone and/or to displace the proximal nerve. Imaging is also useful to exclude other causes of hemifacial spasm such as brainstem pathology or a mass associated with the facial nerve along its course.

Case 7.9

A 48-year-old male presents with long-standing right CN VII palsy (**Figs. 7.45, 7.46, 7.47, 7.48**).

Diagnosis

- Facial nerve schwannoma, tympanic segment

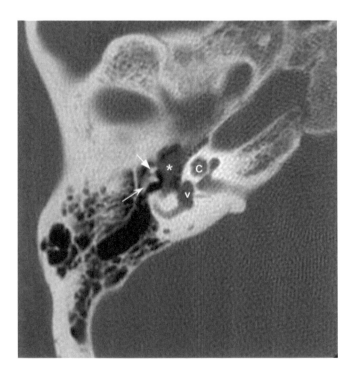

Fig. 7.45 A high-resolution axial CT image through the temporal bone at the level of the incudomalleolar junction, cochlea (C), and vestibule (v) demonstrates an ovoid, homogeneous soft tissue mass (*asterisk*) within the anteromedial aspect of the middle ear cavity along the expected course of the tympanic segment of the facial nerve canal. Malleus (*straight arrow*) and incus (*concave arrow*) are shown.

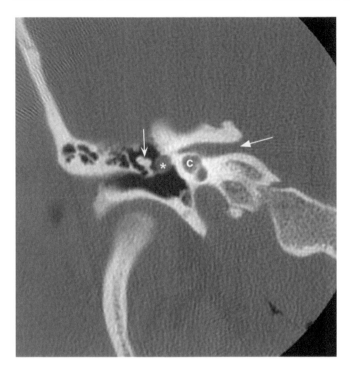

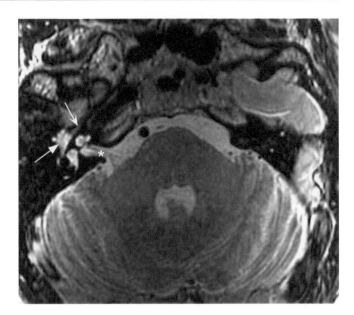

Fig. 7.46 A high-resolution coronal CT image through the right temporal bone at the level of the internal auditory canal (*straight arrow*), cochlea (C), and ossicles (*concave arrow*) shows a rounded, homogeneous soft tissue mass (*asterisk*) centered on the tympanic (horizontal) segment of the right facial nerve canal and emanating from it. There is associated smooth remodeling of adjacent bone. The lesion has no aggressive features and is not associated with any middle ear or mastoid inflammatory changes.

Fig. 7.47 A thin-section, axial, three-dimensional, fast spin echo T2-weighted image through the posterior fossa at the level of the right internal auditory canal (*asterisk*) shows a well-defined, homogeneous, fairly bright mass (*straight arrow*) associated with the tympanic segment of the right facial nerve canal (*concave arrow*).

Clinical Pearl

- A schwannoma may arise anywhere along the course of CN VII. CN VII dysfunction is often surprisingly absent or mild even when these lesions are fairly large, especially if they occur along a segment of the nerve where growth does not lead to compression within a narrow bony canal. Hearing loss may be sensorineural due to impingement on CN VIII in the CPA or IAC or conductive due to middle ear extension and interference with ossicular function.

Imaging Pearl

- CT classically demonstrates an ovoid, tubular mass associated with benign-appearing bony remodeling and enlargement of the facial nerve canal. MR demonstrates a well-circumscribed enhancing tubular mass enlarging the facial canal.

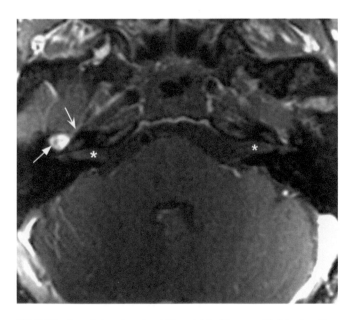

Fig. 7.48 An axial postcontrast T1-weighted image with fat saturation through a similar level (internal auditory canals, *asterisk*) shows slightly heterogeneous enhancement of the smoothly marginated, benign-appearing lesion (*straight arrow*) arising from the tympanic segment of the right CN VII (*concave arrow*). Diagnosis: CN VII schwannoma.

Case 7.10

A 36-year-old female with no history of seizure, headache, or facial nerve weakness underwent middle ear/mastoid exploration for conductive hearing loss. No preoperative imaging was performed. A middle ear and mastoid antral mass was identified intraoperatively, and subsequent imaging was performed (**Figs. 7.49, 7.50**).

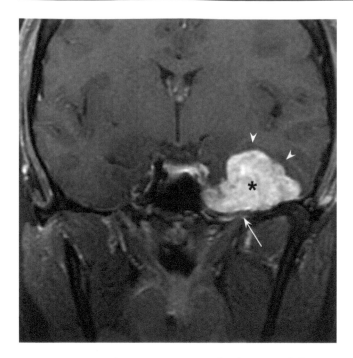

Fig. 7.49 A coronal postcontrast T1-weighted image with fat saturation demonstrates an intensely enhancing intracranial mass (*asterisk*) located in the left middle cranial fossa. The mass is clearly extraaxial as it has a sharp interface (*arrowheads*) with the adjacent left temporal lobe and displaces the cortex as well as the underlying white matter. The mass overlies foramen ovale (*concave arrow*) but does not extend into it.

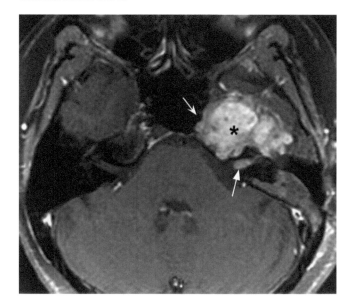

Fig. 7.50 An axial postcontrast T1-weighted image with fat saturation in the same patient again demonstrates the enhancing mass (*asterisk*) centered in the left middle cranial fossa and extending to the cavernous sinus, where it abuts the left internal carotid artery flow void (*concave arrow*). The tumor can now be seen to extend into the left internal auditory canal (*straight arrow*) via the geniculate ganglion, consistent with this being a large CN VII schwannoma. The lesion was subsequently removed with facial nerve grafting and reconstruction.

Diagnosis

- CN VII schwannoma extending into middle cranial fossa

Clinical Pearl

- CN VII schwannoma involving the middle cranial fossa is uncommon, and its accurate noninvasive diagnosis can be difficult. Clinically the patient may have no facial nerve dysfunction as the tumor has effectively "auto-decompressed" into the middle fossa. On imaging studies these lesions are often mistaken for more common middle cranial fossa lesions such as meningiomas. If the connection to the facial nerve (typically at the level of the geniculate ganglion) is not recognized preoperatively, then the facial nerve may be injured at the time of surgery. Surgical intervention for CN VII schwannomas can range from simple drainage of cystic components to aggressive tumor resection and facial nerve reconstruction.

Imaging Pearl

- The imaging features are similar to schwannomas elsewhere in that these masses are typically rounded and well-circumscribed. They are usually intermediate in signal intensity on T1-weighted images, mildly hyperintense on T2-weighted images, and enhance moderately postgadolinium. Areas of intratumor cystic degeneration are common, and areas of hemorrhage may sometimes be seen. The key feature to suggest that a middle cranial fossa mass might represent a CN VII schwannoma is clear extension back to the facial nerve canal, with a connection typically at the geniculate ganglion level and then extension proximally into the IAC or distally along the tympanic and mastoid segments of the nerve.

Case 7.11

A 49-year-old female presents with a 10-year history of a left parotid mass and left CN VII paresis (**Figs. 7.51, 7.52, 7.53, 7.54**).

Diagnosis

- Left intraparotid CN VII schwannoma

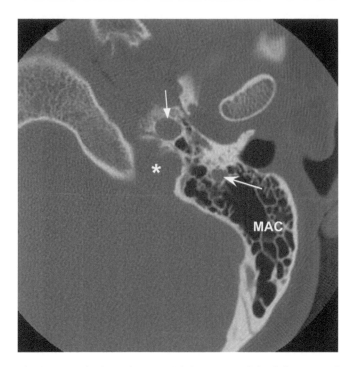

Fig. 7.51   A high-resolution axial CT image of the left temporal bone at the level of the jugular foramen (*asterisk*) demonstrates smooth enlargement of the descending mastoid segment of the facial nerve canal (*arrow*). Mastoid air cells (MAC) and petrous internal carotid artery canal (*concave arrow*) are shown.

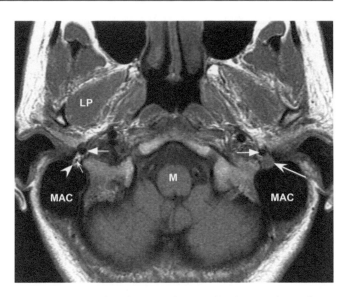

Fig. 7.52   More inferiorly, an axial T1-weighted image shows abnormal soft tissue within an expanded left stylomastoid foramen (*curved arrow*). Normal fat signal is noted within the right stylomastoid foramen (*concave arrowhead*) surrounding a normal CN VII (*small concave arrow*). Rounded, low signal intensity structures (*straight white arrows*) just anterior to the stylomastoid foramina represent the styloid processes. (LP, lateral pterygoid muscle; M, medulla; MAC, mastoid air cells.)

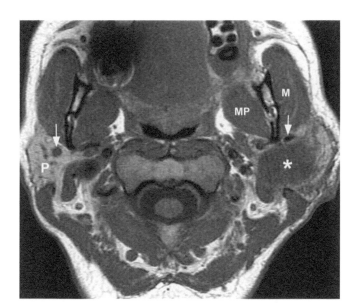

Fig. 7.53   More inferiorly, an axial T1-weighted image through the upper neck shows an intermediate signal intensity mass (*asterisk*) involving both the deep and superficial portions of the left parotid gland with anterior displacement of the left retromandibular vein (*arrows*). Normal hyperintense fat signal is noted throughout the normal right parotid gland (P). Medial pterygoid (MP) and masseter (M) muscles are shown.

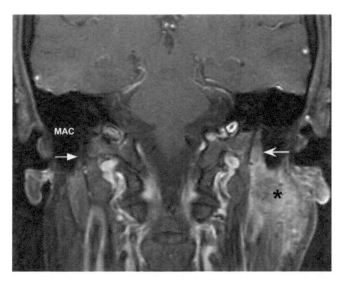

Fig. 7.54   A coronal postcontrast T1-weighted image with fat saturation through the stylomastoid foramen shows an enhancing mass (*asterisk*) centered in the left parotid gland. Abnormal enhancement extends superiorly through an expanded stylomastoid foramen and along the mastoid segment of the left CN VII (*concave arrow*). Normal signal is noted along the barely visible right CN VII (*straight arrow*). Mastoid air cells (MAC) are shown. Diagnosis: CN VII schwannoma involving intraparotid and mastoid segments of the facial nerve.

Clinical Pearl

• Intraparotid facial nerve schwannoma is a rare presentation of facial nerve schwannoma. This benign, slow-growing, well-circumscribed tumor mimics other more common benign parotid lesions such as pleomorphic adenoma, and resection of this mass by an unwary surgeon may result in unnecessary facial nerve paralysis. Extension back toward the stylomastoid foramen should be carefully sought for any parotid mass, and extension proximally along the descending facial nerve canal with smooth remodeling of the canal is strong supportive evidence for the diagnosis of intraparotid facial nerve schwannoma.

Case 7.12

A 38-year-old patient with a history of vertigo, as well as left-sided sensorineural hearing loss and mild facial weakness, is referred for stereotactic radiosurgical treatment of "acoustic neuroma" (**Figs. 7.55, 7.56, 7.57, 7.58, 7.59**).

Diagnosis

• Facial nerve hemangioma

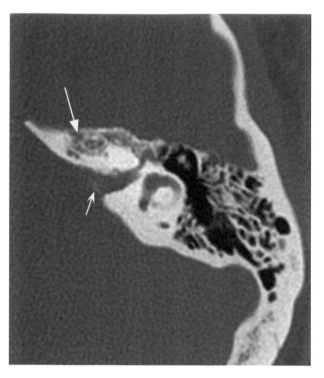

Fig. 7.55 An axial noncontrast CT image through the left temporal bone demonstrates faint calcification or ossification (*concave arrow*) within the internal auditory canal, as well as permeative lucency within the dense bone of the petrous apex (*straight arrow*).

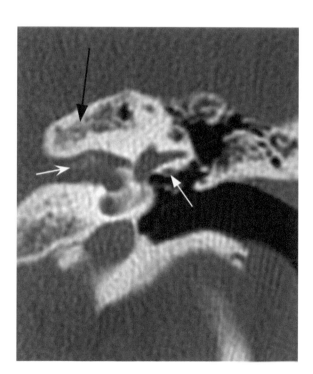

Fig. 7.56 A coronal noncontrast CT image through the left temporal bone in the same patient again demonstrates faint calcification or ossification (*white concave arrow*) within the internal auditory canal as well as permeative changes within the dense bone of the petrous apex (*black arrow*). The normal tympanic segment of the left CN VII (*white straight arrow*) coursing superolateral to the oval window and inferior to the horizontal semicircular canal is demonstrated.

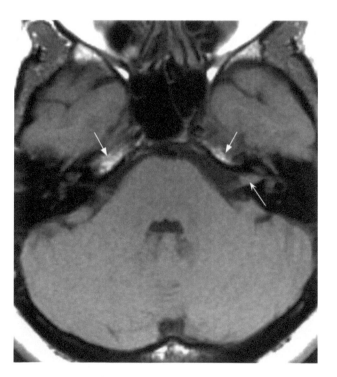

Fig. 7.57 An axial T1-weighted image through the posterior fossa in the same patient demonstrates an intermediate signal intensity lesion within the left internal auditory canal (*concave arrow*). Hyperintensity within the bilateral petrous apices represents normal fatty marrow signal (*straight arrows*), but there is less fat in the abnormal left apex.

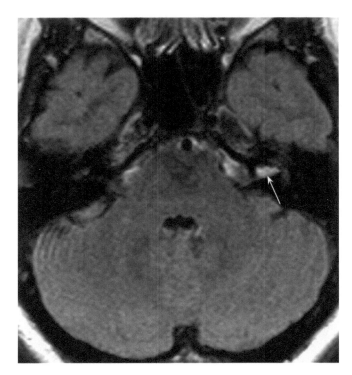

Fig. 7.58 An axial fluid-attenuated inversion recovery (FLAIR) image in the same patient at a similar level shows high signal intensity within the left internal auditory canal mass (*arrow*).

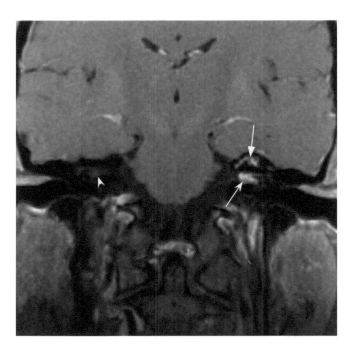

Fig. 7.59 A coronal postcontrast T1-weighted image with fat saturation in the same patient demonstrates intense focal enhancement within the left internal auditory canal (*concave arrow*) as well as irregular enhancement within the left petrous apex (*straight arrow*). Normal signal is noted in the right internal auditory canal (*concave arrowhead*). Diagnosis: ossifying hemangioma with involvement of the internal auditory canal and petrous apex.

Clinical Pearl

- A facial nerve hemangioma is a rare, benign, vascular tumor that originates from the capillary bed of the epineurium surrounding the facial nerve. It occurs most commonly at the level of the geniculate ganglion, but may also occur in the IAC or along the descending mastoid segment of the nerve. The lesion frequently involves the bone adjacent to the involved segments of the facial nerve.

Imaging Pearl

- On CT, the lesion often displays subtle ossification ("honeycomb" matrix), and this is a very helpful clue to the diagnosis. On MR, the lesions tend to be relatively bright on T2-weighted images and to enhance intensely postcontrast. CT and MRI are generally complementary in making the noninvasive diagnosis of ossifying facial nerve hemangioma.

Case 7.13

Two different patients present with hearing loss and facial palsy after severe head trauma (**Figs. 7.60, 7.61**).

Diagnosis

- Temporal bone fractures with posttraumatic facial palsy

Clinical Pearl

- The facial nerve is the most commonly injured motor CN. In the past, temporal bone fractures were classified as transverse or longitudinal (see below) based on their relationship to the long axis of the petrous bone. Longitudinal fractures are most common (>80%), run parallel to the long axis of the petrous temporal bone, and often result in disruption of the ossicles (associated with conductive hearing loss). Transverse fractures run perpendicular to the petrous temporal bone and are more often associated with facial nerve injury. Overall, facial nerve injury has been said to complicate ~50% of transverse and ~20% of longitudinal temporal bone fractures. The most common sites of injury are at the geniculate ganglion or along the descending mastoid segment of the facial canal. Proximal interruption leads to unilateral complete facial paralysis, ageusia over the anterior two thirds of the tongue, and loss of lacrimation. A newer classification of temporal bone fractures describes them as otic capsule-sparing or otic capsule-violating. Patients with otic capsule-violating fractures are more likely to develop facial paralysis, more likely to develop CSF leak, and more likely to experience profound posttraumatic hearing loss. They are also more likely to sustain intracranial complications such as epidural hematoma and subarachnoid hemorrhage.

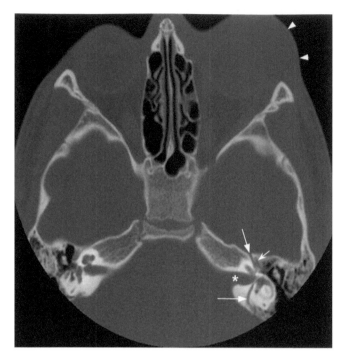

Fig. 7.60 An axial CT image in bone window through the skull base demonstrates a transverse temporal bone fracture (*straight arrows*) that traverses the fundus of the left internal auditory canal (*) and the fallopian canal and extends to the geniculate fossa (*concave arrow*). This otic capsule-involving fracture clearly crosses the path of CN VII. Note the presence of left periorbital soft tissue swelling (*arrowheads*), compatible with recent trauma.

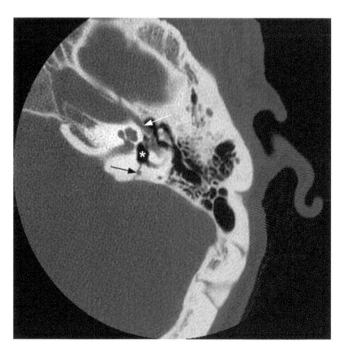

Fig. 7.61 An axial CT image in bone window in a different patient shows a transverse left temporal bone fracture (*black arrow*) that extends into the vestibule (*asterisk*). The presence of air in the vestibule is known as pneumolabyrinth. The fracture also extends to the tympanic segment of CN VII (*white arrow*), resulting in facial palsy.

Imaging Pearl

- High-resolution temporal bone CT is the imaging study of choice for assessment of temporal bone fractures and for classification as otic capsule-sparing or otic capsule-violating. Temporal bone fractures can be subtle. A good clue to the potential presence of a temporal bone fracture is unilateral opacification of the mastoid air cells or EAC on a routine noncontrast head CT in a patient who has had significant head trauma. Extension of a fracture into the inner ear may result in pneumolabyrinth (air within the membranous labyrinth). Pneumolabyrinth is identified most commonly in the vestibule and is usually accompanied by severe sensorineural hearing loss.

Case 7.14

An elderly female with a history of multiple skin cancers presents with a progressive right CN VII palsy (**Fig. 7.62**).

Diagnosis

- Squamous cell carcinoma of right face with perineural extension of tumor

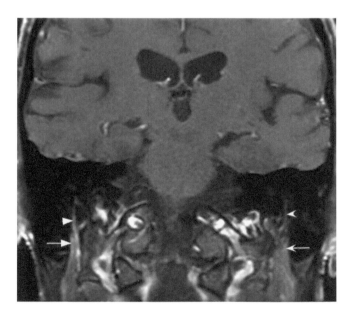

Fig. 7.62 A coronal postcontrast T1-weighted image with fat saturation through the mastoid air cells and along the course of the mastoid segment of CN VII as it passes into the stylomastoid foramen and parotid gland. Asymmetric enhancement is noted within the right stylomastoid foramen (*straight arrow*) as compared with the left (*concave arrow*). There is abnormal thickening, nodularity, and enhancement involving the mastoid segment of the right CN VII (*straight arrowhead*). The left stylomastoid foramen (*concave arrow*) and left CN VII (*concave arrowhead*) are normal. Findings on the right are highly suspicious for perineural extension of tumor along CN VII, and this was subsequently confirmed by tissue sampling.

- Perineural extension of tumor is a well-described complication of many head and neck malignancies, including squamous cell carcinoma of the skin or mucosal surfaces, adenoid cystic carcinoma, cutaneous or mucosal melanoma, and lymphoma, among other pathologies. Perineural spread of tumor most commonly occurs along branches of the trigeminal nerve and the facial nerve, but other CNs can also be involved. Some patients may be clinically asymptomatic even when they have gross spread of disease by imaging or histopathology; others may initially be misdiagnosed with "benign" conditions such as trigeminal neuralgia or Bell's palsy. A clinical index of suspicion for perineural spread of tumor must be high in any patient with a history of head and neck cancer and new CN palsy.

- Recognition of perineural spread of tumor at MRI often changes treatment goals from curative to palliative and can therefore significantly affect patient management. Imaging features of perineural spread of disease include enlargement, asymmetric enhancement, and nodularity of CNs; enlargement of skull base foramina; effacement of fat planes along the course of CNs; and denervation changes in muscles innervated by involved CNs. Though some of these features may be appreciated on CT scans, MRI is generally indicated in the assessment of a patient suspected of having perineural extension of tumor.

Case 7.15

A 54-year-old female underwent a craniotomy for assessment of a "cavernous sinus meningioma" after she presented with multiple CN palsies, including CN V and CN VII. Pathology demonstrated adenocarcinoma rather than meningioma. At that point a head and neck examination was performed, and the preoperative MR scan was re-reviewed (**Figs. 7.63, 7.64**).

Diagnosis

- Adenocarcinoma of the palate with perineural spread from CN V to CN VII along right GSPN

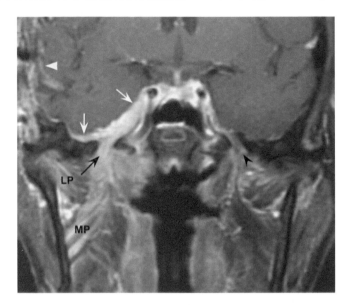

Fig. 7.63 A coronal postcontrast T1-weighted image with fat saturation shows abnormal enhancement and widening of the right foramen ovale (*black arrow*) and right V₃ compared with the normal left side (*black arrowhead*). Enhancing soft tissue extends intracranially to infiltrate the dura along the floor and medial aspect of the right middle cranial fossa (*white arrows*). Note the postoperative changes (*white arrowhead*) related to a prior right temporal craniotomy to approach what was thought to be a meningioma of the cavernous sinus. Volume loss and asymmetric enhancement of the right pterygoid muscles compared with the left are due to denervation change. Medial pterygoid (MP) and lateral pterygoid (LP) muscles are shown.

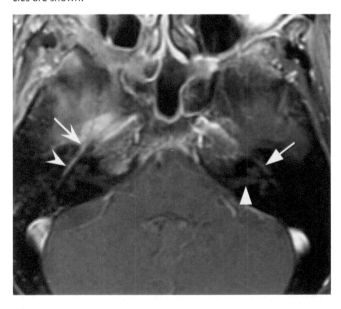

Fig. 7.64 An axial postcontrast T1-weighted image with fat saturation at the level of the internal auditory canals (*straight arrowhead on left*) shows abnormal enhancement along the right greater superficial petrosal nerve (*concave arrow*), extending from the level of Meckel's cave/foramen ovale anteriorly to the horizontal segment of CN VII (*concave arrowhead*) posteriorly. Note the normal minimally enhancing tympanic segment of the left CN VII (*straight arrow*). Diagnosis: perineural spread of adenocarcinoma along the right greater superficial petrosal nerve.

Clinical Pearl

- The GSPN serves as a potential connection between CNs V and VII. Recall that the GSPN passes deep to the trigeminal ganglion in Meckel's cave. Tumor involving CN V can therefore access CN VII at the level of Meckel's cave and may then spread posterolaterally along the GSPN to the temporal bone and proximal segments of the facial nerve.

Imaging Pearl

- CN VII should be carefully scrutinized in any patient with perineural extension of tumor along CN V, and vice versa. High-resolution, thin-section, post-gadolinium T1-weighted imaging with fat saturation should cover the courses of both CN V and CN VII in any patient with perineural extension along either of these nerves. The GSPN, extending from the level of Meckel's cave to the geniculate ganglion, should be assessed for enlargement and/or asymmetric enhancement.

Case 7.16

A 56-year-old male with a history of squamous cell carcinoma of the skin overlying the left parotid gland presents with progressive facial palsy and chin numbness (**Figs. 7.65, 7.66.**)

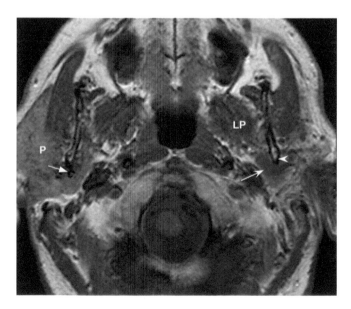

Fig. 7.65 An axial T1-weighted image demonstrates surgical absence of the left parotid gland. There is abnormal soft tissue (*curved arrow*) posterior to the neck of the left mandible (*concave arrowhead*), which represents perineural spread of tumor along the auriculotemporal nerve. Note the normal right parotid gland (P) and right retromandibular vein (*straight arrow*). Only vessels are seen posterior to the neck of the mandible on the normal right side. (LP, lateral pterygoid muscle.)

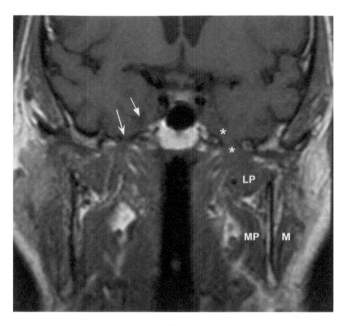

Fig. 7.66 A coronal T1-weighted image shows asymmetric soft tissue thickening of CN V_3 (*asterisk*) as it courses superiorly through a markedly widened left foramen ovale toward Meckel's cave. Note the normal right foramen ovale (*concave arrow*) and right Meckel's cave (*straight arrow*). Mild fatty atrophy of the left-sided muscles of mastication is seen. Lateral pterygoid muscle (LP), medial pterygoid muscle (MP), and masseter muscle (M) are shown.

A 76-year-old man previously treated with surgery and radiation for adenoid cystic carcinoma of the left parotid gland presents with progressive facial palsy, numbness of the left lower face, and difficulty chewing (**Figs. 7.67, 7.68, 7.69**).

Diagnosis

- Two different patients with perineural spread of tumor between CNs V and VII via the auriculotemporal nerve

Clinical Pearl

- The auriculotemporal nerve is formed by two rootlets of CN V_3 (see Chapter 5). The middle meningeal artery courses between the rootlets, which coalesce to form a short trunk. This trunk courses behind the neck of the mandible, and its multiple branches then intermingle with CN VII in the parotid gland. Involvement of the auriculotemporal nerve by tumor is frequently accompanied by periauricular pain and TMJ pain or dysfunction.

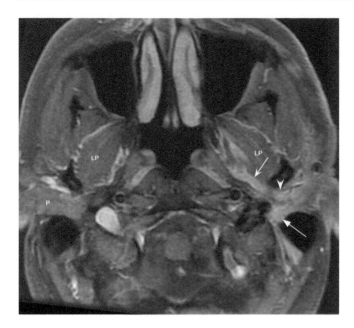

Fig. 7.67 An axial postcontrast T1-weighted image with fat saturation through the upper neck at the parotid level demonstrates infiltrative enhancing soft tissue within the left parotid resection bed and extending posterior to the mandible (*arrowhead*) at the expected location of the auriculotemporal nerve. Abnormal enhancing tissue also extends more posteriorly into the stylomastoid foramen (*straight arrow*) and anteromedially toward the main trunk of CN V₃ (*concave arrow*). Normal right parotid gland (P) and lateral pterygoid muscles (LP) are shown. The left LP and other muscles of mastication are mildly atrophic compared with the contralateral side.

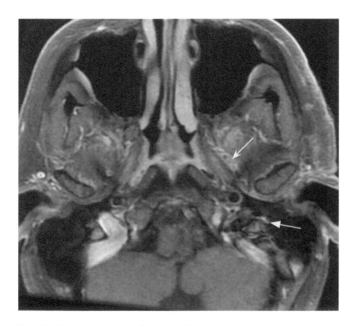

Fig. 7.68 More superiorly, an axial postcontrast T1-weighted image with fat saturation demonstrates abnormal enhancement of left CN VII within the mastoid (*straight arrow*) and along the third division of the trigeminal nerve (CN V₃) (*concave arrow*), compatible with perineural spread of tumor in this patient with known adenoid cystic carcinoma of the left parotid gland.

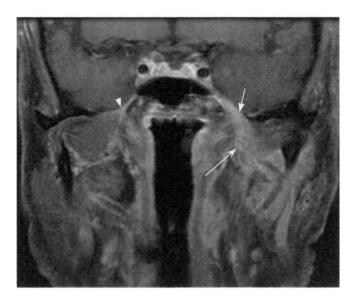

Fig. 7.69 A coronal postcontrast T1-weighted image with fat saturation in the same patient demonstrates abnormal enhancing tissue extending superiorly along a thickened left CN V₃ (*concave arrow*) through the foramen ovale (*straight arrow*). Right foramen ovale (*arrowhead*) is normal. The muscles of mastication on the left are mildly atrophic and mildly enhancing secondary to subacute denervation change.

Imaging Pearl

• Asymmetric soft tissue posterior to the neck of the mandible is often seen in patients with perineural spread of tumor along the auriculotemporal nerve. This tissue can range from subtle to more obvious and mass-like, and it is often most easily appreciated on axial T1-weighted images as it is seen in contrast to the normally fatty tissue of the adult parotid gland. CN VII and CN V₃ should be carefully scrutinized in these cases for the findings of perineural extension of disease already reviewed above.

Case 7.17

A 74-year-old male with chronic right CN VII palsy after prior treatment for right parotid mucoepidermoid carcinoma presents for surveillance imaging (**Fig. 7.70**).

Diagnosis

• Denervation change of muscles of facial expression

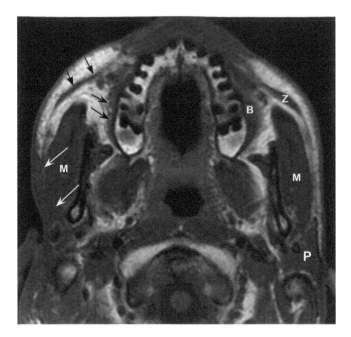

Fig. 7.70 An axial T1-weighted image through the midface and upper neck demonstrates atrophy of the right zygomaticus major muscle (*straight black arrows*) and right buccinator muscle (*black concave arrows*), both of which are innervated by right CN VII. These changes are subtle, as would be expected in such small muscles. This patient has undergone prior surgery for parotid cancer and has a chronic CN VII palsy. Abnormal soft tissue infiltrating the subcutaneous tissues overlying the right masseter muscle (M) is consistent with treatment-related change versus persistent/progressive tumor. Normal left parotid gland (P), zygomaticus major muscle (Z) and buccinator muscle (B) are shown.

Clinical Pearl

- Injury to a motor nerve, whether due to trauma, tumor, or other etiologies, results in denervation change in the muscle(s) innervated by that nerve. Patients may have symptoms related to muscle dysfunction such as difficulty chewing (CN V_3) or facial weakness (CN VII), or they may be relatively asymptomatic.

Imaging Pearl

- Denervation changes evolve through acute, subacute, and chronic stages, and each stage is characterized by specific imaging findings. Acute denervation (days to weeks or a few months) leads to muscle edema (T2 hyperintensity) and post-gadolinium enhancement, but no loss of bulk or fatty infiltration. As denervation becomes subacute over months to a year or so, the T2 changes and post-gadolinium enhancement may persist, but the muscle begins to lose bulk. In the chronic stages of many months to years of denervation, the T2 hyperintensity and post-gadolinium enhancement resolve, while significant atrophy and often fatty infiltration set in (see also **Table 12.2**).

8 Vestibulocochlear Nerve

Functions

- Special sensory afferent (SA) for balance (via superior and inferior vestibular nerves) and hearing (via cochlear nerve).

Anatomy: Vestibular System

Vestibular Nerves (Figs. 8.1, 8.2)

- SA. Vestibular components of membranous labyrinth (three *semicircular canals, utricle,* and *saccule*) provide information to two vestibular nerves (superior and inferior vestibular nerves).
- *The superior vestibular nerve* (from utricle and superior and horizontal semicircular canals) and the *inferior vestibular nerve* (from inferior semicircular canal and saccule) connect with cell bodies in the *vestibular ganglion* (Scarpa ganglion), which lies near the fundus of the internal auditory canal.
- The vestibular nerves, joined by the cochlear nerve, form the vestibulocochlear nerve, which enters the pontomedullary junction near the lateral recess of the fourth ventricle. Whereas the cochlear fibers split *dorsally* to reach the cochlear nuclei, the vestibular fibers split *ventrally* to terminate in
  1. Vestibular nuclei (*superior, lateral, medial,* and *inferior*) (see below).
  2. Cerebellum (flocculonodular lobe). The flocculonodular lobe functions with the semicircular canals to detect rapid changes in direction.
  3. Reticular formation. The reticular formation is an area of interspersed small nuclei and fibers that spans the brainstem (see Appendix A, The Brainstem for more information).
- The vestibular system has three functions:
  1. Provides information about movement of the head and changes in head position. This aids in coordinating the position of the eyes, head, and neck and in providing a sense of balance.
  2. Increases tone in antigravity extensors to support the body against the pull of gravity.
  3. Holds eyes on target while the head moves (vestibular impulses counter-roll the eyes against the direction of head movements to maintain fixation).

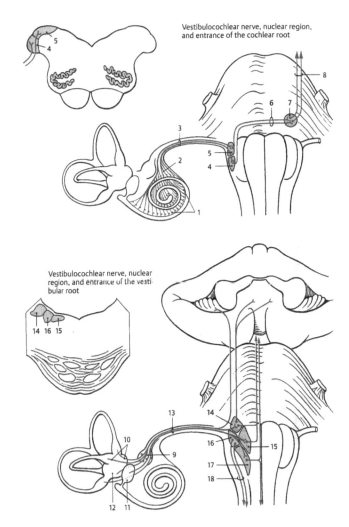

Fig. 8.1 Vestibulocochlear nerve: cochlear and vestibular roots. (1, spiral ganglion; 2, spiral tract; 3, cochlear root; 4, ventral cochlear nucleus; 5, dorsal cochlear nucleus; 6, trapezoid body; 7, trapezoid nuclei; 8, lateral lemniscus; 9, vestibular (Scarpa) ganglion; 10, semicircular ducts; 11, saccule; 12, utricle; 13, vestibular root; 14, superior vestibular nucleus; 15, medial vestibular nucleus; 16, lateral vestibular nucleus; 17, inferior vestibular nucleus; 18, vestibulospinal tract.)

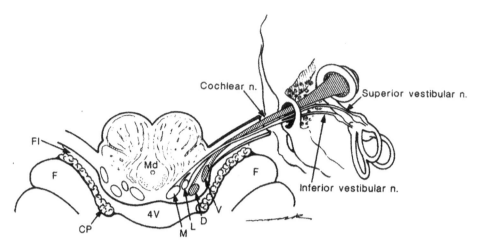

Fig. 8.2 Vestibular and cochlear nuclei. Axial drawing of upper medulla (Md) shows medial (M) and lateral (L) vestibular nuclei and dorsal (D) and ventral (V) cochlear nuclei. Both nuclear groups are located in the lateral aspect of the inferior cerebellar peduncle. (Fl, foramen of Luschka; 4V, fourth ventricle; CP, choroid plexus; F, cerebellar flocculus.) (From Harnsberger HR. Handbook of Head and Neck Imaging (2nd ed.). St. Louis, MO: Mosby, 1995. Reprinted with permission.)

Vestibular Sensory Organs (Figs. 8.3, 8.4)

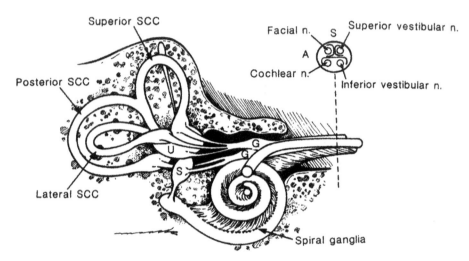

Fig. 8.3 Inner ear. Hearing-related structures include the cochlea, spiral ganglia, and cochlear nerve. Balance-related structures include the superior, posterior, lateral semicircular canals (SCC); utricle (U) and saccule (S); vestibular ganglion (G); and superior and inferior vestibular nerves. A cross-section of the apex of the IAC is shown at upper right. (A, anterior; S, superior.) (From Harnsberger HR. Handbook of Head and Neck Imaging (2nd ed.). St. Louis, MO: Mosby, 1995. Reprinted with permission.)

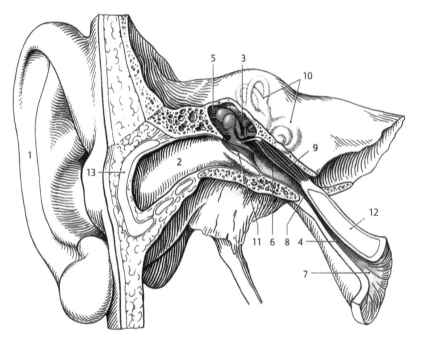

Fig. 8.4 View of the middle and inner ear. 1, auricle. 2, external acoustic meatus. 3, tympanic cavity. 4, auditory (Eustachian) tube. 5, epitympanic recess. 6, tympanic opening into auditory tube. 7, pharyngeal opening into auditory tube. 8, isthmus of auditory tube. 9, tensor tympani muscle. 10, bony labyrinth. 11, tympanic membrane. 12, auditory tube cartilage. 13, continuation of auricular cartilage.

- *Macula.* Sensory organ of utricle and saccule. Contains hair cells with cilia embedded in gelatinous layer containing calcium carbonate *otoliths.* When the head moves in a given direction, otoliths move relatively in the opposite direction because they have more inertia than the surrounding fluid. The hair cells (each with 50–70 stereocilia and one large kinocilium) face in various directions, are stimulated by otolith movement thereby altering their firing rate, and synapse with the vestibular nerve.
- Based on their orientation, the utricle senses *horizontal linear acceleration* and the saccule senses *vertical linear acceleration.*
- The three *semicircular canals* (superior, posterior, and horizontal or lateral) are at right angles to one another and so detect motion in any combination of three planes (i.e., in any direction).
  - *Ampulla.* Dilation at the end of each semicircular canal filled with *endolymph.* Contains *crista ampullaris* (sensory organ of semicircular canals), which has hair cells with cilia that project into the gel cup (cupula).
  - *Cristae* of semicircular canals detect *angular acceleration* because fluid in the ducts stays relatively still from inertia despite head rotation.
- Blood supply of membranous labyrinth is from the *labyrinthine artery* (also called *internal auditory artery;* usually a branch of the anterior inferior cerebellar artery [AICA], or less commonly of the basilar artery). Labyrinthine artery branches into (1) *anterior vestibular artery,* to superior and horizontal semicircular canals and utricle; (2) *posterior vestibular artery,* to posterior semicircular canal, saccule, and part of cochlea; and (3) *cochlear artery.*

Vestibular Nuclei (see also Appendix A)

- There are four vestibular nuclei:
  1. Superior vestibular nucleus (of Bechterew)
  2. Medial vestibular nucleus (of Schwalbe)
  3. Lateral vestibular nucleus (of Deiters)
  4. Inferior vestibular nucleus (of Roller)
- The vestibular nuclei straddle the pontomedullary junction and contain the cell bodies of the second-order neurons of the vestibular pathways.
- An *interstitial nucleus of the vestibular nerve,* located among the fibers of the vestibular root, has also been described, but its functional significance is unclear.
- Inputs to the vestibular nuclei include the following:
  1. Vestibular portion of cranial nerve (CN) VIII (details below)
  2. Cerebellovestibular tracts. The fastigial nucleus (a deep cerebellar nucleus) projects bilaterally to lateral and inferior vestibular nuclei. Uncrossed fastigial fibers project through the *juxtarestiform body* (a sub-

division of the inferior cerebellar peduncle); crossed fastigial fibers project through the *uncinate fasciculus of Russell,* which travels along the superior cerebellar peduncle (see Appendix A).
  3. Reticulovestibular tracts.
- Outputs from vestibular nuclei include the following:
  1. *Cerebellum (vestibulocerebellar* pathways). Inferior and medial vestibular nuclei project via juxtarestiform body to ipsilateral cortex of flocculonodular lobe, uvula, and fastigial nucleus (vestibulocerebellum). This is a reciprocal connection for maintenance of posture.
  2. *Medial longitudinal fasciculus* (MLF). All vestibular nuclei contribute to the MLF. Only the superior vestibular nucleus projects to the ipsilateral MLF; other nuclei send fibers to the contralateral MLF. The MLF interconnects the nuclei of CN III, IV, VI, the PPRF, the superior colliculus, and the interstitial nucleus of Cajal (a mesencephalic nucleus considered to be an important premotor center for eliciting vertical and rotatory eye and head movements) (see Appendix B).
  3. *Medial vestibulospinal tract.* Medial vestibular nucleus to cervical and upper thoracic levels of contralateral spinal cord.
  4. *Lateral vestibulospinal tract.* Lateral vestibular nucleus *(Deiters' nucleus)* to ipsilateral lateral vestibulospinal tract to innervate antigravity extensors.
  5. *Reticular formation (vestibuloreticular* pathways). Vestibuloreticular fibers mediate the nausea, vomiting, pallor, and hypotension that accompany vestibular disorders (e.g., motion sickness).
  6. Vestibular hair cells for feedback control.
- *Superior (Bechterew) and medial (Schwalbe) vestibular nuclei.* Involved with eye reflexes (vestibuloocular reflexes) and coordination of eye movements with head movements. Receive afferent input from the semicircular canals and have efferent fibers to the MLF for eye movement and to the medial vestibulospinal tract for head and neck movement. The *medial vestibular nucleus* is the largest vestibular nucleus and sends crossed fibers to all nuclei involved with control of extraocular muscles and to the cerebellum. The *superior vestibular nucleus* sends uncrossed fibers by way of the MLF to the CN III and IV nuclei.
- *Lateral vestibular nucleus (Deiters' nucleus).* Involved with posture. Afferent input is from the utricle (via the superior vestibular ganglion) and direct inhibitory input is from Purkinje cells in the cerebellar vermis. Efferent fibers to the *lateral vestibulospinal tract* serve to elicit lower limb extension for posture control.
- *Inferior vestibular nucleus (of Roller).* Integrates input from the vestibular system and the cerebellum. Afferent input from the saccule (from the inferior vestibular ganglion). Efferent fibers to the cerebellum and reticular formation.

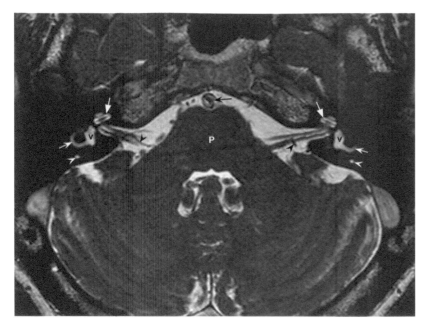

Fig. 8.8 An axial three-dimensional fast imaging employing steady-state acquisition (FIESTA) image through the posterior fossa at the level of the pons (P) demonstrates branches of CN VIII within the bilateral internal auditory canals. The cochlear nerves are present anteriorly within the IACs, and the inferior vestibular nerves are present posteriorly. Vascular flow voids representing AICA (*black concave arrowheads*) are seen in close proximity to the nerves. Cochleae (*white straight arrows*), vestibule (v). Horizontal (*white concave arrows*) and posterior (*white concave arrowheads*) semicircular canals are seen. The basilar artery is also seen (*black concave arrow*).

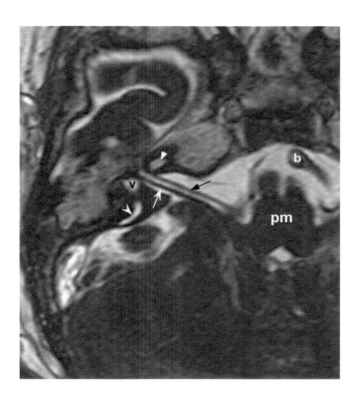

Fig. 8.9 An axial three-dimensional FIESTA image from a different patient at the level of the pontomedullary junction (pm) and through the upper aspect of the right internal auditory canal (IAC) demonstrates the course of the right CNs VII and VIII traversing the cerebellopontine angle and entering the IAC. CN VII (the facial nerve, *black straight arrow*) is seen anteriorly and the superior vestibular nerve (branch of CN VIII, *white concave arrow*) is seen posteriorly. The cochlea (*straight arrowhead*), vestibule (v), and posterior semicircular canal (*concave arrowhead*) are partially shown. Basilar artery flow void (b) is seen at its junction with the left vertebral artery.

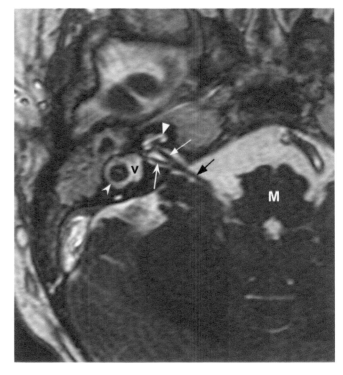

Fig. 8.10 More inferiorly, an axial three-dimensional FIESTA image in the same patient at the level of the upper medulla (M) and lower part of the right internal auditory canal (IAC) demonstrates the vestibulocochlear nerve (*black arrow*) branching into the more anterior cochlear nerve (*white straight arrow*) and the more posterior inferior vestibular nerve (*white concave arrow*). The cochlear branch is seen entering the cochlea (*white straight arrowhead*). The normal vestibule (v) and horizontal semicircular canal (*white concave arrowhead*) are demonstrated.

Fig. 8.11 A coronal T2-weighted image through the level of the pons (P) shows branches of CN VII and VIII within the internal auditory canals (IACs) (*white straight arrows*). Fluid signal is present within the semicircular canals: horizontal (*white concave arrows*) and superior (*arrowheads*). CN V cisternal segments are also indicated bilaterally (*black arrows*) on either side of the pons, just above the level of the IAC.

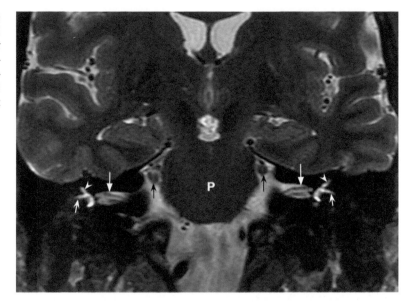

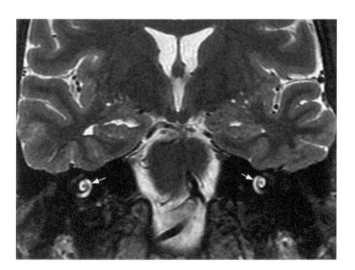

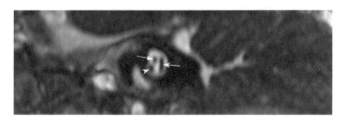

Fig. 8.13 A sagittal three-dimensional FIESTA image at the level of the mid internal auditory canal shows the facial nerve anterosuperiorly (*straight arrow*) and the cochlear nerve anteroinferiorly (*concave arrowhead*). More posteriorly, the branch point of the CN VIII superior and inferior vestibular nerves is seen (*concave white arrow*).

Fig. 8.12 More anteriorly, a coronal T2-weighted image shows fluid signal with the normal turns of the snail-like bilateral cochleae (*arrows*).

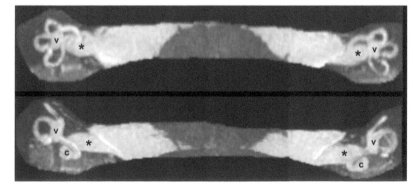

Fig. 8.14 Three-dimensional MIP (maximum intensity projection) an axial FIESTA images demonstrate the internal auditory canals (*) and also show the normal relationship of the cochleae (c), vestibules (v), and three semicircular canals in different projections.

Vestibular Lesions

Evaluation

- Patients with suspected vestibular dysfunction should have a detailed neurologic evaluation including a detailed CN examination, evaluation of hearing, examination of ocular movements, cerebellar testing, and evaluation of vestibular control of balance and movement.
- *Romberg test* is usually positive in unilateral vestibular dysfunction. A positive Romberg test is when a patient is unable to maintain balance while standing upright with feet together and eyes closed. The patient tends to fall to the side of vestibular hypofunction.
- Vestibular reflexes
  - *Decerebrate reflex (decerebrate rigidity).* Described by Sherrington in 1896. Due to anatomical or functional transection of the brainstem above the vestibular nuclei but below the red nucleus. All four extremities become tonically extended. Arises from combined effects of tonic activity in vestibulospinal and pontine reticulospinal neurons (innervating extensors).
  - *Decorticate reflex (decorticate rigidity).* When the brainstem is functionally lesioned above the red nucleus, posture is regulated by the rubrospinal tract, which opposes vestibulospinal and reticulospinal pathways. In humans, lower extremity (LE) extensors and upper extremity (UE) flexors contract steadily (because the rubrospinal tract in humans only projects as far as the cervical region and only counteracts vestibulospinal activity in UEs but not LEs).
  - *Vestibuloocular reflex* (VOR). A reflex eye movement that keeps the visual image still during head movement by producing coordinated eye movements in the direction opposite to head movement. Head rotation causes motion in the membranous labyrinth and ipsilateral horizontal semicircular canal → increases activity in ipsilateral CN VIII → information conveyed to vestibular nuclei → reciprocal alteration in activity in brainstem nuclei that control ipsilateral and contralateral eye movements → compensatory movement of the eyes → stabilization of the visual image on the retina with head movement. The VOR is one of the fastest reflexes in the body, and eye movements lag head movements by < 10 milliseconds. In comatose patients, the VOR is tested as the *oculocephalic reflex* or "doll's eye" reflex when the physician turns the head and examines compensatory eye movements. Absent oculocephalic reflexes indicate brainstem dysfunction.
  - *Caloric testing (oculovestibular reflex).* Useful largely for determining the presence/absence of brainstem function in comatose patients rather than for diagnosis of vestibular dysfunction. Cold water irrigation into the external ear canal causes a decrease in CN VIII firing rate in the ipsilateral utricle, which leads to nystagmus with the fast component away from the stimulus. The mnemonic "COWS" (cold—opposite, warm—same) refers to the direction of the fast component of nystagmus induced by water irrigation.

Clinical Manifestations

- Nystagmus (oscillating eye movements)
- Oscillopsia (a sense of oscillation of objects viewed)
- Autonomic effects (nausea, vomiting, pallor, sweating, hypotension)
- Vertigo
  - Vertigo is an illusory sensation of movement associated with disease of the labyrinth or its central connections (CN VIII, vestibular nuclei).
  - Usually the movement is described as a "spinning" but can also be a "tilting."
  - May be associated with nausea/vomiting (activation of medullary area postrema), pallor, sweating, nystagmus.
  - Differentiate from faintness, lightheadedness, presyncope (caused by decreased cerebral blood flow), dysequilibrium (unsteadiness when walking), nonspecific dizziness.
  - Categorized into *central* causes (dysfunction of vestibular connections), *peripheral* causes (vestibular labyrinthine disease), and *systemic* causes (other diseases/drugs/toxins).
    - *Central causes of vertigo*
      - More likely to be chronic or permanent compared with peripheral vestibulopathies.
      - Associated brainstem findings are more prominent, whereas auditory involvement is less frequent.
      - Vascular.
        1. Transient ischemic attacks (TIAs). Vertebrobasilar ischemia is often accompanied by vertigo. It may be part of a *subclavian steal syndrome* (stenosis of subclavian artery proximal to the origin of the vertebral artery associated with flow reversal in the vertebral artery especially during arm exercise).
        2. *Wallenberg syndrome* (lateral medullary syndrome). Caused by occlusion of the intracranial vertebral artery or PICA and leads to vertigo by ischemic injury to the vestibular nuclei. It is associated with some or all of the following findings: ipsilateral facial hypalgesia and thermoanesthesia, contralateral trunk and extremity hypalgesia and thermoanesthesia, ipsilateral vocal cord paralysis, dysphagia, dysarthria, ipsilateral Horner syndrome, nausea, vomiting, ipsilateral cerebellar signs/symptoms, diplopia, and hiccups. See also Case 9.1, Chapter 9 and Appendix A.

3. Basilar migraine (vertigo followed by suboccipital headache and vomiting).

4. Cerebellar infarction/hemorrhage (often accompanied by vertigo and ataxia).

- Inflammatory. Multiple sclerosis (MS) (~20% of patients with MS experience vertigo at some point).
- Vestibular epilepsy (vertigo may be an aura for temporal lobe epilepsy).

• *Peripheral causes of vertigo.* Due to lesion of semicircular canals and/or otolith organs. Patient usually lies with affected ear uppermost, slow phase of nystagmus is toward lesion, and Romberg test is positive (falls toward lesion).

- The three most common peripheral causes of vertigo are benign paroxysmal positional vertigo, viral infection/inflammation, and Meniere disease.
- *Benign paroxysmal positional vertigo* (BPPV). Most common single cause of vertigo (~20% of all cases). Usually idiopathic but may be caused by trauma or other ear diseases. Generally considered to be caused by an abnormality of the posterior semicircular canal otoliths. After head tilt toward affected ear or after head extension, rotational vertigo and nystagmus occur. The *Dix-Hallpike maneuver* (also known as the *Nylén-Bárány maneuver*) is the standard test for BPPV and involves moving the patient rapidly from a sitting to a supine position with the head turned 45 degrees to the right or left; after 20–30 seconds, the patient is returned to the sitting position. The finding of rotatory nystagmus with limited duration is considered pathognomonic. Treatments include conservative therapy, vestibulosuppressants (e.g., meclizine), and canalith repositioning procedures (e.g., Semont or Epley maneuvers). Surgery (e.g., posterior canal occlusion) is limited to intractable cases.
- *Vestibular neuritis.* Typically affects young to middle-aged adults, with no gender preponderance. There is often a history of upper respiratory infection, and the etiology is thought to be viral in most cases. Vestibular neuritis is characterized by acute severe vertigo, nausea/vomiting, abnormal caloric testing, and falling to ipsilateral side. No tinnitus or deafness is present. It generally resolves within several weeks, and can be treated with antihistamines and/or antiemetic agents.
- *Acute labyrinthitis.* Like vestibular neuritis, but with associated tinnitus and hearing loss. May follow systemic or middle ear infections or use of ototoxic drugs (toxic labyrinthitis).
- *Labyrinthine hemorrhage* or *stroke* secondary to thrombosis of the labyrinthine (internal auditory) artery. If the cochlear branch is involved, then deafness may occur as well.

- *Meniere disease.* Recurrent *vertigo* with fluctuating unilateral *tinnitus* and *low-tone sensorineural hearing loss* (these are more likely later in the disease course). Typical onset at age 40 years, no gender preponderance. Onset abrupt, and episode may last minutes to hours. Usually unilateral, but can be bilateral in 20% of cases. Also sensation of fullness around affected ear. Horizontal nystagmus is contralateral (occurs during an acute attack) and falling is ipsilateral. Pathology thought secondary to *endolymphatic hydrops* (distension of the endolymphatic duct with rupture into the perilymph, dumping K^+ that paralyzes the vestibular apparatus and may cause nerve degeneration over time).
- *Vestibular schwannoma* (acoustic neuroma). May also cause vertigo secondary to CN VIII involvement, but hearing loss and tinnitus are far more common presenting symptoms.
- *Perilymphatic fistula.* Pathologic communication between the fluid-filled space of the inner ear and the air-filled space of the middle ear (e.g., after trauma or barotrauma, postsurgical or idiopathic). Associated with sudden or progressive sensorineural hearing loss and vertigo. Surgical repair is often necessary.
- *Systemic causes of dizziness/vertigo*
- *Dizziness* is a subjective term variably used to connote lightheadedness, faintness, and disequilibrium among other things, whereas *vertigo* refers specifically to an illusory sensation of movement (often described as spinning sensation).
- Cardiovascular disease (usually dizziness/syncope).
- Vasculitides (e.g., Cogan syndrome—vertigo, tinnitus, hearing loss, keratitis).
- Hematologic disorders (hyperviscosity or anemia can both cause dizziness).
- Hypoglycemia (dizziness).
- Hypothyroidism (associated with lightheadedness, dizziness, and occasionally vertigo).
- Hyperventilation (dizziness, circumoral paresthesiae).
- Ototoxic drugs (e.g., aminoglycoside antibiotics).

Auditory Pathway Lesions

Types

Cortical Lesions

• Unilateral damage to primary auditory cortex (Heschl gyri, area 41) causes a subtle impairment in spatial localization of sound.

- Damage to auditory association areas causes sound agnosia (difficulty identifying sounds).
- Bilateral temporal lesions affecting Heschl gyri and/or their interconnections may cause the syndrome of *pure word deafness* (auditory verbal agnosia).

Brainstem Lesions

- Brainstem lesions above the cochlear nuclei do not cause complete deafness.
- Lesion of the lateral lemniscus causes bilateral partial deafness, greater in the contralateral ear.
- Localization of auditory brainstem lesions can be assisted with brainstem auditory evoked responses (BAERs).

Cerebellopontine Angle and Peripheral Lesions

- Usually cause sensorineural hearing loss (deficit in perceiving tones or speech).
- Often associated with tinnitus (see below).
- Causes include the following:
  1. Cerebellopontine angle (CPA)/IAC mass lesions. Typically cause unilateral high-pitched tinnitus and progressive sensorineural hearing loss. Include tumors or tumor-like lesions (e.g., schwannomas, epidermoids, meningiomas, arachnoid cysts) and vascular lesions such as AICA aneurysms.
  2. Trauma (basal skull fracture with temporal bone involvement). Conductive hearing loss is classically associated with longitudinal fractures and sensorineural hearing loss with transverse fractures, but fractures are often complex and components of each may occur.
  3. Infection (e.g., suppurative labyrinthitis, meningitis, syphilis).
  4. Ototoxic drugs (e.g., aminoglycoside antibiotics).
  5. Inflammatory/autoimmune disease (e.g., Cogan syndrome, Wegener granulomatosis, polyarteritis nodosa, temporal arteritis, Buerger disease (thromboangiitis obliterans), systemic lupus erythomatosis).
  6. Cochlear hemorrhage.
  7. Noise-induced (prolonged exposure to loud noise causes hair cell loss).
  8. Congenital anomalies such as cochlear aplasia or dysplasia. *Michel aplasia* is characterized by complete inner ear (labyrinthine and cochlear) aplasia. A *Mondini malformation* refers to cochlear hypoplasia, with development of only 1½ of the normal 2½ turns of the cochlea. A Mondini malformation may be isolated or may be part of more widespread inner ear dysplasia.
  9. Aging (presbycusis). Most common overall cause of sensorineural hearing loss, age-related and mostly affects high frequencies.
- May be bilateral and progressive (e.g., presbycusis, ototoxic drugs), unilateral and progressive (e.g., Meniere disease, vestibular schwannoma), or unilateral and acute (e.g., cochlear infarction or hemorrhage, viral infection).
- Aging (presbycusis) and vestibular schwannomas typically cause high-pitched hearing loss and tinnitus.
  ○ Hearing tests
    - *Weber test.* Vibration over midline. Sensorineural loss: louder in normal ear. Conductive loss: louder in affected ear.
    - *Rinne test.* Air conduction (AC) versus bone conduction (BC). Normal: AC > BC (positive Rinne). Sensorineural loss: AC > BC. Conductive loss: BC > AC.
    - *Schwabach test.* Compare the examiner's bone conduction over mastoid with patient. If examiner's is better, sensorineural loss is suspected.
    - In sensorineural hearing loss, Weber lateralizes to normal ear, Rinne positive, Schwabach abnormal.
    - In conductive hearing loss, Weber lateralizes to affected ear, Rinne negative, Schwabach normal.
  ○ Tinnitus
    - Tinnitus is a perception of noise (often but not always described as "ringing") that appears to originate from the ear or head.
    - Any cochlear nerve lesion may be associated with tinnitus.
    - Tinnitus is more frequent with peripheral than central lesions.
    - *Low roaring tinnitus.* Associated with cochlear hydrops (tinnitus, aural fullness, and fluctuating hearing loss *without* vertigo, also sometimes called atypical Meniere disease).
    - *High-pitched tinnitus.* Associated with presbycusis, vestibular schwannoma.
    - *Pulsatile tinnitus.* May be caused by a vascular tumor such as glomus jugulare or the rare endolymphatic sac tumor, or a vascular lesion such as aneurysm, arteriovenous malformation (AVM), dural AV fistula, dural sinus stenosis, or persistent stapedial artery. May also be seen in patients with either intracranial hypertension (increased intracranial pressure) or spontaneous intracranial hypotension (SIH). Addition of vascular imaging (computed tomography angiography [CTA]; magnetic resonance angiography [MRA]/magnetic resonance venography [MRV]; possibly catheter angiography) to routine anatomical imaging is often useful in this setting.
    - *Gaze-evoked tinnitus.* May occur following removal of CPA tumors (thought to occur secondary to abnormal interaction between vestibular and cochlear nuclei).
    - Miscellaneous causes of tinnitus. Subjective, temporomandibular joint (TMJ) disease, Paget disease, labyrinthitis, brainstem lesions, drugs (e.g., aspirin, aminoglycosides, quinine), stenotic arterial disease, arterial dissection, high cardiac output, palatal myoclonus.

Vestibulocochlear Nerve: Pathologic Images

Case 8.1

Case 8.1 demonstrates congenital anomalies. Two patients present for evaluation of bilateral congenital deafness.

Patient 1 (Figs. 8.15, 8.16)

Diagnosis

Congenital cochlear dysplasia and CN VIII aplasia

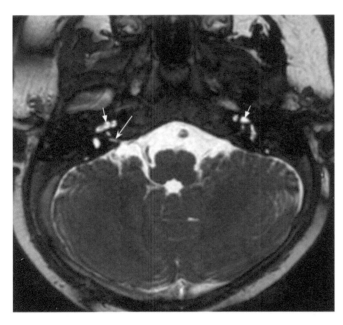

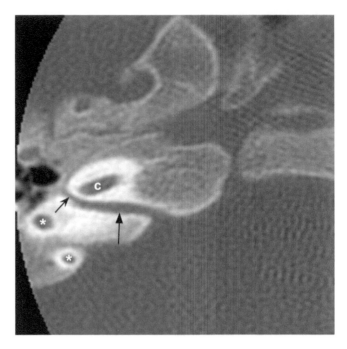

Fig. 8.16 A thin-section high-resolution axial CT image in bone window through the right internal auditory canal (IAC) in the same patient shows a diminutive right IAC. This patient has congenital aplasia of CN VIII, and only the facial nerve traverses the narrow IAC (*straight arrow*). Note the fallopian segment of the facial nerve canal (*concave arrow*) arising from the fundus of the IAC. (c, cochlea; *, anterior and posterior limbs of superior semicircular canal.)

Patient 2 (Figs. 8.17, 8.18, 8.19, 8.20, 8.21)

Diagnosis

Cochlear nerve deficiency associated with bilateral inner ear malformation

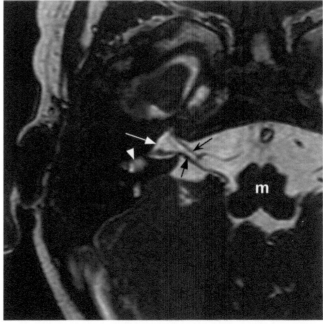

Fig. 8.15 An axial three-dimensional FIESTA high-resolution image through the posterior fossa at the level of the inner ear structures demonstrates marked hypoplasia of the internal auditory canals (thin linear hyperintensity on the right, *concave arrow*) and severe deformity of the bilateral cochleae (*straight arrows*).

Fig. 8.17 An axial three-dimensional FIESTA image through the posterior fossa at the level of the upper medulla (m) shows abnormal morphology of the right internal auditory canal (IAC) (*white straight arrow*) consistent with congenital deformity. The right vestibular nerve (*black straight arrow*) courses posteriorly toward a dysplastic vestibule (*arrowhead*). The right facial nerve (*black concave arrow*) is seen in the anterior aspect of the IAC.

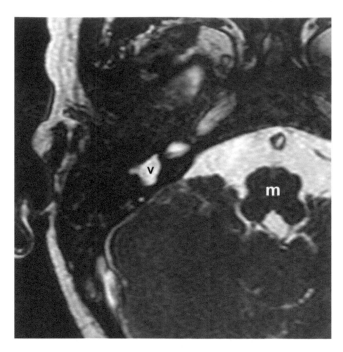

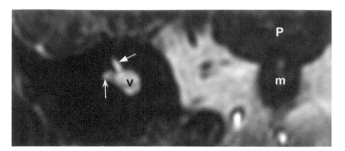

Fig. 8.19 A coronal three-dimensional FIESTA reformatted image in the same patient shows the bulbous deformity of the right vestibule (v) and blunting of the horizontal semicircular canal (*concave arrow*). The superior semicircular canal is also small and deviates laterally. (medulla; P, pons.)

Fig. 8.18 More inferiorly, an axial three-dimensional FIESTA image shows bulbous enlargement of the right vestibule (v). (m, medulla.)

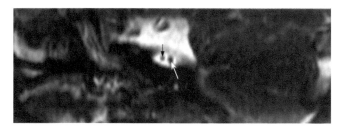

Fig. 8.20 A sagittal oblique three-dimensional an axial FIESTA image at the level of the porus acusticus (entrance to the internal auditory canal) demonstrates the facial nerve anteriorly (*straight arrow*) and CN VIII vestibular nerve posteriorly (*concave arrow*). No cochlear nerve is seen inferior to the facial nerve.

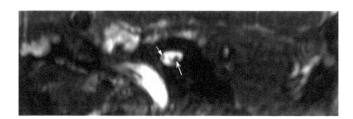

Fig. 8.21 More laterally, another sagittal oblique three-dimensional FIESTA image in the same patient shows the facial nerve anteriorly (*straight arrow*) and the vestibular nerve posteriorly (*concave arrow*) but still no visualization of the cochlear nerve in this patient with cochlear nerve aplasia.

Clinical Pearl

The term *cochlear nerve deficiency* refers to situations in which the nerve is either small or absent on magnetic resonance imaging (MRI). It occurs as a result of failure of the nerve to develop either partially (hypoplasia) or completely (aplasia or agenesis) or as a result of postdevelopmental degeneration. Cochlear nerve deficiency has been described in association with inner ear malformation, IAC stenosis, and occasionally in the presence of a normal IAC morphology. Profound hearing loss usually accompanies cochlear nerve agenesis. The status of the cochlear nerve should be addressed on all MRI scans performed prior to cochlear implantation.

Imaging Pearl

Hypoplasia or aplasia of the cochlear nerve may be associated with an abnormally small IAC on computed tomography (CT) imaging, but the IAC may also be normal in size. On MRI, however, the cochlear nerve can be directly assessed on thin-section heavily T2-weighted images. Oblique parasagittal reformations through the IAC normally demonstrate the facial nerve in its anterosuperior position, the cochlear nerve in its anteroinferior position, and the superior and inferior divisions of the vestibular nerve in the posterior aspect of the IAC. A small or absent cochlear nerve is best appreciated on these images, which may also show malformations of the cochlea, vestibule, and semicircular canals.

Case 8.2

A 72-year-old male presents with acute right-sided hearing loss as well as ataxia (**Figs. 8.22, 8.23**).

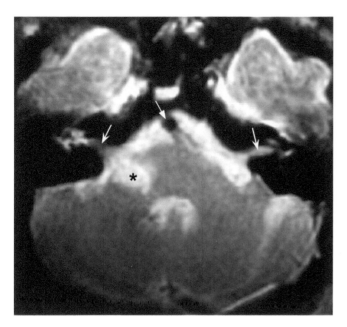

Fig. 8.22 An axial T2-weighted image through the posterior fossa at the level of the internal auditory canals (*concave arrows*) demonstrates focal intraparenchymal hyperintensity within the lateral aspect of the midpons and right middle cerebellar peduncle (*). Subtle bulging of the ventral margin of the peduncle is consistent with swelling in the setting of an acute process. This lesion involves the expected course of the right CN VIII pathway prior to its exiting the brainstem in this patient with acute onset hearing loss. The flow void of the basilar artery is seen (*straight arrow*) and is patent. Apparent low signal intensity in the right IAC is related to volume averaging.

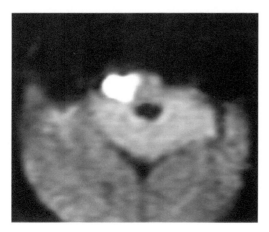

Fig. 8.23 An axial DWI at a similar level in the same patient shows marked hyperintensity of the right pontine/middle cerebellar peduncle lesion due to reduced diffusion in the setting of acute ischemia. This is consistent with an acute infarct in the right anterior inferior cerebellar artery (AICA) territory. It is unclear whether the hearing loss observed in this case related to the brain injury or, more likely, to occlusion of the labyrinthine artery, a branch of the AICA.

Diagnosis

AICA infarct with involvement of the labyrinthine artery

Clinical Pearl

The labyrinthine (internal auditory) artery arises from the AICA and supplies the inner ear. Clinically, sequelae of AICA infarction may mimic acute labyrinthitis, vestibular neuritis, or Meniere disease and may include vertigo, tinnitus, nystagmus, facial weakness, and/or ataxia. Sensorineural hearing loss can be present with other symptoms or an isolated finding and is usually due to dysfunction of the cochlea resulting from inner ear ischemia.

Imaging Pearl

Current imaging techniques are unable to detect ischemia/infarction of the inner ear. Diffusion-weighted imaging (DWI), however, may demonstrate acute ischemia in the brain parenchyma supplied by the AICA. The vascular territory of the AICA generally includes the ipsilateral middle cerebellar peduncle, anterior inferior cerebellum, and lateral pons. CTA or MRA may show AICA occlusion or stenosis.

Case 8.3

A 37-year-old female presents with a one-week history of acute left-sided hearing loss (**Figs. 8.24, 8.25**).

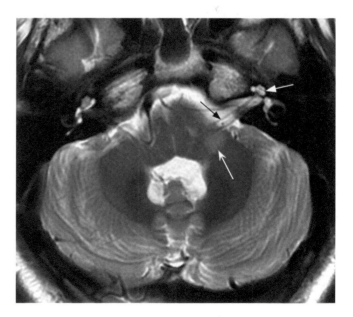

Fig. 8.24 An axial T2-weighted image through the posterior fossa at the level of the pontomedullary junction demonstrates a faint focus of high signal intensity (*white concave arrow*) within the left middle cerebellar peduncle, along the course of CN VIII. Left CN VIII nerve roots are seen entering the brainstem just anterior to this lesion. The left cochlear nerve (*black arrow*) is seen traversing the internal auditory canal (IAC) to enter the cochlea (*white straight arrow*).

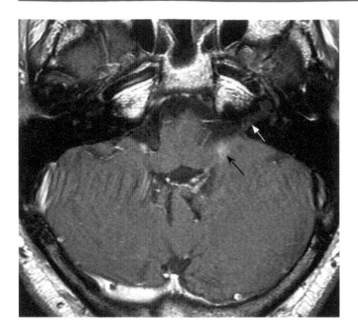

Fig. 8.25 An axial postcontrast T1-weighted image through a similar level shows ill-defined enhancement within the left middle cerebellar peduncle lesion (*black arrow*) at the CN VIII nerve root entry zone at the level of the left internal auditory canal (*white arrow*). In this patient with known underlying multiple sclerosis, these findings are characteristic of acute demyelination.

Diagnosis

Multiple sclerosis (MS). See Case 6.1, Chapter 6 for further discussion of MS.

Case 8.4

A 45-year-old male presents with bilateral sensorineural hearing loss and a remote history of ependymoma resection (**Fig. 8.26**).

Diagnosis

Superficial siderosis

Imaging Pearl

T2*-weighted (gradient echo, for example) imaging is the preferred MRI sequence to demonstrate a low signal intensity "rim" or "outline" along the surface of the cerebrum, brainstem, cerebellum, spinal cord, and CNs (notably CN I, II, and VIII). This finding is diagnostic of superficial siderosis.

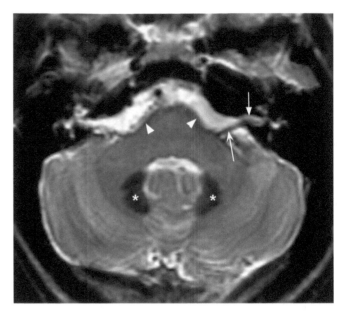

Fig. 8.26 An axial T2*-weighted image through the posterior fossa at the level of the midpons demonstrates a thin low signal intensity rim along the surfaces of the brainstem and cerebellum, best seen along the ventral brainstem (*arrowheads*) and left CN VIII (*concave arrow*) as it traverses the cerebellopontine angle and internal auditory canal (IAC) (*straight arrow*). This is consistent with susceptibility due to hemosiderin deposition in this patient with superficial siderosis. Note the dark signal within the cerebellar dentate nuclei (*); this is common in middle-aged and older patients and is typically due to iron deposition and/or calcification.

Clinical Pearl

Superficial siderosis is a condition in which hemosiderin is deposited in the leptomeninges, subpial tissues, and subependyma of the brain and spinal cord. It is caused by repeated or chronic subarachnoid hemorrhage. The conditions most commonly associated with superficial siderosis include central nervous system (CNS) vascular malformations, CNS tumors, and prior trauma, including traumatic nerve root avulsion. The classic clinical triad of superficial siderosis is bilateral sensorineural hearing loss, ataxia, and myelopathy; dementia may also ensue. Superficial siderosis only occurs where there is central myelin. CN VIII is prominently affected because in this nerve the transition from central to peripheral myelin (*Obersteiner-Redlich zone*) is 10–15 mm away from the root entry zone. The other CNs and spinal nerve roots have a very proximal transition from central to peripheral myelin. Treatment is directed at ablating or removing the source of bleeding.

Case 8.5

A 59-year-old male presents with right-sided sensorineural hearing loss (**Figs. 8.27, 8.28, 8.29**).

Diagnosis

Vestibular schwannoma

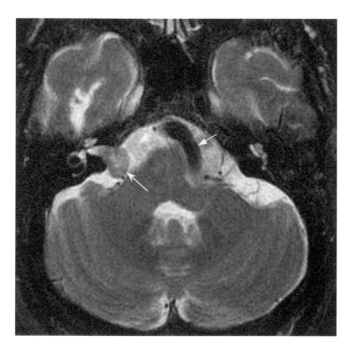

Fig. 8.27 An axial T2-weighted image with fat saturation through the posterior fossa demonstrates a slightly heterogeneous mass within the right cerebellopontine angle (*concave arrow*) that extends into the internal auditory canal (IAC). Though the contralateral side is not visible on the image for comparison, the right IAC is mildly expanded by the mass, and in particular the porus acusticus is widened. Dolichoectasia (dilatation and tortuosity) of the basilar artery (*straight arrow*) is incidentally noted; this is a common finding in older hypertensive individuals.

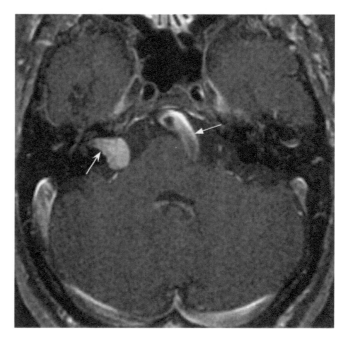

Fig. 8.28 An axial postcontrast T1-weighted image with fat saturation through a similar level shows intense homogeneous enhancement of the right internal auditory canal mass (*concave arrow*) that extends into the cerebellopontine angle. This appearance is consistent with a vestibular schwannoma. The dolichoectatic basilar artery (*straight arrow*) is again seen.

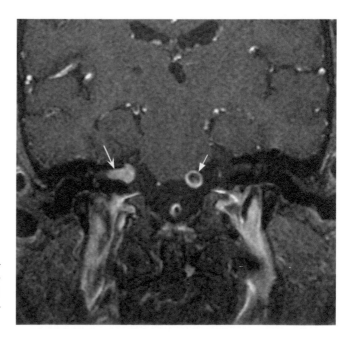

Fig. 8.29 A coronal postcontrast T1-weighted image with fat saturation through the posterior fossa in the same patient again shows the enhancing mass (*concave arrow*) within the right internal auditory canal (IAC) "dumbbelling" through the porus acusticus into the cerebellopontine angle. The basilar artery (*straight arrow*) is also seen.

Clinical Pearl

See Case 3.3, Chapter 3 for more details regarding epidemiology, clinical presentation, imaging, pathology, and treatment of schwannomas. Intracranially, the most common site of origin of schwannomas is the *superior vestibular nerve*. Hence, although these tumors have often been called "acoustic neuromas," the preferred term is *vestibular schwannoma*. Vestibular schwannomas are the most common CPA tumor. They usually present with unilateral high-pitched tinnitus and progressive sensorineural hearing loss, and less commonly with vertigo. Treatment includes observation, surgery, or radiosurgery. Surgical approaches include translabyrinthine, retrosigmoid, and middle fossa and differ by approach corridor and degree of hearing and facial nerve preservation.

Imaging Pearl

Vestibular schwannomas are centered on the IAC and typically have intermediate T1 and T2 signal; they enhance after contrast administration (see also **Table 8.1**). When the cisternal (CPA) portion is larger than the intracanalicular portion, then the tumor may present a classic "ice cream cone" appearance. Larger vestibular schwannomas are associated with bony expansion/remodeling of the IAC, and this can help differentiate them from other masses (e.g., meningiomas) that usually do not cause widening of the IAC. Large tumors often show cystic change and hemorrhage; they frequently abut the dura and may demonstrate a "dural tail" (a finding more often associated with meningioma). Optimal imaging of the IAC requires a dedicated protocol with thin-section images through the IAC, typically with high-resolution heavily T2-weighted sequences and fat-saturated postcontrast T1-weighted images. Bilateral vestibular schwannomas are diagnostic of neurofibromatosis type 2 (NF-2).

Table 8.1   Imaging Differential Diagnosis of CPA Masses

Lesion	Imaging Characteristics
Vestibular schwannoma	Enhancing mass centered in IAC with bony remodeling/expansion.
Meningioma	Dural tail; IAC extension less common
Epidermoid cyst	Cyst-like on most sequences but with marked DWI hyperintensity
Arachnoid cyst	Follows CSF on all sequences, including DWI; typically asymptomatic
Facial nerve schwannoma	Less common than vestibular schwannoma; look for extension into fallopian segment of facial nerve canal ("labyrinthine tail")

Case 8.6

Cases 8.6 through 8.12 are intended to demonstrate the spectrum of imaging appearances of vestibular schwannomas.

A 19-year-old male undergoing imaging assessment of juvenile angiofibroma had another lesion incidentally noted. The patient had no clinical complaint referable to his hearing (**Figs. 8.30, 8.31**).

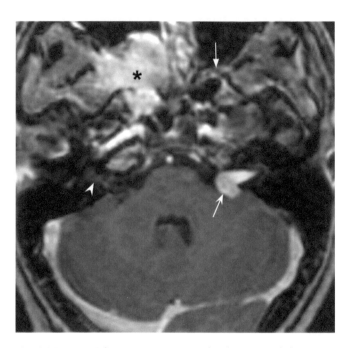

Fig. 8.30   An axial postcontrast T1-weighted image with fat saturation demonstrates a homogeneously enhancing mass within the left internal auditory canal (IAC) that "mushrooms" or "dumbbells" into the cerebellopontine angle (*concave arrow*), giving it the appearance of an ice cream cone. The left IAC is widened compared with the normal right side (*arrowhead*). Note the intensely enhancing mass (***) centered at the right posterolateral nasal cavity that extends into the pterygopalatine fossa, sphenoid sinus, and skull base, representing the patient's juvenile angiofibroma. The left pterygopalatine fossa (*straight arrow*) is normal.

Diagnosis

Vestibular schwannoma

Case 8.7

A 50-year-old male presents with 2 months of hearing decline, as well as a slight feeling of being off balance (**Figs. 8.32, 8.33, 8.34**).

Diagnosis

Vestibular schwannoma

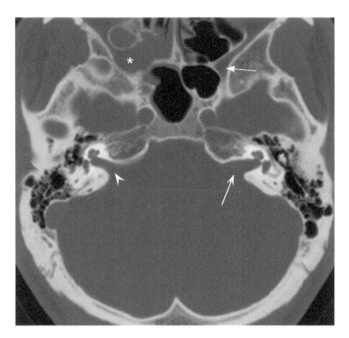

Fig. 8.31 An axial CT image in bone window through a similar level demonstrates smooth bony remodeling of the widened left internal auditory canal (*concave arrow*) when compared with the normal right side (*arrowhead*), due to the underlying vestibular schwannoma. There is also expansion of the right pterygopalatine fossa (*) and abnormal soft tissue in the right posterolateral nasal cavity, consistent with the juvenile angiofibroma. The upper aspect of the left pterygopalatine fossa (*straight arrow*) at the level of the inferior orbital fissure and foramen rotundum is normal. The vestibular schwannoma was an incidental finding in this patient who was being imaged for preoperative assessment of his juvenile angiofibroma.

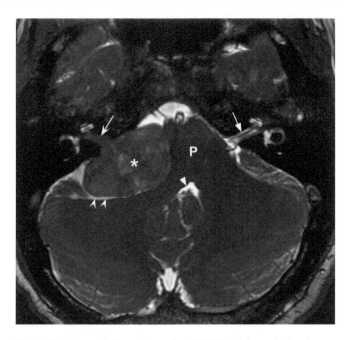

Fig. 8.32 An axial three-dimensional FIESTA high-resolution image through the posterior fossa at the level of the internal auditory canals demonstrates a fairly homogeneous extraaxial mass (*) centered in the right cerebellopontine angle (CPA) with mass effect upon the pons (P) and middle cerebellar peduncle and with shift of the fourth ventricle (*straight arrowhead*) to the left. The mass extends into the right IAC (*concave arrow*) but does not widen it, a feature which is atypical for a large vestibular schwannoma. Note the thin cleft of CSF signal along the posterolateral margin of the mass (*concave arrowheads*), clearly separating it from the cerebellum and confirming its extraaxial nature.

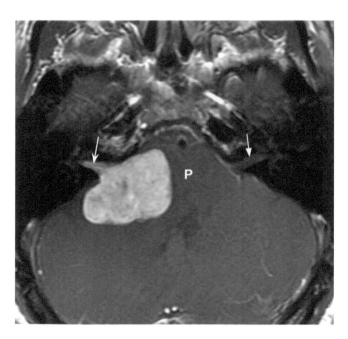

Fig. 8.33 An axial postcontrast T1-weighted image at a similar level shows relatively homogeneous and intense enhancement of the right cerebellopontine angle mass, which extends into the internal auditory canal (IAC) (*concave arrow*). Though the IAC is not much widened in this patient with a vestibular schwannoma, the porus acusticus is clearly seen to be eroded and widened on this image. The normal left IAC is indicated for comparison (*white straight arrow*).

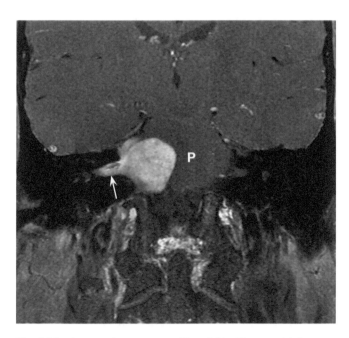

Fig. 8.34 A coronal postcontrast T1-weighted image with fat saturation through the level of the pons (P) in the same patient again depicts the large right cerebellopontine angle mass with extension into the internal auditory canal (*arrow*) and mass effect on the pons. No dural tail is present, and the cerebellopontine angle component of the mass is round and lobulated, rather than having the semicircular or half-moon appearance typical of meningioma.

Case 8.8

A 55-year-old male presents with headaches for one month and progressive loss of balance and coordination. He also notes that his hearing on the left has been reduced for some time (**Fig. 8.35**).

Diagnosis

Vestibular schwannoma

Case 8.9

A 48-year-old male with decreased hearing on the right presents with sudden onset headache and dizziness (**Fig. 8.36**).

Diagnosis

Vestibular schwannoma with hemorrhage

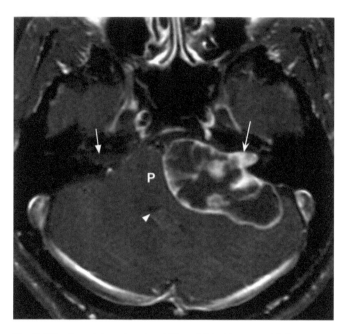

Fig. 8.35 An axial postcontrast T1-weighted image with fat saturation through the posterior fossa at the level of the internal auditory canals (IAC) shows a large heterogeneously enhancing extraaxial mass centered in the left cerebellopontine angle (CPA). The areas of nonenhancement within the mass are consistent with areas of cystic degeneration within this large vestibular schwannoma. The mass extends into and widens the left IAC (*concave arrow*). There is significant mass effect on the pons (P), middle cerebellar peduncle, and cerebellum. Additionally, the fourth ventricle (*arrowhead*) is compressed and shifted to the right. Note the normal right IAC (*straight arrow*).

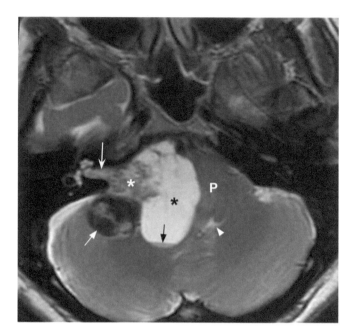

Fig. 8.36 An axial T2-weighted image through the posterior fossa demonstrates a large complex right cerebellopontine angle mass that extends into the internal auditory canal (IAC) (*white concave arrow*). Mixed signal intensity within the mass is due to both solid (*white asterisk*) and cystic (*black asterisk*) components. The mass-like region of darker signal posterolaterally is consistent with focal hemorrhage (*white straight arrow*). A fluid level (*black straight arrow*) is noted layering dependently in the large cyst, consistent with prior hemorrhage into the cyst. Marked mass effect is seen upon the pons (P) and fourth ventricle (*arrowhead*). At surgery this was a complex cystic and solid vestibular schwannoma with areas of internal hemorrhage.

Case 8.10

Two patients present with right-sided sensorineural hearing loss and tinnitus.

Patient 1 (Figs. 8.37, 8.38)

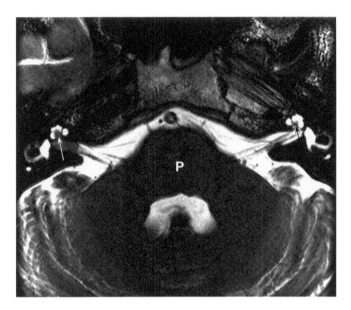

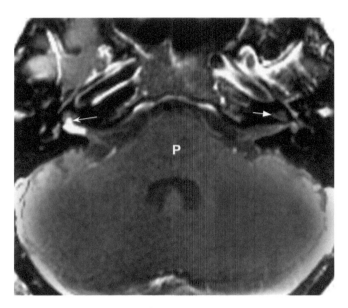

Fig. 8.37 An axial three-dimensional FIESTA high-resolution image through the posterior fossa at the level of the midpons (P) and internal auditory canals demonstrates a homogeneous mass within the right IAC that extends beyond the fundus of the IAC into the cochlea (*white arrow*). This represents intracochlear extension of tumor. The left cochlea shows the expected appearance of a normal modiolus (*black arrow*).

Fig. 8.38 An axial postcontrast T1-weighted image with fat saturation at a similar level shows an intensely enhancing mass within the right internal auditory canal and confirms the intracochlear transmodiolar extension (*white concave arrow*). Note the normal left cochlea for comparison (*white straight arrow*). (P, pons.)

Patient 2 (Figs. 8.39, 8.40)

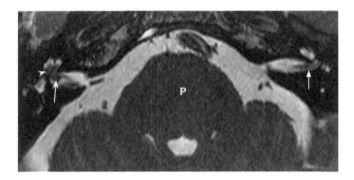

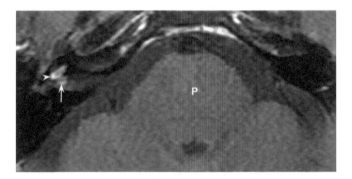

Fig. 8.39 An axial three-dimensional FIESTA high-resolution image in a different patient through the pons (P) and internal auditory canals demonstrates asymmetric soft tissue within the fundus of the right IAC (*white concave arrow*), which extends into the basal turn and central aspect of the right cochlea (*arrowhead*). Normal nerve roots are present within the left IAC (*white straight arrow*), and the left cochlea has normal signal intensity.

Fig. 8.40 An axial postcontrast T1-weighted image with fat saturation through a similar level shows enhancement within the fundus of the right internal auditory canal (IAC) (*arrow*) extending into the cochlea (*arrowhead*), consistent with a vestibular schwannoma with intracochlear transmodiolar extension. (P, pons.)

Diagnosis

Vestibular schwannoma with intracochlear (transmodiolar) extension

Clinical Pearl

Eighth nerve and facial schwannomas of the IAC that extend to the fundus of the IAC may leave the confines of the IAC and extend into inner ear structures. This results in a lesion with a "dumbbell" morphology. It is important to differentiate these lesions from simple intracanalicular schwannomas, as surgical approaches and prognostic implications are distinct.

Imaging Pearl

Dumbbell schwannomas of the eighth nerve may be transmodiolar (extending into the cochlea), transmacular (extending into the vestibule), and combined transmodiolar/transmacular types. Dumbbell schwannomas of the facial nerve extend along the labyrinthine segment of the facial nerve, often to the level of the geniculate ganglion. High-resolution T2-weighted MRI and thin-section postcontrast T1-weighted images with fat saturation are necessary to evaluate the full extent of these lesions.

Case 8.11

Two different patients present with progressive hearing loss and vertigo.

Patient 1 (Figs. 8.41, 8.42)

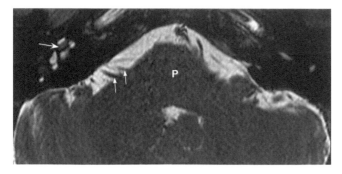

Fig. 8.41   An axial three-dimensional FIESTA high-resolution image through the posterior fossa at the level of the pons (P) demonstrates abnormal soft tissue within the middle turn of the right cochlea (*white concave arrow*), suggesting the possibility of an intracochlear mass. Note the proximal portions of CNs VII and VIII (*white straight arrows*) as they traverse the right cerebellopontine angle.

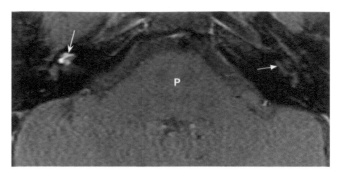

Fig. 8.42   An axial postcontrast T1-weighted image at a slightly different angle and level shows abnormal enhancement involving the middle and apical turns of the right cochlea (*white concave arrow*), compatible with an intracochlear schwannoma. The normal left cochlea does not enhance (*white straight arrow*). Although an inflammatory labyrinthitis could be considered in the differential diagnosis of this lesion, the mass-like appearance on the T2-weighted image makes neoplasm far more likely. When there is a dilemma regarding neoplasm versus inflammation, then a follow-up MRI can be useful because a mass should remain stable or enlarge, whereas an inflammatory process would be expected to improve over time. (P, pons.)

Patient 2 (Figs. 8.43, 8.44)

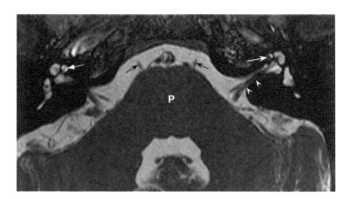

Fig. 8.43   An axial three-dimensional FIESTA high-resolution image through the posterior fossa at the level of the pons (P) demonstrates abnormal soft tissue signal intensity within the scala tympani of the basal turn of the left cochlea (*white concave arrow*), which replaces the normal fluid signal intensity. The right cochlea is normal (*white straight arrow* on scala tympani). CNs VII and VIII (*arrowheads*) are noted within the left internal auditory canal (IAC). Bilateral CN VI nerves are also seen traversing the prepontine cistern (*black arrows*).

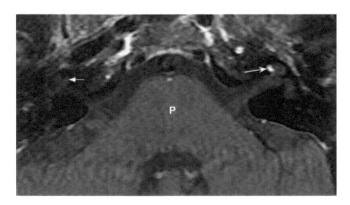

Fig. 8.44 An axial postcontrast T1-weighted image with fat saturation through a similar level confirms an intensely enhancing mass in the scala tympani of the basal turn of the left cochlea (*concave arrow*) consistent with an intracochlear schwannoma. Normal right cochlea is again shown for comparison (*straight arrow*). (P, pons.)

Diagnosis

Intralabyrinthine schwannoma (specifically intracochlear)

Clinical Pearl
Intralabyrinthine schwannomas arise from the intralabyrinthine branches of the vestibulocochlear nerve and at least initially have no component in the IAC. These lesions typically present with hearing loss and/or vertigo. Tumor growth tends to be slow but can result in progressive hearing loss and/or intractable tinnitus.

Imaging Pearl
Intralabyrinthine schwannomas can be identified on heavily T2-weighted, thin-section imaging studies as focal mass lesions that are in low signal intensity compared with the bright fluid that is normally present in the cochlea, vestibule, and semicircular canals. These lesions enhance post-gadolinium and can extend extensively within the confines of the bony labyrinth. These lesions can sometimes be difficult to distinguish from labyrinthitis, and serial imaging follow-up can be helpful to assess for progression over time.

Case 8.12

Patient 1

A 71-year-old male with long-standing right-sided sensorineural hearing loss presents with more recent left-sided sensorineural hearing loss (**Fig. 8.45**).

Diagnosis

Bilateral vestibular schwannomas, diagnostic of NF-2. Please see Case 5.6, Chapter 5 for a full discussion of NF-2.

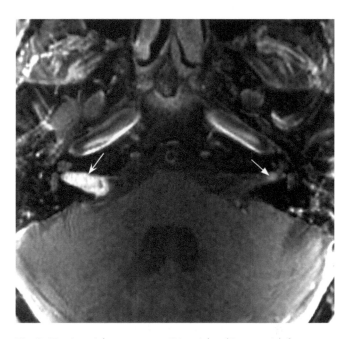

Fig. 8.45 An axial postcontrast T1-weighted image with fat saturation at the level of the pons demonstrates an intensely enhancing mass (*concave arrow*) within an expanded right internal canal (IAC) that extends from the fundus to the porus acusticus and bulges slightly into the cerebellopontine angle (CPA). A much more subtle enhancing lesion (*straight arrow*) is also present at the fundus of the left IAC. These are consistent with bilateral vestibular schwannomas in the setting of neurofibromatosis type 2 (NF-2).

Patient 2

A 48-year-old female presents with bilateral sensorineural hearing loss (**Fig. 8.46**).

Diagnosis

Bilateral vestibular schwannomas in the setting of NF-2. Intracochlear extension on the left.

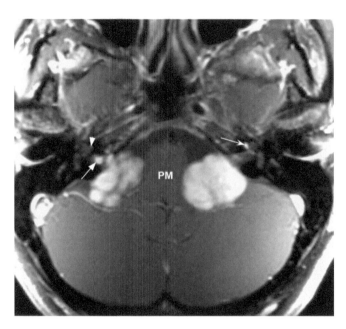

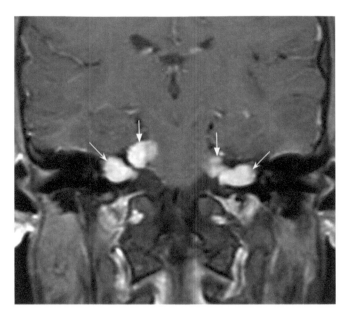

Fig. 8.47 A coronal postcontrast T1-weighted image in another patient with NF-2 demonstrates bilateral vestibular schwannomas (*concave arrows*). Additional CN V schwannomas are seen bilaterally, with the right larger than the left (*straight arrows*).

Diagnosis

CPA meningioma

Fig. 8.46 An axial postcontrast T1-weighted image in a different patient at the level of the pontomedullary junction (PM) and the internal auditory canals (IACs) demonstrates enhancing bilateral cerebellopontine angle masses. Extension into the IAC is well seen on the right (*straight arrow*). In addition, a small enhancing nodule is noted within the basal turn of the left cochlea (*concave arrow*) when compared with the right cochlea (*arrowhead*), consistent with intracochlear extension of vestibular schwannomas in this patient with known neurofibromatosis type 2 (NF-2).

Patient 3

A 32-year-old female presents with bilateral sensorineural hearing loss. She has no other CN symptoms (**Fig. 8.47**).

Diagnosis

Bilateral vestibular schwannomas with multiple additional schwannomas in the setting of NF-2.

Case 8.13

Patient 1

A 72-year-old female presents with sensorineural hearing loss (**Fig. 8.48**).

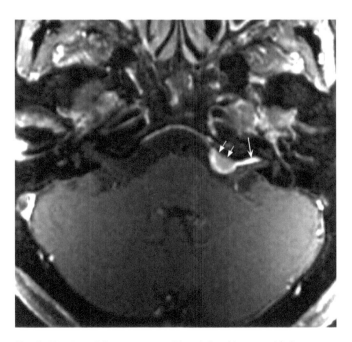

Fig. 8.48 An axial postcontrast T1-weighted image with fat saturation demonstrates a left cerebellopontine angle extraaxial mass. The mass, centered anteromedial to the left internal auditory canal, has a "half moon" shape and a broad dural base (*straight arrows*). Thin linear enhancement (*concave arrow*) along the anterior wall of the left IAC represents a "dural tail." The presence of a dural tail is characteristic of, though not pathognomonic for, meningioma.

CPA meningiomas may grow to a large size before causing symptoms related to brainstem and cerebellar compression and/or hydrocephalus. Growth in the CPA may lead to palsies of CNs VII and VIII, especially if the meningioma grows into the IAC. Inferior extension, notably into the jugular foramen, may lead to palsies of CNs IX and X. Superior extension may result in palsy of CN V and other upper CNs.

Patient 2

A 53-year-old female presents with progressive left-sided hearing loss, left facial palsy, and vestibular dysfunction (**Figs. 8.49, 8.50, 8.51**).

Diagnosis

CPA meningioma

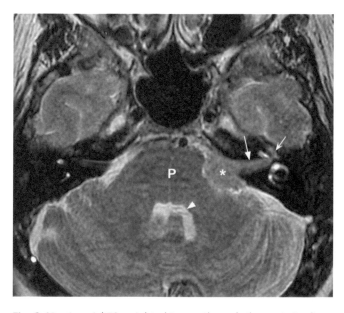

Fig. 8.49 An axial T2-weighted image through the posterior fossa demonstrates an intermediate signal intensity soft tissue mass (*) centered within the left cerebellopontine angle with minimal mass effect upon the adjacent pons (P) and fourth ventricle (*arrowhead*). The mass extends into the left internal auditory canal (*straight arrow*), which may be slightly widened compared with the opposite side. There is a suggestion of subtle intermediate soft tissue signal within the left cochlea and extending along the horizontal (tympanic) segment of the left facial nerve canal (*concave arrow*).

On occasion the CPA meningioma may truly mimic a vestibular schwannoma, but more typically the CPA meningioma has a broad base against the dural surface and a characteristic dural tail. Meningiomas are typically isointense to brain on noncontrast CT images and T1- and T2-weighted MRI, and they enhance intensely and homogeneously postcontrast. Meningiomas of the CPA may extend into the IAC, but they generally do not widen the IAC or erode the porus acusticus. Meningiomas of the CPA may be large and may be associated with brain compression and edema, calcification, and cysts. See **Table 8.1**.

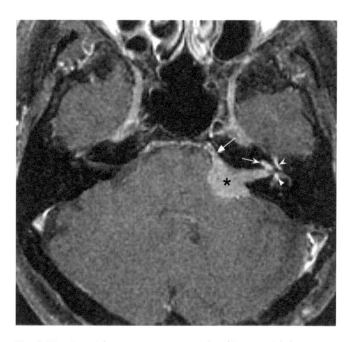

Fig. 8.50 An axial postcontrast T1-weighted image with fat saturation in the same patient at a similar level shows a homogeneously enhancing left cerebellopontine angle mass (*) that extends into the internal auditory canal (IAC). Linear enhancement extending anteriorly is consistent with a dural tail (*straight arrow*). Abnormal enhancement is noted within the basal turn of the left cochlea (*concave arrow*) and within the vestibule (*concave arrowhead*), consistent with inner ear involvement. Additional extension is noted along the horizontal (tympanic) segment of the facial nerve canal (*straight arrowhead*).

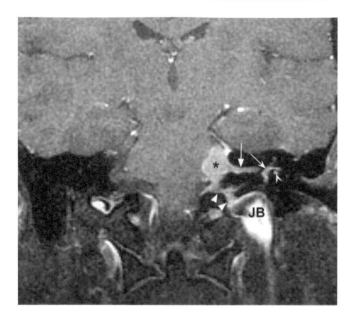

Fig. 8.51 A coronal postcontrast T1-weighted image with fat saturation in the same patient as in **Figs. 8.49** and **8.50** again shows the left cerebellopontine angle mass (*) extending into what appears here to be a nonenlarged internal auditory canal (*straight arrow*). Abnormal inner ear enhancement is noted with the vestibule (*concave arrow*) and semicircular canals. Additional enhancement is seen along the horizontal (tympanic) segment of the facial nerve canal (*concave arrowhead*). There is also extension inferolaterally into the left jugular foramen (pars nervosa, *straight arrowheads*). Heterogeneous signal related to turbulent flow is noted in the adjacent jugular bulb (JB). The findings are consistent with an unusual skull base meningioma that has extended into the inner ear.

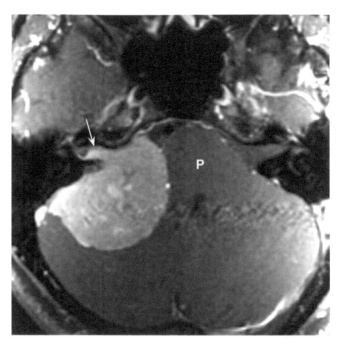

Fig. 8.52 An axial postcontrast T1-weighted image with fat saturation through the posterior fossa at the level of the internal auditory canals (IACs) demonstrates a large enhancing extraaxial mass in the right cerebellopontine angle with mass effect upon the pons (P), middle cerebellar peduncle, and cerebellum. The mass has a broad dural base and extends into the adjacent IAC (*arrow*), but the IAC is not expanded. The imaging features of this mass are typical of a meningioma.

Patient 3

A 42-year-old female presents with right-sided hearing loss (**Figs. 8.52, 8.53**).

Diagnosis

CPA meningioma

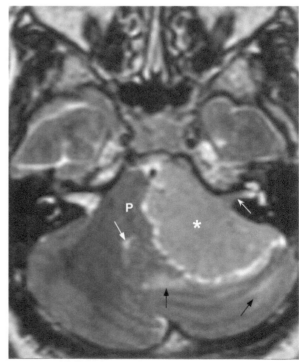

Fig. 8.53 An axial T2-weighted image in a different patient with the same diagnosis as **Fig. 8.52** (meningioma) shows a large left cerebellopontine angle mass (*) with mass effect upon the pons (P) and adjacent structures. The fourth ventricle is compressed and shifted to the right (*white straight arrow*). The mass is quite homogeneous and similar in signal intensity to gray matter. Although the mass is extraaxial, mild parenchymal edema is seen as patchy areas of hyperintensity within the left cerebellum (*black arrows*). Extension of the mass into a nonexpanded left IAC is noted (*white concave arrow*).

Patient 4

A 60-year-old female presents with bilateral progressive hearing loss, as well as headache and ataxia (**Fig. 8.54**).

Diagnosis

Bilateral CPA meningiomas

Case 8.14

A 45-year-old female with a known underlying diagnosis presents with progressive left-sided hearing loss and facial palsy (**Figs. 8.55, 8.56, 8.57, 8.58**).

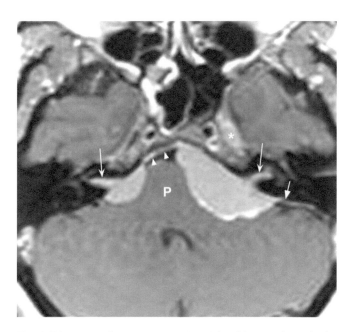

Fig. 8.54 An axial postcontrast T1-weighted image through the posterior fossa and internal auditory canals (IACs) demonstrates bilateral homogeneously enhancing cerebellopontine angle (CPA) masses with mass effect and compression of the pons (P). Extension is noted into both IACs (*concave arrows*), which are not expanded. Both masses have a broad dural base. Thin linear enhancement posterolateral to the left-sided mass (*straight arrow*) is consistent with a dural tail. Also note enhancement within the left Meckel cave (*) consistent with extension of the left-sided mass. Additional thin linear enhancement anteromedial (*arrowheads*) to the masses behind the clivus likely represents a dural tail as well, though this could also represent a normal retroclival venous plexus. Bilateral CPA/IAC meningiomas are very uncommon, though multiple meningiomas in general are not uncommon and often occur in association with NF-2.

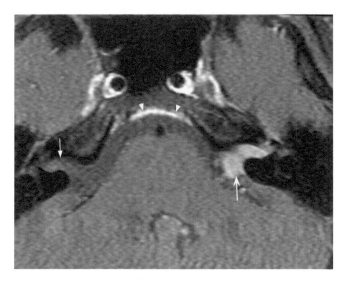

Fig. 8.55 An axial postcontrast T1-weighted image with fat-saturation through the posterior fossa demonstrates a homogeneously enhancing mass within the left internal auditory canal (IAC) that bulges slightly into the cerebellopontine angle (*concave arrow*). There is slight widening of the porus acusticus but no definite expansion of the left IAC. In addition, no enhancing dural tail is seen. The right IAC (*straight arrow*) is normal. Thin retroclival enhancement is due to the normal retroclival venous plexus (*arrowheads*).

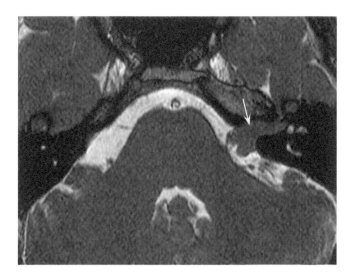

Fig. 8.56 An axial three-dimensional FIESTA high-resolution image at a similar level shows a homogeneous soft tissue mass (*concave arrow*) filling the left internal auditory canal (IAC). It protrudes into the cerebellopontine angle and has a lobulated medial margin. The imaging characteristics are nonspecific and a differential diagnosis at this point would include vestibular schwannoma and meningioma as well as other masses.

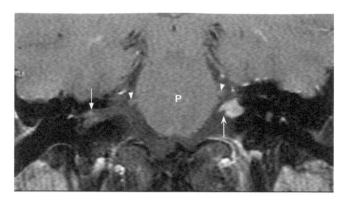

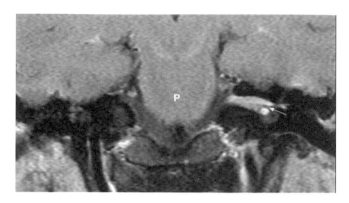

Fig. 8.57 A coronal postcontrast T1-weighted image with fat saturation at the level of the pons (P) in the same patient shows the left cerebellopontine angle component of the mass (*concave arrow*). The lobulated irregular medial margin is atypical for vestibular schwannoma, whereas the lack of a dural tail is atypical for meningioma. The right internal auditory canal (*straight arrow*) and cerebellopontine angle are normal. Normal trigeminal nerves (CNs V) are seen bilaterally (*arrowheads*).

Fig. 8.58 More anteriorly, another coronal postcontrast T1-weighted image with fat saturation shows the internal auditory canal (IAC) component of the mass, which extends to the fundus. Enhancement is noted above and below the crista falciformis (*straight arrow*), as if the lesion is tracking along nerves; this is different from the round or ovoid homogeneous mass that is typical of eighth nerve schwannoma. This patient had known lymphoma, and this mass resolved following chemotherapy. Lymphoma is an uncommon cause of an enhancing IAC/CPA mass as compared with vestibular schwannoma and meningioma.

Diagnosis

Lymphoma involving the IAC

Clinical Pearl

Lymphoma originating in the IAC may present with hearing loss, tinnitus, and/or vertigo. It is clinically indistinguishable from other more common tumors of the same region such as vestibular schwannoma, though the symptoms may progress more rapidly. Lymphoma of the IAC may present as a primary extranodal mass, or may occur in the context of diffuse leptomeningeal involvement by lymphoma; in the latter case, the involvement is usually bilateral and accompanied by more diffuse leptomeningeal enhancement over the surface of the brain and spinal cord.

Imaging Pearl

Lymphomatous masses are typically isointense to brain on T1-weighted images and enhance homogeneously postcontrast. They are intermediate in T2 signal intensity due to their high cellularity, and may also show mildly reduced diffusion due to their high nuclear-to-cytoplasmic ratio. They may be associated with additional sites of CN or leptomeningeal involvement. A solitary mass in the IAC or CPA can be difficult to distinguish from other more common lesions of these regions, but the lymphomatous mass is often more irregularly marginated, tracks along CNs, and may be associated as mentioned above with additional sites of CN or meningeal involvement.

Case 8.15

Patient 1

A 38-year-old female presents with left-sided hearing loss (**Figs. 8.59, 8.60, 8.61**).

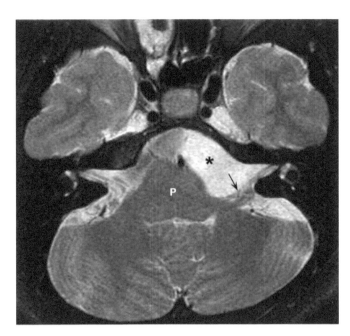

Fig. 8.59 An axial T2-weighted image through the posterior fossa demonstrates asymmetric widening of the left cerebellopontine angle (CPA) (*). There is homogeneous hyperintense signal in the left CPA, whereas relatively low signal intensity in the right CPA cistern and prepontine cistern is consistent with dephasing and signal loss due to CSF flow. Minimal mass effect is noted upon the pons (P) which is shifted slightly to the right. Additional evidence of mass effect is seen as the traversing left CNs VII and VIII (*concave arrow*) are displaced posteriorly prior to entering the left internal auditory canal.

Diagnosis

Epidermoid cyst

Epidermoid Cyst

- *Epidemiology.* Accounts for ~1% of primary brain tumors. Peak age is 30–50 years, no gender predominance. The most common intracranial location is the CPA, and it is the third most common CPA lesion after vestibular schwannoma and meningioma.
- *Clinical presentation.* Most commonly presents as a skull base lesion with progressive cranial neuropathies ± hydrocephalus. Cyst rupture may be associated with recurring aseptic meningitis in some patients.
- *Imaging.* Nonenhancing mass lesion that may be lobulated or scalloped with mass effect upon adjacent structures. CT shows well-defined, hypodense, lobulated mass with CSF density. Calcification is uncommon. On T1- and

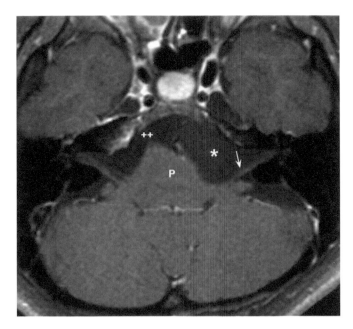

Fig. 8.60 An axial postcontrast T1-weighted image with fat saturation at a similar level again shows widening of the cerebellopontine angle (CPA) and mild mass effect upon the pons (P) and traversing left CNs VII and VIII (*concave arrow*). No enhancing mass is seen. Note, however, subtle increased signal intensity within the left CPA (*) when compared with the normal hypointensity of CSF (++) in the right prepontine cistern. These imaging characteristics are consistent with either an arachnoid or epidermoid cyst.

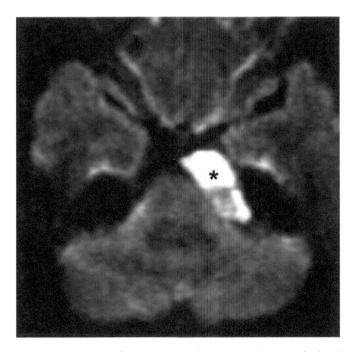

Fig. 8.61 An axial diffusion-weighted image (DWI) at a similar level in the same patient shows very high signal intensity within the left cerebellopontine angle mass (*). This finding is characteristic of an epidermoid cyst. An arachnoid cyst is isointense to CSF on DWI and would have low signal intensity.

9 Glossopharyngeal Nerve

Functions

- Special visceral efferent (SVE). Branchial motor to stylopharyngeus muscle.
- General visceral efferent (GVE). Visceral motor (parasympathetic) to the parotid gland (via lesser superficial petrosal nerve, LSPN).
- General sensory afferent (GSA). Somatic sensory from posterior external ear, tragus, posterior one third of the tongue, soft palate, nasopharynx, tympanic membrane, eustachian tube, and mastoid region.
- Visceral afferent (VA). Visceral sensory from carotid body (O_2, CO_2 chemoreceptors) and carotid sinus (baroreceptors).
- Special afferent (SA). Special sensory for taste from posterior one third of tongue.

Anatomy

- The glossopharyngeal nerve leaves the medulla between the olive ventrally and the inferior cerebellar peduncle dorsally (postolivary sulcus) as the most rostral three to five of the group of rootlets that will form cranial nerve (CN) IX, X, and the cranial root of XI (**Figs. 9.1, 9.2, 9.3**). In its short (~15 mm) subarachnoid course, it traverses the cerebellomedullary cistern. The nerve sends off a tympanic branch (*tympanic nerve* or *Jacobson nerve*) to the middle ear before exiting the skull through the jugular foramen. In the jugular foramen, it lies anterior (in the *pars nervosa*) to CNs X and XI (which lie posterior in the *pars vascularis*). The superior and inferior (*petrosal*) glossopharyngeal ganglia are located in the jugular foramen. The nerve exits the jugular foramen posteromedial to the styloid process, then descends lateral to the pharynx between the internal carotid artery (ICA) and IJV (internal jugular vein) in the carotid space. It supplies the stylopharyngeus muscle and then penetrates the pharyngeal constrictor muscles (above the level of the middle constrictor) to reach the posterior aspect of the tongue.

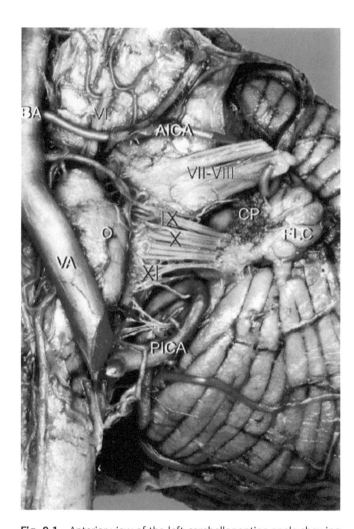

Fig. 9.1 Anterior view of the left cerebellopontine angle showing the origin of CN IX at the postolivary sulcus of the medulla. (AICA, anterior inferior cerebellar artery; BA, basilar artery; CP, choroid plexus; FLC, flocculus; PICA, posterior inferior cerebellar artery; O, olive; Roman numerals, cranial nerves; [VA], vertebral artery.) (From Ozveren MF, Ture U, Ozek MM, et al. Anatomic landmarks of the glossopharyngeal nerve: a microsurgical anatomic study. Neurosurgery 2003;52:1400-1410. Reprinted with permission.)

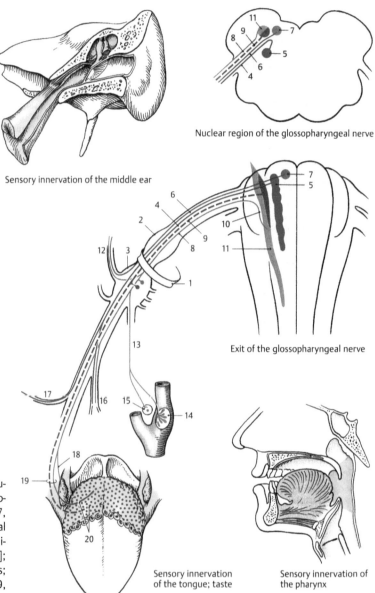

Fig. 9.2 Glossopharyngeal nerve. (1, jugular foramen; 2, superior ganglion; 3, inferior [petrosal] ganglion; 4, branchial motor fibers; 5, nucleus ambiguus; 6; parasympathetic fibers; 7, inferior salivatory nucleus; 8, visceral sensory fibers; 9, special sensory fibers [taste]; 10, tractus solitarius; 11, nucleus solitarius; 12, tympanic nerve; 13, carotid sinus nerve [of Hering]; 14, carotid sinus; 15, carotid body; 16, pharyngeal branches; 17, nerve to stylopharyngeus muscle; 18, tonsillar branches; 19, lingual branches; 20, taste fibers.)

Nuclear region of the glossopharyngeal nerve

Sensory innervation of the middle ear

Exit of the glossopharyngeal nerve

Sensory innervation of the tongue; taste

Sensory innervation of the pharynx

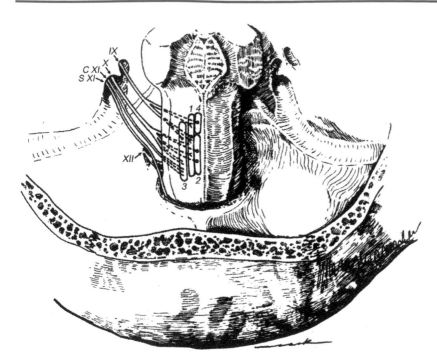

Fig. 9.3 Origin and cisternal courses of glossopharyngeal, vagus, spinal accessory, and hypoglossal nerves. Note that the glossopharyngeal nerve is made up of three to five rootlets (only two shown on this schematic). The glossopharyngeal nerve passes through the more anterior part of the jugular foramen (*pars nervosa*), whereas the vagus and spinal accessory nerves pass through the posterior part (*pars vascularis*). The hypoglossal nerve passes through the more inferiorly located hypoglossal canal. (1, nucleus solitarius; 2, dorsal motor nucleus of X; 3, nucleus ambiguus; 4, superior salivatory nucleus; C XI, cranial root of CN XI; S XI, spinal root of CN XI.) (From Harnsberger HR. Handbook of Head and Neck Imaging (2nd ed.) St. Louis, MO: Mosby, 1995. Reprinted with permission.)

Distinct Branches of the Glossopharyngeal Nerve (Fig. 9.4)

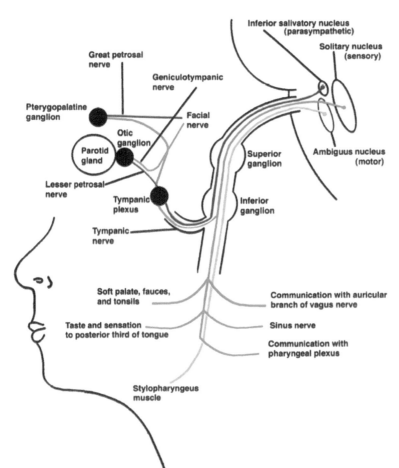

Fig. 9.4 Schematic drawing demonstrating the portions and branches of the glossopharyngeal nerve. (From Ozveren MF, Ture U, Ozek MM, et al. Anatomic landmarks of the glossopharyngeal nerve: a microsurgical anatomic study. Neurosurgery 2003;52:1400-1410. Reprinted with permission.)

- Tympanic nerve (*Jacobson's nerve*) (parasympathetic + sensory). Parasympathetic innervation of parotid gland and sensory information from tympanic membrane and eustachian tube. The tympanic nerve arises from the inferior ganglion within the jugular foramen and reaches the tympanic cavity through a small canal (inferior tympanic canaliculus) on the undersurface of the petrous temporal bone. There it divides into branches that, together with the superior and inferior caroticotympanic nerves (from the ICA sympathetic plexus), create the *tympanic plexus*. The tympanic plexus in turn gives off (1) the LSPN; (2) a branch to join the greater superficial petrosal nerve (GSPN); and (3) sensory branches to the mucous membranes of the tympanic cavity, mastoid air cells and eustachian tube.
- Motor branch to stylopharyngeus muscle.
- Carotid sinus nerve (*Hering's nerve*). To carotid sinus and carotid body (visceral sensory).
- Pharyngeal branches. To oro- and nasopharynx.
- Tonsillar branches. To palatine tonsil and soft palate.
- Lingual branch. To posterior one third of the tongue (sensory and taste).

Functional Pathways of the Glossopharyngeal Nerve

- The glossopharyngeal nerve is complex, supporting five separate functions with a complex anatomical course. It is helpful to think of each pathway and its associated anatomy separately as detailed here.
- *SVE (branchial motor) pathway.* The rostral portion of the *nucleus ambiguus* (in medulla) innervates the stylopharyngeus muscle and part of the superior pharyngeal constrictor.
- *GVE (visceral motor) pathway.* Parasympathetic preganglionic fibers from the *inferior salivatory nucleus* in the rostral medulla travel with CN IX and join the tympanic nerve to enter the tympanic plexus (no synapse here), from which the LSPN arises. The LSPN reenters the cranium through a small canal in the petrous temporal bone lateral to the canal for the GSPN, then travels back out through the foramen ovale to synapse in the *otic ganglion* (below the foramen ovale). Postganglionic fibers then travel with the auriculotemporal nerve (branch of CN V_3) to the parotid gland to cause salivation and vasodilation.
- *GSA (somatic sensory) pathways.* Sensation from the back of the ear, tragus, posterior one third of the tongue, soft palate, oro- and nasopharynx (e.g., for gag reflex) travels via lingual, tonsillar, and pharyngeal branches to the *superior* ganglion (location of cell bodies of sensory neurons) and then to the caudal spinal trigeminal nucleus. Sensation from the tympanic membrane, eustachian tube, and mastoid region travels via the tympanic plexus to the tympanic nerve to the *inferior* ganglion to the spinal trigeminal nucleus.

- *VA (visceral sensory) pathway.*
  1. Baroreceptors in *carotid sinus.* Baroreceptors at the carotid bifurcation sense an increase in blood pressure that travels via the carotid sinus nerve to the inferior (petrosal) ganglion to the tractus solitarius and then to the caudal nucleus solitarius (site of synapse). Interneurons then synapse on the *dorsal nucleus of CN X* to cause a vagal response (decreased blood pressure and heart rate and force of cardiac contraction) (*carotid sinus reflex*).
  2. Chemoreceptors in *carotid body.* Carotid body chemoreceptors detect blood O_2 and CO_2 concentrations, and transmit information via Hering's nerve to the inferior (petrosal) ganglion to the tractus solitarius and to the caudal nucleus solitarius. Interneurons then synapse on the respiratory center in the medulla to control respiratory rate and depth.
- *SA (special sensory) pathway.* Taste fibers in the *posterior one third of the tongue*, posterior pharynx and eustachian tube transmit information to the inferior (petrosal) ganglion to the rostral nucleus solitarius to the reticular formation and via the central tegmental tract to the contralateral thalamic VPM.

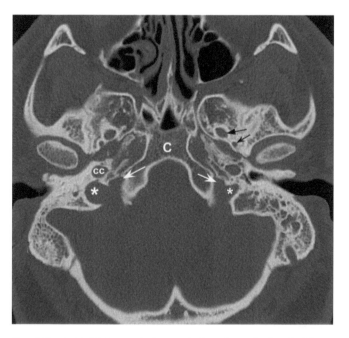

Fig. 9.5 Axial CT image in bone window through the skull base demonstrates normal jugular foramina bilaterally. The jugular vein and CN X and XI exit via the pars vascularis (*). The glossopharyngeal nerves pass through the pars nervosa (*white arrows*), which is located anteromedially. The right jugular foramen is larger than the left, a typical and normal finding. The normal carotid canals are seen just anteriorly (CC). Note the normal clivus (C), foramen ovale, and foramen spinosum (*straight black arrow* and *concave black arrow*, respectively).

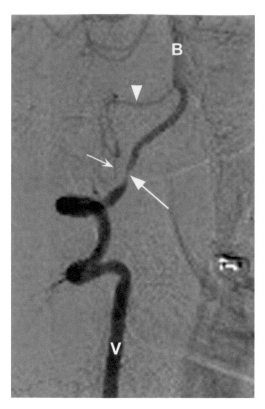

Fig. 9.10 A catheter angiographic image during contrast injection of the right vertebral artery (V) demonstrates focal stenosis (*straight arrow*) of the distal vertebral artery at the origin of the posterior inferior cerebellar artery (PICA) (*concave arrow*). A large right anterior inferior cerebellar artery (AICA) arises from a normal caliber basilar artery (B). Diagnosis: atherosclerotic disease of the vertebral artery and PICA resulting in lateral medullary infarction (Wallenberg syndrome).

Diagnosis

Wallenberg syndrome (lateral medullary syndrome)

Imaging Pearl

• Posterior fossa (cerebellum and brainstem) ischemia is best evaluated with magnetic resonance imaging (MRI). Reduced diffusion on diffusion-weighted sequences is most sensitive for detection of acute ischemia. Ischemia/infarction of the medulla will generally go undetected on computed tomography (CT) examination unless concomitant cerebellar involvement is present.

Clinical Pearl

• Lateral medullary syndrome (Wallenberg syndrome) is caused by occlusion of the intracranial vertebral artery or PICA and leads to some or all of the following findings: ipsilateral facial hypalgesia and thermoanesthesia (spinal CN V nucleus), contralateral trunk and extremity hypalgesia and thermoanesthesia (spinothalamic tract), ipsilateral vocal cord paralysis, dysphagia, dysarthria (nucleus ambiguus), ipsilateral Horner syndrome (descending sympathetic fibers), vertigo, nausea, vomiting (CN VIII) (involvement of vestibular nuclei), ipsilateral cerebellar signs/symptoms (inferior cerebellar peduncle, cerebellum), sometimes accompanied by hiccups (involvement of respiratory center) and diplopia (involvement of pons). Other oculomotor abnormalities can be seen including dysfunction of ocular alignment (skew deviation due to damage to vestibular nuclei), nystagmus, smooth pursuit and gaze-holding abnormalities, and abnormalities of saccades (saccadic dysmetria). See Appendix A, Brainstem.

Case 9.2

A 43-year-old female presents with excruciating lancinating pain in the right ear (**Figs. 9.11, 9.12**).

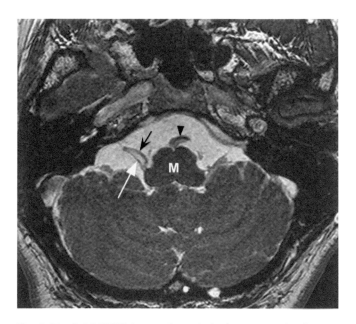

Fig. 9.11 Axial FIESTA image through the lower posterior fossa at the level of the medulla (M) shows a large tortuous segment of the posterior inferior cerebellar artery (PICA) (*concave black arrow*) adjacent to the right glossopharyngeal nerve (*straight white arrow*) as it exits the dorsolateral medulla. Note the prominent flow void of a tortuous basilar artery (*black arrowhead*) ventral to the medulla.

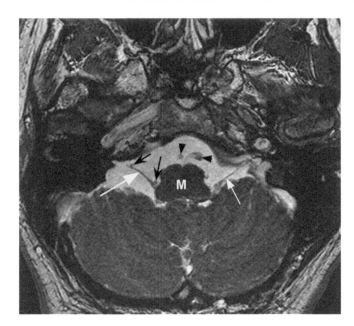

Fig. 9.12 Just inferiorly, the posterior inferior cerebellar artery (*concave black arrows*) clearly contacts and slightly displaces the right glossopharyngeal nerve (*large straight white arrow*) in this patient with glossopharyngeal neuralgia due to neurovascular compression. Ventral to the medulla, both vertebral arteries (*black straight arrowheads*) are seen just below the basilar artery. At surgery, compression of the right glossopharyngeal nerve by PICA was observed, and decompression resulted in pain relief.

Diagnosis

Glossopharyngeal neuralgia. At operation, branches of the PICA were found to be compressing the right CN IX, and relief of neurovascular compression provided effective pain relief.

Glossopharyngeal Neuralgia

- *Epidemiology.* Peak onset 40 to 60 years of age. Seventy to 100 times less common than trigeminal neuralgia. Occurs more in females and equally on left and right.
- *Clinical presentation.* Unilateral, lancinating, paroxysmal pain in *tonsillar fossa* ("pharyngeal type") or *ear* ("tympanic type") or both. Often precipitated by swallowing, coughing, chewing, talking, yawning, or touching the earlobe. May be associated with *syncope* and *bradycardia*.
- *Imaging.* Imaging may demonstrate a tortuous vessel, vascular loop, or aneurysm in the region of the CN IX root entry zone, or may be normal. Dedicated skull base MRI with thin cuts and/or MR angiography may identify compressive vascular structures. Other vascular pathologies such as dural arteriovenous fistulae may occasionally be demonstrated. Demyelinating plaques or compressive or infiltrative neoplastic lesions may also be identified.
- *Pathology.* Etiologies include vascular compression (most cases), neoplasm, perineural spread of tumor, and demyelination. Some cases are idiopathic.

- *Treatment.* Medical treatment with carbamazepine and phenytoin can be attempted. Surgical treatments include microvascular decompression (usually PICA), division of CN IX and the upper part of CN X, or tumor resection (if applicable).

Case 9.3

A 33-year-old HIV+ male presents with fever, stiff neck, and right facial weakness including inability to close the right eye. He had a recent tick bite while hiking in Connecticut (**Fig. 9.13**).

Diagnosis

Lyme disease

Lyme Disease

- *Epidemiology.* Most common vector-borne disease in the United States (~15,000 cases/year). Caused by *Borrelia burgdorferi*, a tick-borne spirochete now endemic in more than 15 states as well as in parts of Europe and Asia. Transmitted by the deer tick (*Ixodes* spp.). In the United States, most frequently seen in three areas: Northeast from Maine to Maryland, Midwest in Wisconsin and Minnesota, and in the West in northern California and Oregon.
- *Clinical presentation.* Within days after initial inoculation, 80% of humans will develop a rash (*erythema chronicum migrans*) and flu-like symptoms (*Stage 1*). In

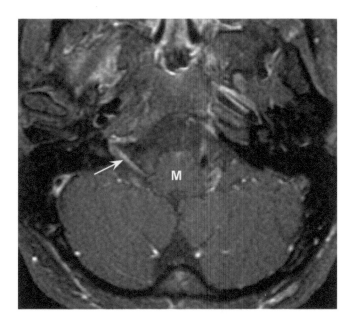

Fig. 9.13 Axial postcontrast fat-saturated T1-weighted image through the lower skull base at the level of the medulla (M) shows an enlarged and smoothly enhancing right glossopharyngeal nerve (*arrow*). This patient was confirmed to have Lyme disease.

the next few weeks (*Stage 2*), systemic involvement may ensue, affecting the nervous system, heart, and joints in particular. Approximately 15% of patients develop neurologic abnormalities ("neuroborreliosis") such as aseptic meningitis, *cranial neuritis* (especially unilateral or bilateral CN VII palsy), encephalitis, myelitis, radiculitis, and peripheral neuropathy. Weeks to months after infection (*Stage 3*), ~60% of people will experience intermittent arthritis attacks and 5% will develop chronic neurologic manifestations ("chronic neuroborreliosis"), including chronic polyneuropathy, encephalomyelitis or encephalopathy.

- *Imaging.* Imaging may show parenchymal lesions involving subcortical white matter, brainstem, and deep gray nuclei, generally better appreciated on MRI than on CT. The parenchymal lesions may be indistinguishable from demyelinating diseases such as multiple sclerosis (MS) or ADEM. MRI may also demonstrate leptomeningeal abnormalities as well as CN enlargement and/or enhancement. Differential considerations for enhancement of multiple CNs include perineural or leptomeningeal spread of malignancy, atypical infectious processes such as tuberculosis (TB) or fungal infections, sarcoidosis, autoimmune processes, syphilis, and Lyme disease. The presence of single or multiple

parenchymal abnormalities in combination with meningeal or CN enhancement in the appropriate clinical setting (endemic area, history of rash) should suggest Lyme disease, and confirmatory serologic testing should be undertaken.

- *Pathology.* Spirochetal infection leads to complex immunological response against both spirochetal and host antigens, resulting in diffuse inflammatory response. Diagnosis is usually based on clinical findings, polymerase chain reaction (PCR) of affected fluid (e.g., joint fluid or cerebrospinal fluid [CSF]) and serologic tests.
- *Treatment.* Options include doxycycline, amoxicillin, and cefuroxime. Intravenous ceftriaxone is often given for documented neurologic abnormalities because of good blood–brain barrier penetration.

Case 9.4

A 53-year-old female presents with hoarseness (**Figs. 9.14, 9.15, 9.16**).

Diagnosis

CN IX schwannoma

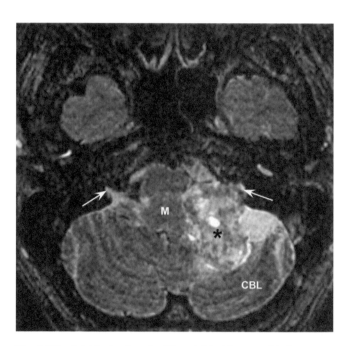

Fig. 9.14 Axial fast spin echo T2-weighted image with fat saturation demonstrates a heterogeneous extraaxial mass (*) centered in the left cerebellomedullary angle with mass effect upon the adjacent medulla (M) and left cerebellar hemisphere (CBL). The mass extends laterally into the left pars nervosa, which is widened compared with the normal right side (*concave arrows*).

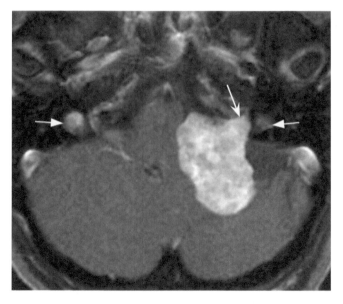

Fig. 9.15 Axial postcontrast fat-saturated T1-weighted image at the same level demonstrates intense homogeneous enhancement of the mass extending into the pars nervosa of the left jugular foramen (*concave arrow*). Normal enhancement is seen within the jugular bulbs bilaterally (*straight arrows*).

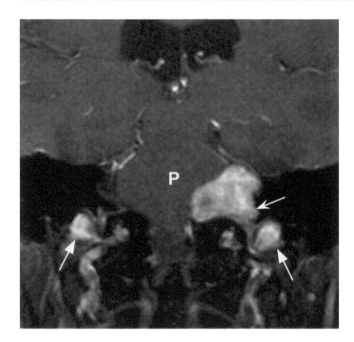

Fig. 9.16 Coronal postcontrast fat-saturated T1-weighted image through the posterior fossa at the level of the pons (P) also shows extension into the left jugular foramen (*concave arrow*). Imaging is suggestive of a nerve sheath tumor, and the lesion was found to be a schwannoma arising from CN IX at surgery. Again note the normal enhancement of the jugular bulbs bilaterally (*straight arrows*).

Case 9.5

A 32-year-old male with supratentorial primitive neuroectodermal tumor (PNET) diagnosed 10 months ago presents with multiple cranial neuropathies and is found to have CSF spread of tumor by cytology (**Figs. 9.17, 9.18**).

Diagnosis

PNET with leptomeningeal spread to multiple CNs

Primitive Neuroectodermal Tumors

* *Epidemiology.* PNETs are the most common primary brain tumors in children, typically occurring in the posterior fossa before the age of 15 years. Locations (in descending order of frequency) include the superior medullary velum/cerebellar vermis, cerebellar hemispheres (older children and young adults), pineal gland, cerebral hemispheres, spinal cord, and brainstem. Types of PNETs include: *medulloblastoma* (most common type, occurring in the superior medullary velum and cerebellar hemispheres), *retinoblastoma, esthesioneuroblastoma, pineoblastoma, ependymoblastoma,* and *neuroblastoma.*
* *Clinical presentation.* Related to size and location (e.g., infratentorial vs. supratentorial), as well as the presence

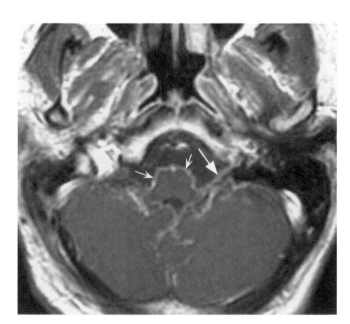

Fig. 9.17 Axial postcontrast T1-weighted image at the level of the medulla demonstrates smooth linear enhancement (*small concave arrows*) over the surface of the medulla consistent with leptomeningeal spread of tumor in this patient with a supratentorial PNET. Enhancement is also noted along the left glossopharyngeal nerve (*straight arrow*).

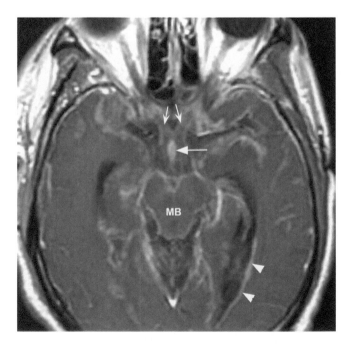

Fig. 9.18 More superiorly, an axial postcontrast image shows diffuse leptomeningeal enhancement surrounding the midbrain (MB) as well as along the bilateral optic nerves (*concave arrows*) at the level of the chiasm. Diffuse ependymal enhancement is also present along the lateral ventricles (*arrowheads*) and in the anterior recess of the third ventricle (*straight arrow*), just posterior to the optic chiasm.

or absence of hydrocephalus. Most medulloblastomas present with symptoms and signs of hydrocephalus, and may present with cerebellar signs (truncal or appendicular ataxia) and/or cranial neuropathies depending on size and location.

- *Imaging.* Typically well-defined tumors, hyperdense on noncontrast CT and iso- or hypointense on T2-weighted image due to their high cellularity. "Atypical" features may be seen in up to 60% of cases on CT, including calcification in 20% and cystic or necrotic regions in 50%. Hemorrhage is rare. Enhancement is seen in more than 90% of medulloblastomas, most commonly diffuse, but may be patchy. In addition, when the tumor arises in the posterior fossa, hydrocephalus is present in ~95% of patients at the time of presentation. Screening MRI with contrast of the spine is indicated at the time of presentation for most PNETs to rule out dissemination given the propensity of this tumor for CSF spread.
- *Pathology.* PNETs are densely cellular with small round cells with large nuclei and scant cytoplasm. They are thought to arise from cells capable of differentiating into glia, neurons, or mesenchymal cells. *Homer-Wright rosettes* (around central granulofibrillar material with radially arranged nuclei) and *pseudorosettes* (around blood vessels) are typical. *Flexner-Wintersteiner rosettes* are a pattern of columnar cells with a small lumen seen with retinoblastomas and pineoblastomas. For medulloblas-

tomas, local extension into the cerebellar hemisphere, infiltration of the floor of the fourth ventricle, and subarachnoid seeding into the CSF are common.

- *Treatment.* Surgery (tumor resection ± ventriculoperitoneal shunt) + craniospinal radiation therapy ± chemotherapy. Treatment is often complicated by recurrence at the primary site, CSF seeding, and distant metastases. Peritoneal spread may occur via the ventriculoperitoneal shunt and PNET is the *most common cause of shunt-related metastasis*. The five-year survival rate is 50 to 70% with treatment. Factors associated with good prognosis include gross total resection, no metastasis, desmoplastic histology, and high trkC (tropomyosin-related kinase C) expression. Factors associated with poor prognosis include younger age, subtotal resection, metastasis, large-cell anaplastic histology, elevated *ErbB2* expression, and loss of heterozygosity on chromosome 17p.

Case 9.6

A 49-year-old female presents with dysphagia and sharp right parotid pain (**Figs. 9.19, 9.20**).

Diagnosis

Eagle syndrome

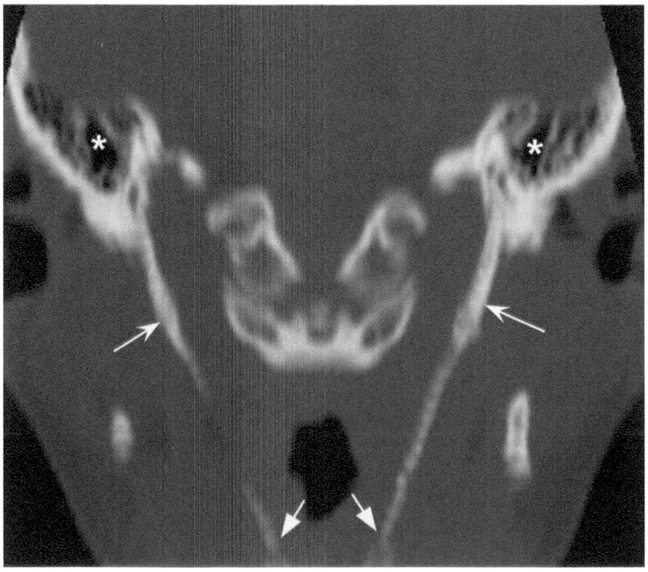

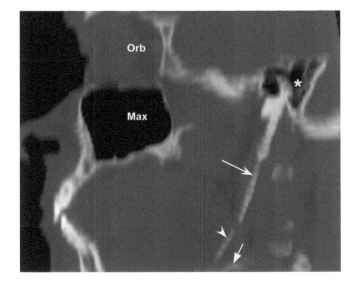

Fig. 9.19 Coronal CT image through the face and pneumatized mastoid air cells (*) in bone windows demonstrates abnormal ossification and/or calcification along the styloid process and stylohyoid ligaments bilaterally. Proximally, the styloid processes are abnormally elongated (*concave arrows*) and distally, there is calcification/ossification of the stylohyoid ligaments to the level of the hyoid bone (*straight arrows*).

Fig. 9.20 Parasagittal CT image in the same patient at the level of the maxillary sinus (Max), orbit (Orb), and temporal bone shows the elongated styloid process (*concave arrow*) arising from the pneumatized mastoid bone (*) and calcification/ossification of the stylohyoid ligament (*arrowhead*) as it extends inferiorly to the level of the hyoid bone (*straight arrow*) in this patient with Eagle syndrome.

Clinical Pearl

- *Eagle* syndrome is an entrapment syndrome of the extracranial portion of CN IX caused by an elongated or calcified styloid process and/or stylohyoid ligament. May occur unilaterally or bilaterally and variably results in symptoms of pain in throat and/or ear, pain on rotation of the neck or extension of the tongue, dysphagia, headache, change in voice, and a sensation of hypersalivation. Treatment is conservative but if necessary styloid resection can be performed.

Imaging Pearl

- The normal styloid process is 2.5 cm or less and is considered elongated when greater than 3 cm. In Eagle syndrome, an elongated styloid process as well as calcification or ossification of the stylohyoid ligament may be observed.

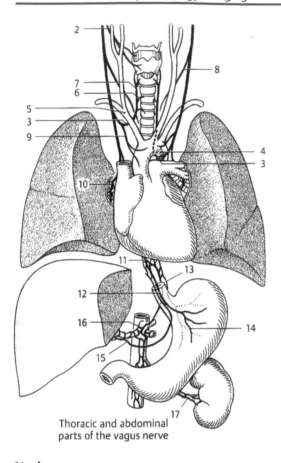

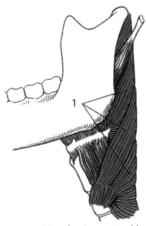

Muscles innervated by
the vagus nerve

Fig. 10.4 Vagus nerve: cervical, thoracic, and abdominal portions. (1, constrictor muscles of the pharynx; 2, superior laryngeal nerve; 3, recurrent laryngeal nerve; 4, arch of the aorta; 5, subclavian artery; 6, tracheal branches; 7, inferior laryngeal nerve; 8, superior cardiac branches; 9, inferior cardiac branches; 10, pulmonary plexus; 11, esophageal plexus; 12, anterior vagal trunk; 13, posterior vagal trunk; 14, anterior gastric branches; 15, posterior gastric branches; 16, celiac branches; 17, renal branches.)

Thoracic and abdominal
parts of the vagus nerve

Neck

- *Pharyngeal ramus.* SVE. Arises from the nodose ganglion, divides into filaments to form *pharyngeal plexus* with branches of CN IX and external laryngeal nerve (see below). Supplies all the muscles of the pharynx and soft palate except stylopharyngeus (CN IX) and tensor veli palatini (CN V), including the superior and middle pharyngeal constrictors, levator veli palatini, salpingopharyngeus, palatopharyngeus, and palatoglossus.
- *Superior laryngeal nerve.* SVE and GSA. Arises just below the nodose ganglion, descends on the side of the pharynx, and divides into the internal and external laryngeal nerves. External branch (*external laryngeal nerve,* smaller, SVE) supplies the inferior pharyngeal constrictor and cricothyroid muscles and communicates with the pharyngeal plexus and *superior cardiac branches.* The internal branch (*internal laryngeal nerve,* larger, GSA) pierces the thyrohyoid membrane along with the superior laryngeal artery and sends sensory fibers to the epiglottis and mucous membranes of the larynx above the vocal folds.
- *Recurrent laryngeal nerves* (at base of neck). SVE and GSA. The right recurrent laryngeal nerve (RLN) arises in front of the subclavian artery and bends upward and medially behind the subclavian artery to ascend in the right tracheoesophageal sulcus. The left RLN arises to the left of the aortic arch and loops beneath the ligamentum arteriosum before ascending in the left tracheoesophageal sulcus. Each nerve passes under the inferior constrictor

and enters the larynx. The RLNs supply *all the intrinsic laryngeal muscles except the cricothyroid* (supplied by the external laryngeal ramus of the superior laryngeal nerve, the cricothyroid swings the thyroid cartilage forward, thereby tensing vocal ligaments and increasing pitch). These include the lateral cricoarytenoid (draws vocal folds together, closes glottis), posterior cricoarytenoid (draws vocal folds apart, opens glottis, deepens pitch), and vocalis (fine adjustments in tension of vocal ligaments). RLNs also supply GSA to the vocal cords and the subglottis, and communicate with the cardiac plexus.
- *Superior cardiac branches.* Several (2–3) branches arising from vagus in the neck, which follow the ICA to the aorta to supply the cardiac plexus.

Thorax

- *Inferior cardiac branches.* Arise from the vagus at the side of the trachea, and from the RLN. Supply the cardiac plexus.
- *Anterior bronchial branches.* Small branches join with sympathetic filaments to form the *anterior pulmonary plexus.*
- *Posterior bronchial nerve.* Larger branches join with sympathetic filaments from thoracic ganglia to form the *posterior pulmonary plexus.*
- *Esophageal branches.* Ramify with branches from the opposite side to form the *esophageal plexus.*

Abdomen

- *Gastric branches.* The right vagus forms the *posterior gastric plexus* (postero-inferior surface of stomach) and the left vagus forms the *anterior gastric plexus* (antero-superior surface).
- *Celiac branches.* From the right vagus, join the celiac plexus.
- *Hepatic nerve.* From the left vagus, join the hepatic plexus.

Functional Pathways of the Vagus Nerve

- *SVE (branchial motor) pathway. Nucleus ambiguus* (in medullary reticular formation medial to spinal trigeminal nucleus) supplies striated musculature of soft palate, pharynx (including pharyngeal constrictors), and larynx (via CN IX, X, and bulbar XI). Supranuclear innervation to the nucleus ambiguus is via corticobulbar fibers originating in the lower precentral gyri (bilateral innervation) and traveling in the genu of the internal capsule.
- *GVE (visceral motor) pathway.* Parasympathetic (GVE) outflow arises from *dorsal motor nucleus of CN X* (located in the floor of the fourth ventricle in the *vagal trigone* lateral to the hypoglossal nucleus). Input to the dorsal motor nucleus of CN X is from the hypothalamus, olfactory system, reticular formation, and nucleus solitarius. Sends preganglionic parasympathetics via the vagus nerve to the thorax and abdomen, innervating abdominal viscera up to the splenic flexure. Secretomotor innervation to pharyngeal mucosa (via pharyngeal plexus), laryngeal mucosa, ganglia in walls of individual thoracic organs, and esophageal, gastric, celiac, and hepatic plexi. *Selective vagotomy* involves partial severing of the right and left gastric nerves to treat persistent/recurrent gastric ulcers. Vagal intestinal branches increase peristalsis and secretion in small intestine, cecum, vermiform appendix, ascending colon, and transverse colon to splenic flexure. Synapses occur in the ganglia of the myenteric (*Auerbach's*) plexus and submucosal (*Meissner's*) plexus.
- *GSA (somatic sensory) pathway.* Somatic sensation from ear, external auditory meatus, tympanic membrane (via Arnold's nerve) and posterior fossa dura (via meningeal branch) to jugular ganglion to spinal trigeminal nucleus.
- *VA (visceral sensory) pathway.* Visceral afferent sensations from pharynx, larynx, trachea, lungs, heart, esophagus, stomach, thoracoabdominal viscera down to the splenic flexure, aortic arch baroreceptors, and aortic body (chemoreceptors) travel via vagal branches to nodose ganglion to tractus solitarius and caudal nucleus solitarius.
- *SA (special sensory) pathway.* Taste information from the epiglottis, hard and soft palates, and pharynx travels to nodose ganglion to rostral nucleus solitarius.
- *Nucleus solitarius* (also sometimes called nucleus of the solitary tract). Rostral nucleus solitarius is gustatory with input mainly from CN VII (geniculate ganglion) and CN IX (petrosal ganglion), but also from CN X. Caudal nucleus solitarius is mainly for visceral sensation (carotid body and carotid sinus from CN IX, and visceral sensation from CN X). Efferent fibers from nucleus solitarius are distributed to thalamic ventroposteromedial nucleus (VPM) (via central tegmental tract), salivatory nucleus (for salivation with taste stimulation), dorsal motor nucleus of CN X (for increased peristalsis), nucleus ambiguus, and hypoglossal nucleus.
- *Medullary respiratory center.* Includes nucleus ambiguus, nucleus solitarius, and the medullary reticular formation. Responds to vagal input and CO_2 accumulation (via carotid body (CN IX) and aortic arch (CN X) chemoreceptors). Medullary vasomotor center is less well defined anatomically.

Vagus Nerve: Normal Images (Figs. 10.5, 10.6, 10.7, 10.8, 10.9, 10.10)

Vagus Nerve Lesions

Evaluation

- *Sensory evaluation.* Difficult to assess separately from other CNs for both somatic sensation (larynx, pharynx,

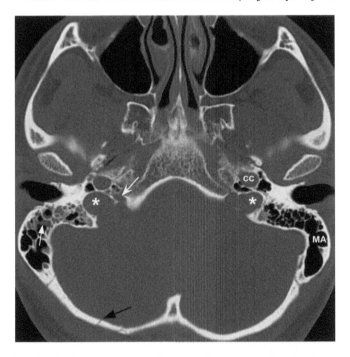

Fig. 10.5 Axial CT image in bone window through the skull base demonstrates normal jugular foramina bilaterally. The jugular vein and CNs X and XI exit via the pars vascularis (*). The glossopharyngeal nerves pass through the pars nervosa (*white concave arrow*), which is located anteromedially. The normal carotid canals (CC) are seen just anterior to the jugular foramina. Note the incidental right occipital skull fracture (*black arrow*). Fluid within the right mastoid (*white straight arrow*) is secondary to an associated temporal bone fracture. On the left, the normal mastoid air cells (MA) are well aerated.

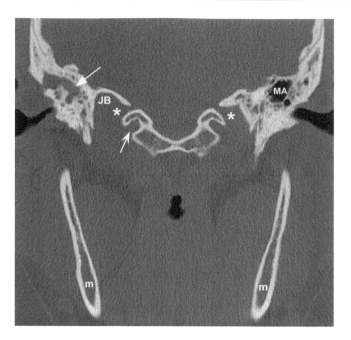

Fig. 10.6 Coronal CT image in bone window of a different patient, at the level of the jugular foramina (*) and mandible (m). The jugular bulb (JB) is more prominent on the right, as is commonly the case. Normal hypoglossal canals (*concave arrow*) are also apparent, just inferomedial to the jugular foramina. Bony erosion with opacification of the right mastoid (*straight arrow*) is secondary to the patient's known cholesteatoma. On the left, the normal mastoid air cells are well aerated.

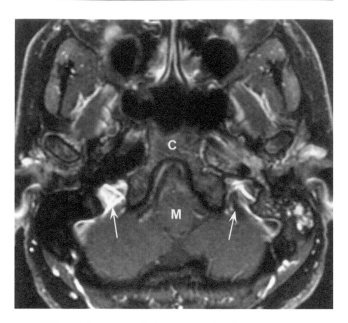

Fig. 10.7 Axial post-gadolinium T1-weighted image with fat saturation through the skull base at the level of the medulla (M) and clivus (C) shows the jugular bulbs within the jugular foramina bilaterally (*arrows*). Note that there is asymmetric and heterogeneous signal (bright on the right and dark on the left) due to variations in flow patterns and variable degrees of enhancement. This can make the diagnosis of jugular foramen lesions difficult, and the normal jugular bulb may be misinterpreted as a mass lesion. It is therefore very important to recognize this normal appearance.

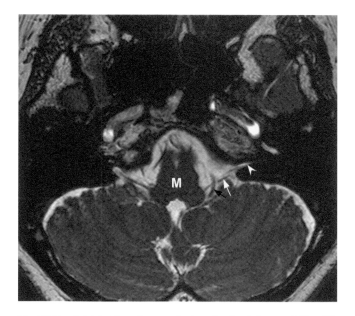

Fig. 10.8 Axial fast imaging employing steady-state acquisition (FIESTA) image through the level of the medulla (M) and pars nervosa (*arrowhead*) demonstrates the bilateral vagal (*straight white arrow*) and left glossopharyngeal nerves as well as an adjacent loop of the left PICA (*straight black arrow*).

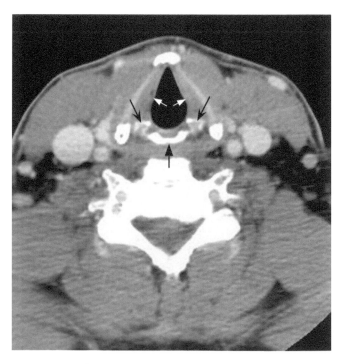

Fig. 10.9 Axial CT image through the larynx at the level of the cricoid cartilage (*straight black arrow*) and arytenoid cartilages (*concave black arrows*). The true vocal cords (*straight white arrows*) are symmetric and normal in position and morphology.

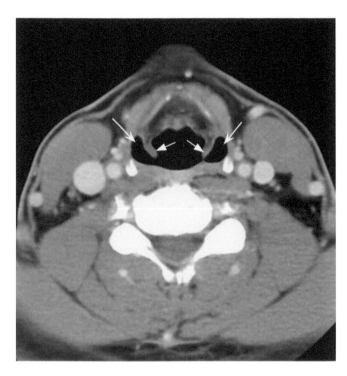

Fig. 10.10 More superiorly, an axial CT image at the supraglottic level shows normal and symmetric aryepiglottic folds (*straight arrows*) and normal pyriform sinuses (*concave arrows*) bilaterally.

pinna, meninges) and taste (epiglottis) as there is considerable overlap with CNs VII and IX.

- *Motor evaluation.* Soft palate and uvula are examined at rest and with phonation; symmetric palatal elevation without uvular deviation is normal. Laryngeal and pharyngeal function can be evaluated with phonation, with swallowing, with respirations and coughing, and by direct laryngoscopy. Unilateral vagal injury may result in failure of palatal elevation, uvular deviation away from the lesion, dysphagia, dysarthria, vocal cord paralysis with hoarseness, and dysphonia. Bilateral vagal injury may result in bilateral palatal paresis, more profound dysphagia, dysphonia or aphonia, dysarthria, and/or paralysis of the esophagus and stomach with pain and emesis.
- *Reflex evaluation.*
  - *Gag reflex.* Light touch to pharynx, tonsillar area, or base of tongue leads to gagging (tongue retraction along with elevation and constriction of pharyngeal muscles). Afferent arc is CN IX sensory (pharynx) to caudal nucleus solitarius. Efferent arc is nucleus ambiguus to CN IX/X to pharyngeal muscles.
  - *Cough reflex.* CN X sensory (usually larynx, trachea, or bronchial tree) to caudal nucleus solitarius to medullary respiratory center leads to forced expiration, and to nucleus ambiguus to CN X to muscles of larynx and pharynx leads to coughing from airway irritation.

- *Vomiting reflex.* CN X sensory to caudal nucleus solitarius to nucleus ambiguus to CN X to close glottis and also to reticulospinal tract to cause contraction of diaphragm and abdominal muscles. May be stimulated by increased intracranial pressure (ICP) and by emetics stimulating the area postrema of the caudal medulla.
- *Autonomic evaluation.* Ipsilateral decreased carotid sinus reflex may be seen because vagal outflow is necessary. Bilateral vagal dysfunction is associated with tachycardia and other signs of sympathetic overactivity.

Types

Supranuclear Lesions

- Lesions causing vagal palsy often involve other CNs (e.g., CN IX, XI, XII) concomitantly.
- If unilateral, no or minor deficit (bilateral corticobulbar input to nucleus ambiguus).
- Bilateral upper motor neuron (UMN) corticobulbar lesions may result in pseudobulbar palsy.

Brainstem Lesions (Nucleus or Fascicular Portion)

- Localization distinguished by presence/absence of other findings (cranial nerve and/or long tract involvement)
- Specific causes:
  - Neoplasm (e.g., brainstem glioma).
  - Inflammatory/demyelinating disease (e.g., acute disseminated encephalomyelitis [ADEM]).
  - Vascular disease (e.g., posterior inferior cerebellar artery (PICA) stroke).
  - Syringobulbia.
  - *Avellis syndrome*, also called laryngeal hemiplegia, is paralysis of the palate and larynx due to a medullary stroke involving the nucleus ambiguus. It may be associated with contralateral hemiparesis/hemihypesthesia.

Lesions in the Jugular Foramen

- Neoplasm (most commonly glomus jugulare, schwannoma, meningioma, skull base metastasis).
- Trauma (basal skull fracture).
- *Vernet syndrome* (jugular foramen syndrome). Due to injury of structures in the jugular foramen (CN IX, X, and XI). It consists of ipsilateral trapezius and sternocleidomastoid (SCM) paresis (CN XI); dysphonia; dysphagia; homolateral vocal cord paresis; loss of taste and sensation on posterior one third of the tongue on involved side; loss of sensation from ipsilateral palate, uvula, pharynx, and larynx; and loss of gag reflex (CN IX, X).

Extracranial Lesions Affecting Specific Vagal Branches

- *Lesions affecting vagus nerve proper.* The trunk of the vagus can be injured in the neck and thorax leading to ipsilateral vocal cord paralysis and laryngeal anesthesia.
  - Iatrogenic injury (typically after thyroid, parathyroid, or cervical disc surgery, but postradiation injury also described)
  - Inflammatory/infectious (e.g., carotid space abscess)
  - Vascular (e.g., ICA dissection)
  - Neoplastic (e.g., schwannoma, neurofibroma, squamous cell carcinoma, thyroid malignancy, non-Hodgkin lymphoma, nasopharyngeal carcinoma, glomus vagale)
- *Lesions in the mediastinum* (especially affecting left CN X).
  - Vascular (e.g., aortic arch aneurysm)
  - Inflammatory/infectious (e.g., mediastinitis, lymphadenopathy, sarcoidosis)
  - Neoplastic (e.g., bronchogenic carcinoma, non-Hodgkin lymphoma)
- *Lesions of superior laryngeal nerve.* Damage (e.g., trauma, surgery, tumor) results in primarily sensory dysfunction, but cricothyroid involvement may cause mild hoarseness.

- *Lesions of the recurrent laryngeal nerve.* Unilateral RLN palsy results in flaccid dysphonia (hoarseness, breathiness) due to paralysis of all laryngeal muscles except cricothyroid. Bilateral RLN palsy (usually after thyroidectomy) leads to inspiratory stridor and aphonia.
  - Iatrogenic (intubation, surgery—e.g. thyroidectomy, anterior cervical discectomy, postradiation)
  - Trauma (blunt laryngeal trauma can damage either superior or recurrent laryngeal innervation)
  - Neoplasm (mediastinal tumors or adenopathy)
  - Vascular (e.g., aortic arch or subclavian artery aneurysms)
  - Idiopathic (unilateral vocal cord paralysis is often idiopathic although many cases are ultimately found to be associated with an underlying neurological condition)

Vagus Nerve: Pathologic Images

Case 10.1

A 55-year-old male presents with hoarseness and dysphagia (**Figs. 10.11, 10.12**).

Diagnosis

CN X schwannoma

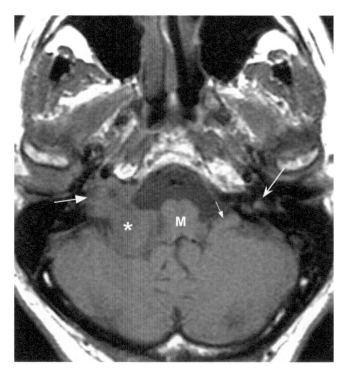

Fig. 10.11 Axial T1-weighted image at the level the jugular foramen demonstrates a homogeneous extraaxial soft tissue mass (*) centered in the right cerebellomedullary angle. There is mass effect upon the medulla (M) and extension into a widened right jugular foramen (*large straight arrow*). Normal signal is seen in the small left jugular bulb (*concave arrow*). On the left, note the normal cerebellar flocculus (*small straight arrow*), which can mimic a cerebellomedullary mass.

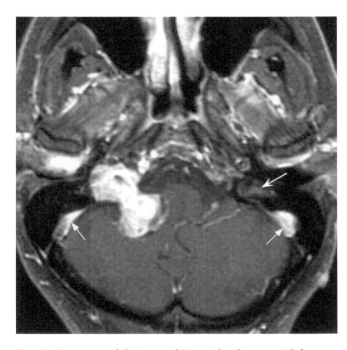

Fig. 10.12 Post-gadolinium axial T1-weighted image with fat saturation at the same level demonstrates intense and fairly homogeneous enhancement of the dumbbell-shaped mass in this patient with a CN X schwannoma. Slightly heterogeneous signal is seen with the normal left jugular bulb (*concave arrow*) due to turbulent flow. Bright signal within the bilateral sigmoid sinuses (*straight arrows*) is normal post-gadolinium vascular enhancement.

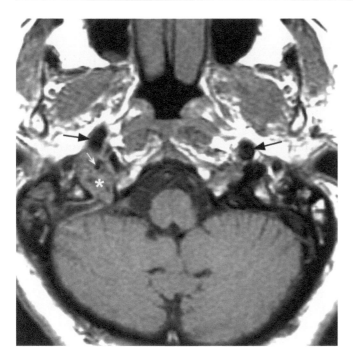

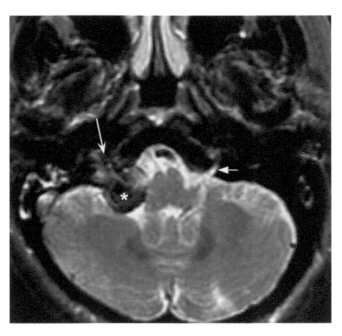

Fig. 10.13 Axial T1-weighted image at the level of the jugular foramina shows a soft tissue mass (*) centered in the right jugular foramen. Scattered flow voids (*concave arrow*) within the mass are typical of a hypervascular lesion such as a paraganglioma. Normal flow voids (*bilateral straight arrows*) are present in the more anteriorly located internal carotid arteries.

Fig. 10.14 Axial T2-weighted image at a slightly superior level demonstrates heterogeneous signal in the right jugular foramen component of the mass (*concave arrow*), as well as within a larger component of the mass centered on the cerebellomedullary angle (*). The very low T2 signal is presumably related to prior hemorrhage. Normal, bright cerebrospinal fluid signal is seen in the pars nervosa of the left jugular foramen.

Case 10.2

A 78-year-old female presents with pulsatile tinnitus (**Fig. 10.13, 10.14, 10.15, 10.16**).

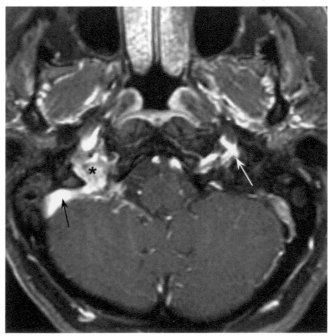

Fig. 10.15 Post-gadolinium axial T1-weighted image with fat saturation at the same level demonstrates intense enhancement of the mass (*). Normal post-gadolinium enhancement is seen in the right sigmoid sinus (*black arrow*) and left jugular vein (*white arrow*). Postcontrast images often show asymmetric enhancement within the jugular bulbs in normal patients due to differences in flow patterns in the often very asymmetrically sized jugular veins. This can make this diagnosis of a mass versus a normal structure difficult without other MR imaging sequences, and small jugular foramen lesions can be missed if only postcontrast images are reviewed.

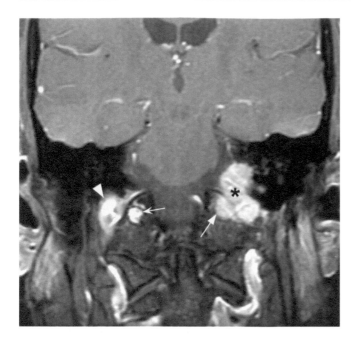

Fig. 10.22 Coronal post-gadolinium image with fat saturation in the same patient shows the intensely enhancing mass (*) centered within the left jugular foramen with extension into the hypoglossal canal and clivus (*straight arrow*). Normal enhancement is seen in the right jugular bulb (*arrowhead*) and right hypoglossal canal (*concave arrow*). Glomus jugulare.

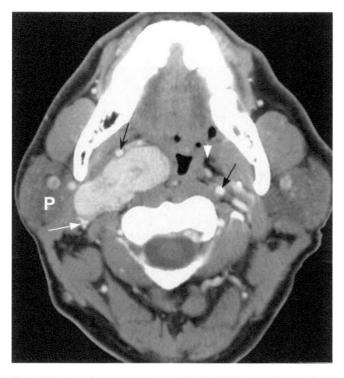

Fig. 10.23 Axial postcontrast CT at the level of the oropharynx demonstrates a large intensely enhancing mass centered in the carotid space between the right internal carotid artery which is displaced anteriorly (*black concave arrow*) and the right internal jugular vein which is compressed posteriorly (*white straight arrow*). The parapharyngeal fat on the right side is effaced (*white arrowhead* shows parapharyngeal fat on the normal left side). There is a well-defined lateral margin with the parotid gland (P), which is uninvolved. The internal carotid artery is in normal position on the left (*straight black arrow*).

Diagnosis

Glomus jugulare

Case 10.4

A 44-year-old male presents with a right neck mass and right vocal cord palsy (**Figs. 10.23, 10.24, 10.25, 10.26**).

Diagnosis

Glomus vagale

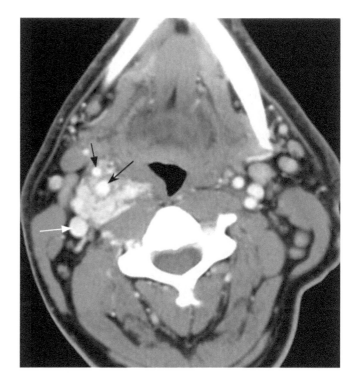

Fig. 10.24 More inferiorly, the mass is seen to displace both the right internal carotid artery (*black concave arrow*) and the right external carotid artery (*black straight arrow*) anteriorly. The right jugular vein (*white arrow*) is displaced posteriorly. Glomus vagale.

Case 10.5

A 48-year-old male presents with hoarseness and dysphagia (**Figs. 10.27, 10.28, 10.29, 10.30**).

Diagnosis

Vagal schwannoma. Pathology demonstrated necrosis and cystic change.

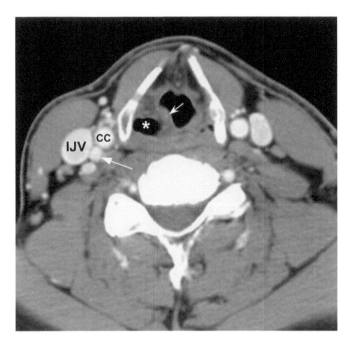

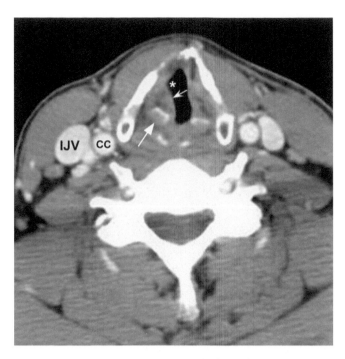

Fig. 10.25 Axial post-contrast CT image in the same patient at the supraglottic level shows that the right aryepiglottic fold deviates anteromedially (*concave arrow*), and the right pyriform sinus (*) is patulous. Asymmetrically increased vascularity (*straight arrow*) is seen adjacent to the right common carotid artery (CC) and internal jugular vein (IJV).

Fig. 10.26 More inferiorly at the level of the glottis, there is anteromedial rotation of the right arytenoid cartilage (*straight arrow*) and medial deviation of the right vocal cord (*concave arrow*) due to loss of muscle tone. There is also prominence of the right laryngeal ventricle (*asterisk*). These findings are consistent with right vocal cord palsy due to the patient's glomus vagale. (CC, common carotid artery; IJV, internal jugular vein.)

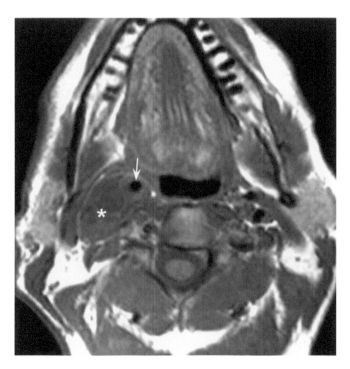

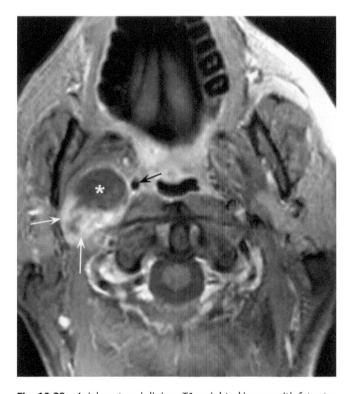

Fig. 10.27 Axial T1-weighted image at the level of the oropharynx demonstrates a somewhat heterogeneous soft tissue mass (*) centered in the right carotid space which displaces the internal carotid artery (*arrow*) anteromedially. A jugular vein flow void is not appreciated and the vein is presumably compressed or occluded.

Fig. 10.28 Axial post-gadolinium T1-weighted image with fat saturation at the same level shows a partly cystic (*) mass with a solid enhancing component posteriorly (*white arrows*). The right internal carotid artery (*black arrow*) is again seen to be displaced anteromedially, and the jugular vein cannot be specifically identified.

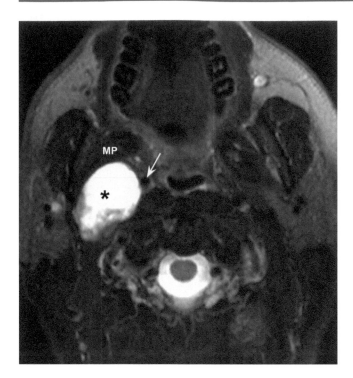

Fig. 10.29   Axial T2-weighted image with fat saturation at the same level confirms a heterogeneous mass with marked hyperintensity in the cystic portion (*). There is mild mass effect upon the adjacent medial pterygoid muscle (MP) and internal carotid artery (*arrow*).

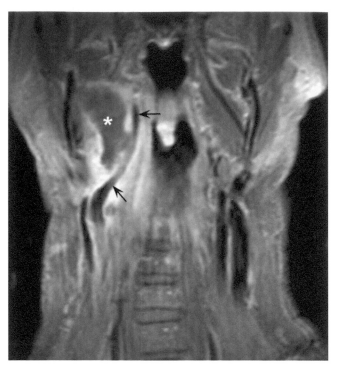

Fig. 10.30   Coronal post-gadolinium T1-weighted image with fat saturation in the same patient shows the cystic component of the mass (*) displacing the internal carotid artery medially (*arrows*). The mass is somewhat oblong in shape and very well circumscribed, which is typical of a nerve sheath tumor. Vagal schwannoma.

Case 10.6

A 56-year-old female presents with progressive hoarseness and is found to have a left vocal cord (VC) palsy (**Fig. 10.31, 10.32, 10.33**).

Diagnosis

Bronchogenic carcinoma with involvement of the left recurrent laryngeal nerve

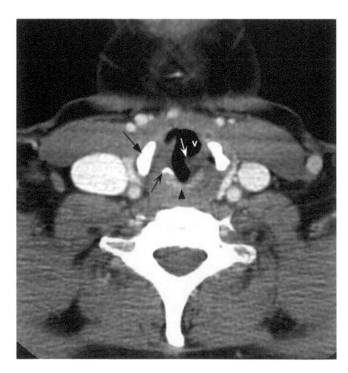

Fig. 10.31   Axial postcontrast CT image through the larynx at the level of the cricoid (*black arrowhead*), right arytenoid (*black concave arrow*) and thyroid (*black straight arrow*) cartilages demonstrates an abnormal left true vocal cord (*white arrow*). The left true vocal cord is medially deviated, the left laryngeal ventricle (v) is dilated, and fatty atrophy of the underlying thyroarytenoid muscle is also noted. The sternocleidomastoid muscles are symmetrical.

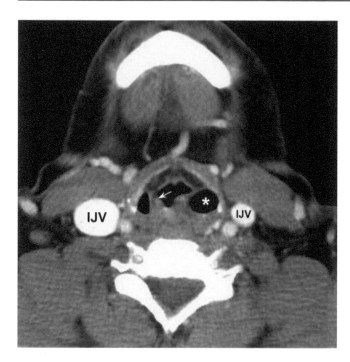

Fig. 10.32 More superiorly, at the level of the aryepiglottic folds (*white arrow* on normal right side), an asymmetric and patulous left pyriform sinus (*) is seen. Note the asymmetric internal jugular veins (IJV), right larger than left, which is a common and normal finding.

Case 10.7

An 85-year-old male presents with progressive hoarseness and is found to have a left VC palsy (**Fig. 10.34**).

Diagnosis

Thoracic aortic aneurysm with involvement of the left recurrent laryngeal nerve

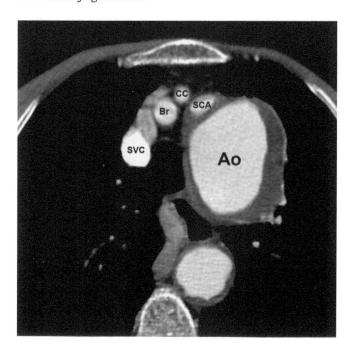

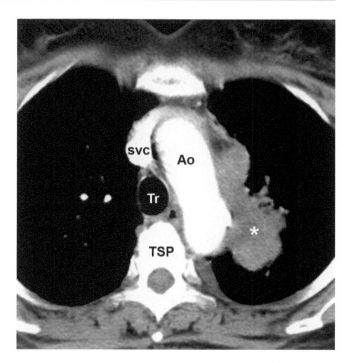

Fig. 10.33 Postcontrast CT image through the superior mediastinum in the same patient demonstrates a focal soft tissue mass within the left upper lobe (*asterisk*) with invasion medially to abut the aortic arch (Ao) in this patient with lung carcinoma. There is presumed invasion of the left recurrent laryngeal nerve (not specifically identified) as it courses through the mediastinum, resulting in the patient's left vocal cord palsy. The superior vena cava (SVC), trachea (Tr), and thoracic spine (TSP) are identified.

Imaging Pearl

Proximal lesions (i.e. above the hyoid bone) of CN X are best imaged with magnetic resonance imaging (MRI) of the suprahyoid carotid space, skull base, and basal cisterns. Excellent soft tissue definition as well as fat-saturation techniques allow superior evaluation of the skull base with MRI as compared with CT. MRI is best for skull base anatomy and CNs. Distal lesions (i.e., below hyoid bone) are often better evaluated with contrast-enhanced CT due to technical limitations of MRI including difficulty with larger spatial coverage (skull base to upper mediastinum) as well as poor fat-saturation techniques at the cervical–thoracic junction. It is important to check both the carotid space (main vagal trunk) and tracheoesophageal groove (RLN). One must image from the hyoid bone to the aortopulmonary window to fully evaluate recurrent laryngeal nerve pathologies.

Fig. 10.34 Postcontrast CT image through the superior mediastinum in a patient with hoarseness and a left vocal cord palsy demonstrates an ascending aortic aneurysm (Ao). There is presumed compression of the left recurrent laryngeal nerve (not specifically identified) as it courses through the mediastinum. The superior vena cava (SVC), brachiocephalic artery (Br), left common carotid artery (CC), and left subclavian artery (SCA) are identified.

11 Spinal Accessory Nerve

Functions

- Special visceral efferent (SVE). Branchial motor to sternocleidomastoid and trapezius muscles.

Anatomy

- The spinal accessory nerve arises from the cervical spinal cord (levels C-1–5) from a column of ventral horn cells that together are called the *accessory nucleus* (**Fig. 11.1**). The spinal accessory rootlets exit the cervical cord and unite to form a single spinal root that ascends posterior to the dentate ligament, enters the cranium via the foramen magnum, and then exits the cranium through the *pars vascularis* of the jugular foramen. The accessory nerve then descends obliquely in the carotid space between the internal carotid artery (ICA) and the internal jugular vein (IJV), across the anterior surface of the atlantal transverse process posterior to the stylohyoid and digastric muscles, to enter the deep aspect of the sternocleidomastoid muscle, which it penetrates and supplies. Emerging lateral to the sternocleidomastoid muscle in close proximity to the great auricular nerve (sensory branch of cervical plexus from C-2/C-3), it crosses the posterior cervical triangle (the most common site of iatrogenic injury) on the surface of the levator scapulae muscle to end in and supply the trapezius muscle (**Fig. 11.2**). The posterior cervical triangle is formed by the anterosuperior border of the trapezius muscle, the posterior border of the sternocleidomastoid muscle, and the middle third of the clavicle.

- The so-called *cranial root* of the accessory nerve has been described as a group of fibers that arise from the caudal portion of the nucleus ambiguus (the more cranial portions of which also supply branchial motor innervation to cranial nerves [CNs] IX and X), and emerge from the medulla as several rootlets in the postolivary sulcus (**Fig. 11.3**). Along with the vagus nerve proper, the cranial root runs laterally in the cerebellomedullary cistern and passes through the *pars vascularis* of the jugular foramen (**Fig. 11.4**). At the level of the superior vagal (*jugular*) ganglion, fibers from the cranial root blend into the vagus nerve and are distributed with the pharyngeal and superior laryngeal branches of CN X to supply the pharynx and larynx. Therefore, it is best to consider the cranial root of the accessory nerve as a part of the vagus nerve and functionally completely separate from the spinal accessory nerve.

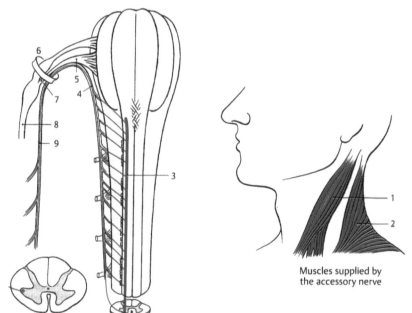

Nuclear region and exit of the accessory nerve

Muscles supplied by the accessory nerve

Fig. 11.1 Spinal accessory nerve, spinal root: spinal nuclear region and root exit. (1, sternocleidomastoid muscle; 2, trapezius muscle; 3, spinal nucleus of the accessory nerve; 4, spinal root; 5, cranial root; 6, jugular foramen; 7, internal branches to vagus nerve; 8, vagus nerve; 9, accessory nerve.)

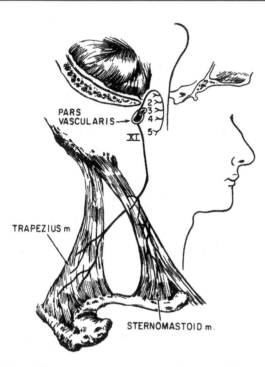

Fig. 11.2 Spinal accessory nerve: distal branches. The spinal accessory nerve receives fibers from cervical levels 1 through 5, ascends through the foramen magnum, and exits the skull base via the *pars vascularis* of the jugular foramen. Extracranial branches supply branchial motor innervation to the sternocleidomastoid and trapezius muscles. (From Harnsberger HR. Handbook of Head and Neck Imaging (2nd ed.) St. Louis, MO: Mosby, 1995. Modified with permission.)

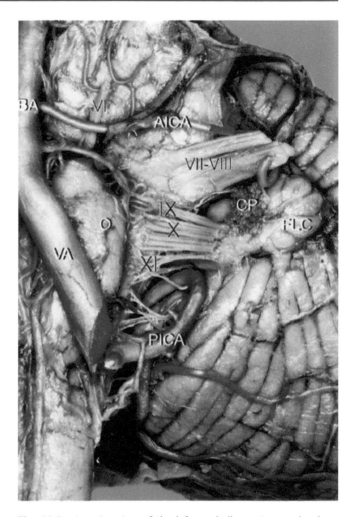

Fig. 11.3 Anterior view of the left cerebellopontine angle, demonstrating the origin of the cranial root of CN XI at the postolivary sulcus of the medulla. Note its position just inferior to the rootlets of CN X. (AICA, anterior inferior cerebellar artery; PICA, posterior-inferior cerebellar artery; BA, basilar artery; CP, choroid plexus; FLC, flocculus; O, olive; VA, vertebral artery; VI–VII, facial and vestibulo-cochlear nerves; IX, glossopharyngeal nerve; X: vagus nerve.) (From Ozveren MF, Ture U, Ozek MM, et al. Anatomic landmarks of the glossopharyngeal nerve: a microsurgical anatomic study. Neurosurgery 2003;52:1400-1410. Reprinted with permission.)

• The sternocleidomastoid muscle consists of two divisions (sternomastoid and cleidomastoid). The sternomastoid (from sternum to mastoid) acts mainly on the atlantoaxial joint to rotate the head toward the contralateral side. The cleidomastoid (from clavicle to mastoid) primarily acts on the cervical joints to tilt the head downward. When the sternocleidomastoid as a whole contracts, the head is drawn toward the ipsilateral shoulder and turned toward the contralateral side. Simultaneous bilateral sternocleidomastoid muscle contraction flexes the head.

• The trapezius muscle retracts the head and also elevates, rotates, and retracts the scapula.

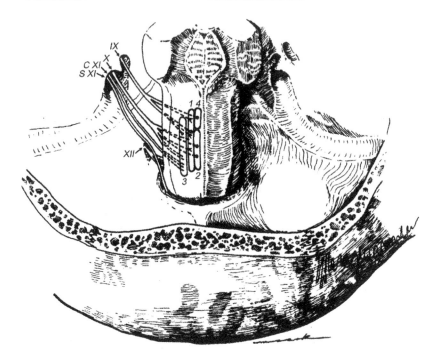

Fig. 11.4 Nuclear origins and cisternal courses of glossopharyngeal, vagus, and spinal accessory nerves. Note that the glossopharyngeal nerve traverses the more anterior part of the jugular foramen (*pars nervosa*), whereas the vagus and spinal accessory nerves pass through the posterior part (*pars vascularis*). The hypoglossal nerve is shown exiting through the more inferiorly located hypoglossal canal. (1, nucleus solitarius; 2, dorsal motor nucleus of CN X; 3, nucleus ambiguus; 4, superior salivatory nucleus; C XI, cranial root of CN XI; S XI, spinal root of CN XI.) (From Harnsberger HR. Handbook of Head and Neck Imaging (2nd ed.) St. Louis, MO: Mosby, 1995. Reprinted with permission.)

Spinal Accessory Nerve Lesions

Evaluation

- *Motor evaluation.* Injury to the spinal accessory nerve results in paresis and/or atrophy of the sternocleidomastoid and trapezius muscles.
  - Sternocleidomastoid paresis. Manifests as weakness in turning the head to the opposite side. Test by observing with inspection and palpation while having the patient rotate the head against resistance. Bilateral sternocleidomastoid paresis results in weak neck flexion.
  - Trapezius paresis. Manifests as shoulder drop, difficulty raising abducted arm above horizontal. Test by observing with inspection and palpation while having the patient shrug the shoulders against resistance. Bilateral trapezius paresis results in weak neck extension. Because of partial innervation of the trapezius from the cervical plexus, lower trapezius function may be spared in pure accessory palsies.

Types

Supranuclear Lesions

- In hemispheric lesions resulting in contralateral hemiplegia, the trapezius muscle contralateral to the lesion is paretic (manifesting as contralateral weakness of shoulder elevation). In contrast, the head is always turned *away from* the plegic side (toward the lesion), indicating paresis of the sternocleidomastoid muscle *ipsilateral* to the lesion. How can this be explained? It is a neuroanatomical pearl that the sternocleidomastoid is

controlled by the *ipsilateral* motor cortex, possibly via a rare double decussation (ipsilateral cortex to contralateral pons to ipsilateral cervical cord). This theory is also supported by the observation that hemispheric seizure foci cause contraction of the *ipsilateral* sternocleidomastoid and cause ictal head deviation *away from* the side of the seizure. Thus the patient looks *away from* the lesion with seizures, and *toward* the lesion with stroke.

Nuclear Lesions

- Rarely cause CN XI palsy in isolation
- High cervical cord or low medullary lesions (e.g., brainstem infarction, brainstem tumor, syringomyelia/syringobulbia)

Foramen Magnum/Jugular Foramen Lesions (Table 11.1)

- Generally also involve adjacent CNs (IX, X, XII) and/or long tracts
- Neoplasms (e.g., glomus tumors, schwannomas, meningiomas)
- Trauma

Extracranial Lesions

- Isolated CN XI palsy may occur at the level of the neck with the following:
  - Iatrogenic. By far the most common etiology of extracranial XI injury. Usually following surgery, e.g., lymph

Table 11.1 Differential Diagnosis of Jugular Foramen Lesions

Lesion	Characteristics
Schwannoma	Homogeneous (except areas of hemorrhage or cyst formation), associated with smooth bony remodeling
Meningioma	Dural-based, often calcified, may cause hyperostosis
Paraganglioma	Heterogeneous, hypervascular with flow voids, irregular margin
Metastasis	Infiltrative, destructive, often associated with pain

node biopsy, neck dissection in the posterior cervical triangle, carotid endarterectomy, IJV cannulation.

○ Trauma. Injury to CN XI in the posterior cervical triangle can occur either by blunt trauma or by penetrating trauma (e.g., stab wound).

○ Postradiation.

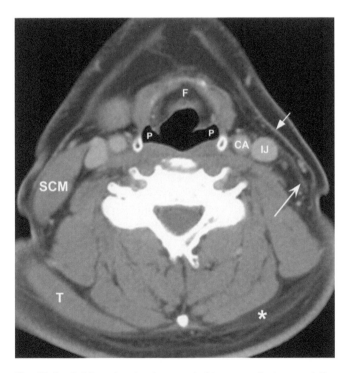

Fig. 11.5 Axial postcontrast computed tomography image at the supraglottic level demonstrates marked atrophy of the left sterno-cleidomastoid (*concave arrow*) and trapezius (*) muscles. Normal sternocleidomastoid (SCM) and trapezius (T) muscles are labeled on the right side. The normal thin and linear left platysma muscle (*straight arrow*) is readily seen superficial to the left common carotid artery (CA), internal jugular vein (IJ), and expected location of the SCM. Note the normal appearance of the preepiglottic fat (F) as well as the bilateral pyriform sinuses (P), which are well aerated. The left pyriform sinus is mildly patulous compared with the right.

Spinal Accessory Nerve: Pathologic Images

Case 11.1

A 48-year-old male presents with left vocal cord palsy, diplophonia, CN IX through XII weakness, recurrent and superior laryngeal nerve palsies, weakness of head turning to right and left, and weakness of shoulder elevation (**Figs. 11.5, 11.6, 11.7, 11.8, 11.9, 11.10, 11.11, 11.12**).

Diagnosis

Jugular foramen schwannoma

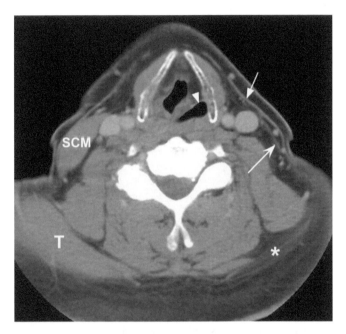

Fig. 11.6 More inferiorly in the same patient, at the midthyroid cartilage level, a clearly asymmetric and patulous left pyriform sinus (*arrowhead*) is seen. In addition, atrophy of the left sternocleidomastoid (*concave arrow*) and trapezius (*) muscles is again appreciated, compatible with denervation changes secondary to CN XI palsy. Normal platysma (*straight arrow*) muscles and normal right sternocleidomastoid (SCM) and trapezius (T) muscles are again indicated.

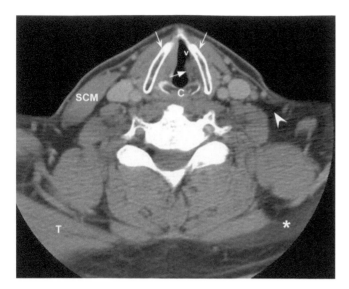

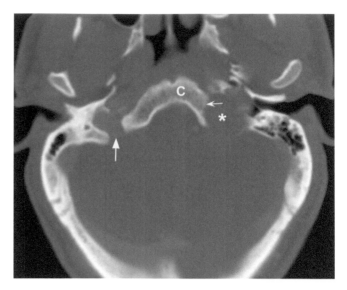

Fig. 11.7 More inferiorly in the same patient, at the level of the cricoid cartilage (C) and lamina of the thyroid cartilage (*concave arrows*), the left vocal cord (*straight arrow*) is decreased in both size and density, consistent with fatty atrophy of the thyroarytenoid muscle. The laryngeal ventricle (v) on the left is also patulous. These changes, along with the patulous pyriform sinus seen in earlier images, are consistent with a chronic left vocal cord paralysis. Atrophy of the left sternocleidomastoid (*arrowhead*) and trapezius (*) muscles is again noted. So in this case, palsies of CN X and XI are both clearly present. Involvement of multiple CNs suggests a lesion above the level of the hyoid bone (from medulla through basal cisterns, jugular foramen, and/or carotid space), and imaging of the brainstem, skull base, and upper carotid space should be pursued.

Fig. 11.8 Axial computed tomography image at the level of the skull base in bone window demonstrates asymmetric widening of the left jugular foramen (*) as compared with the normal right side (*straight arrow*). Additionally, there is smooth bony erosion (*concave arrow*) of the left lateral aspect of the clivus (C). These bony changes suggest a slowly growing mass.

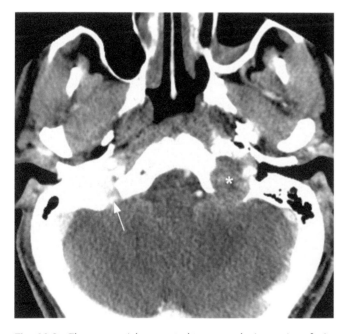

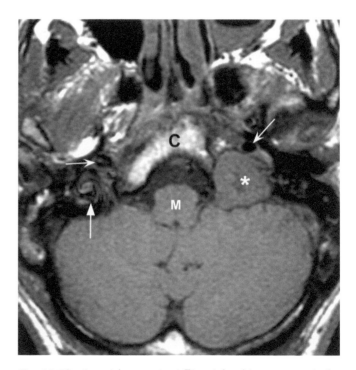

Fig. 11.9 The same axial computed tomography image in soft tissue window shows a mildly enhancing soft tissue mass within the left jugular foramen (*). Enhancement of the right jugular vein is seen within the normal right jugular foramen (*straight arrow*).

Fig. 11.10 An axial precontrast T1-weighted image at a similar level in the same patient demonstrates a relatively homogeneous and well-defined, rounded soft tissue mass (*) centered in the left jugular foramen. This mass displaces the left internal carotid artery (*concave arrow*) anteriorly. The normally positioned right internal carotid is also indicated (*concave arrow*). Heterogeneous signal within the right jugular foramen (*straight arrow*) is typical of normal turbulent flow in the jugular bulb. Remodeling of the left lateral clivus (C) is again appreciated. (M, medulla.)

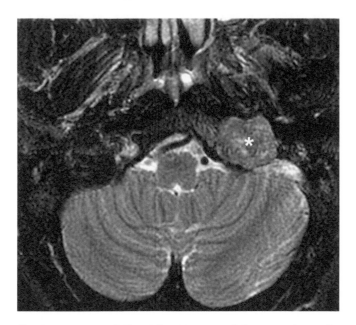

Fig. 11.11 An axial T2-weighted image with fat saturation in the same patient shows a slightly heterogeneous but predominantly intermediate signal intensity mass (*) at the level of the left jugular foramen.

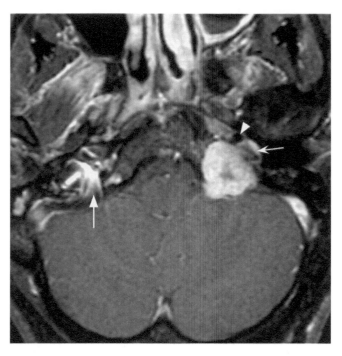

Fig. 11.12 An axial postcontrast T1-weighted image with fat saturation shows a well-circumscribed, slightly lobulated left jugular foramen mass that enhances quite intensely and homogeneously. This appearance is typical of a nerve sheath tumor. Just anterior to the mass, note the normal signal void of the left internal carotid artery (*straight arrowhead*). More laterally, there is enhancement in the displaced and compressed left jugular vein (*concave arrow*). Normal, somewhat heterogeneous jugular vein enhancement is also seen in the right jugular foramen (*straight arrow*). A jugular foramen schwannoma was confirmed at surgery, but the precise lower CN of origin could not be specifically determined.

Case 11.2

A 46-year-old female presents with a 2-year history of progressive hoarseness and dysphagia (**Figs. 11.13, 11.14, 11.15**).

Diagnosis

Jugular foramen meningioma

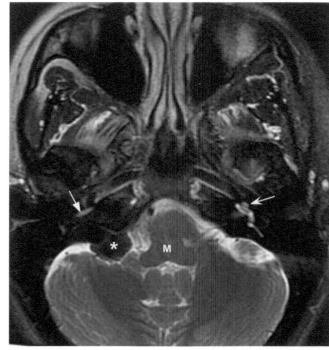

Fig. 11.13 Axial T2-weighted image with fat saturation demonstrates a well-defined, very low signal intensity extraaxial mass (*) in the right cerebellomedullary angle (medulla: M) with a broad dural base against the posterior aspect of the petrous bone. The lesion is located inferior to the internal auditory canal at the level of the basal turn of the right cochlea (*straight arrow*). The cochlea on the left (*concave arrow*) is better seen on this slightly oblique image.

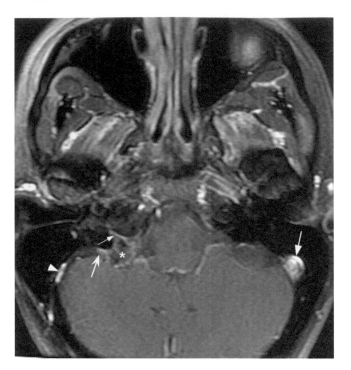

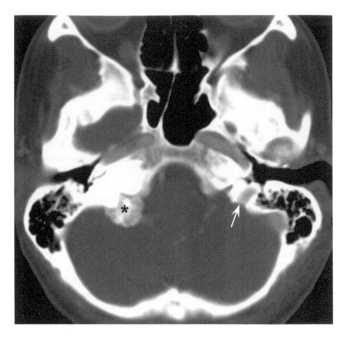

Fig. 11.15 Axial postcontrast computed tomography (CT) image in bone window shows that the mass (*) is heavily calcified. The imaging characteristics on magnetic resonance and CT are consistent with a calcified meningioma. The mass is centered over the upper aspect of the jugular foramen, along the posterior petrous face. The normal *pars vascularis* of the jugular foramen (*arrow*) is labeled on the left.

Fig. 11.14 Axial postcontrast fat-saturated T1-weighted image at the same level shows minimal enhancement of the cerebellomedullary angle mass (*). There is also enhancement along the adjacent posterolateral dura (*concave arrow*), an appearance known as a *dural tail*. Note that the anterior part of the mass is extending into the *pars nervosa* of the jugular foramen (*small straight arrow*). The right sigmoid sinus (*straight arrowhead*) is diminutive, likely secondary to chronic compression more distally by a larger component of the jugular foramen mass (not shown). Normal enhancement is seen in the left sigmoid sinus (*straight arrow*).

Case 11.3

A 72-year-old female presents with palsies of multiple right lower CNs, including IX, X, XI, and XII (**Figs. 11.16, 11.17, 11.18, 11.19, 11.20**).

Diagnosis

Large glomus jugulare tumor

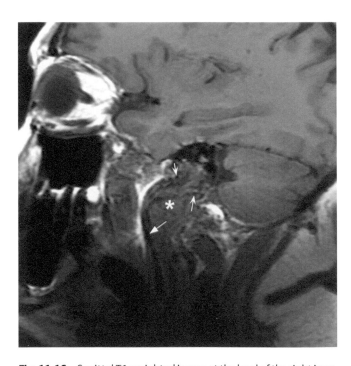

Fig. 11.16 Sagittal T1-weighted image at the level of the right jugular foramen demonstrates a lobulated soft-tissue mass (*) extending from the jugular foramen into the upper carotid space, displacing the internal carotid artery (*straight arrow*) anteriorly. Multiple flow voids (*concave arrows*) are seen within and around the periphery of this mass.

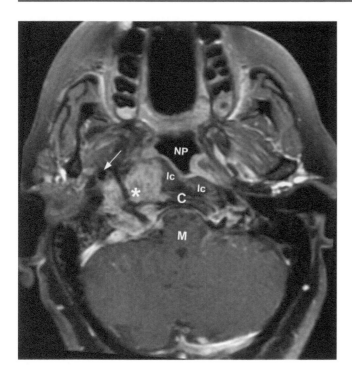

Fig. 11.17 Axial post-gadolinium T1-weighted image with fat saturation demonstrates an intensely enhancing mass (*) centered on the right jugular foramen but extending posteromedially into the cerebellomedullary angle, medially into the clivus (C), and anteromedially to involve and displace the right longus colli muscle and to distort the right nasopharynx. The right internal carotid artery (*straight arrow*) is displaced anterolaterally. (M, medulla; NP, nasopharynx; lc, longus colli muscles.)

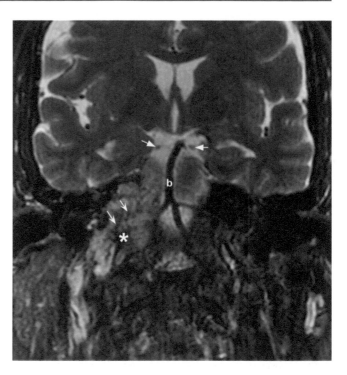

Fig. 11.18 Coronal fast spin echo T2-weighted image with fat saturation demonstrates the lobulated soft tissue mass (*) extending through the right jugular foramen. Multiple flow voids (*concave arrows*) are again well seen within the mass. Basilar artery (b); bilateral third CNs (*straight arrows*).

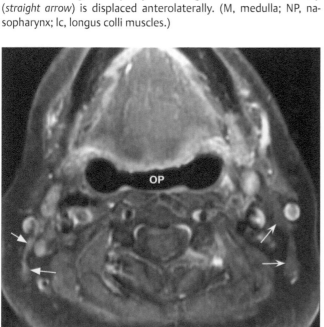

Fig. 11.19 Axial post-gadolinium T1-weighted image with fat saturation in the same patient at the level of the oropharynx (OP) and lower mandible demonstrates atrophy and mild diffuse enhancement of the right sternocleidomastoid muscle (*straight arrows*). The left sternocleidomastoid muscle (*concave arrows*) is normal. Note: the oropharynx has a patulous appearance due to the presence of an esophageal mask as the patient was imaged under anesthesia.

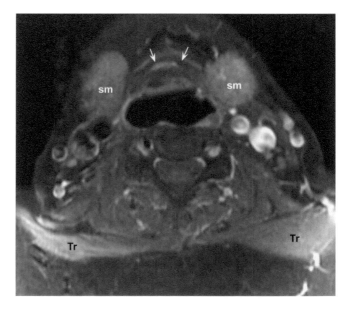

Fig. 11.20 Axial post-gadolinium T1-weighted image with fat saturation in the same patient more inferiorly in the neck shows volume loss and moderate diffuse enhancement of the right trapezius muscle as compared with the left. These changes are consistent with subacute denervation change in the sternocleidomastoid and trapezius muscles in this patient with a large glomus jugulare tumor and lower CN compression. Trapezius muscles (Tr); submandibular glands (sm); and hyoid bone (*arrows*) are identified.

Case 11.4

A 34-year-old female with known liver hemangioendothelioma presents with pain behind the left ear and left jugular foramen syndrome (CNs IX, X, and XI palsies) (**Figs. 11.21, 11.22, 11.23, 11.24**).

Diagnosis

Skull base metastasis

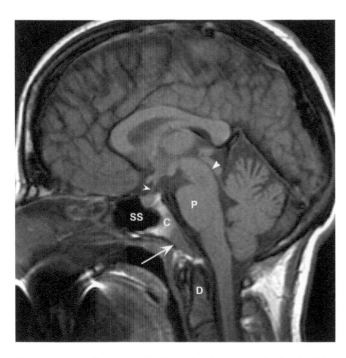

Fig. 11.21 Midline sagittal T1-weighted image at the level of the sella turcica, pituitary stalk (*concave arrowhead*) and aqueduct of Sylvius (*notched arrowhead*) demonstrates abnormal low signal in the inferior aspect of the clivus (*arrow*). Note the normal, bright fatty marrow within the clivus (C) more superiorly. Low signal is also seen in the upper cervical spine including the dens (D) of the C-2 vertebra. These findings are suggestive of marrow infiltration by a neoplastic process such as osseous metastatic disease or lymphoma, or perhaps an infectious or inflammatory process such as chronic osteomyelitis. No nasopharyngeal mass is seen to suggest nasopharyngeal carcinoma. (P, pons; SS, sphenoid sinus.)

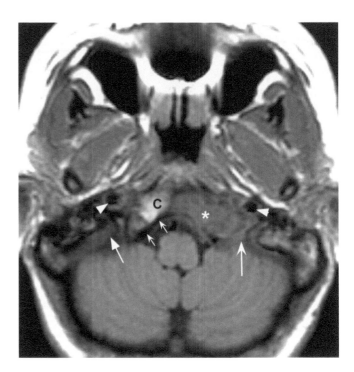

Fig. 11.22 Axial T1-weighted image in the same patient through the skull base at the level of the lower clivus (C) shows an asymmetric soft tissue mass (*) centered in the left clivus and extending into the adjacent left jugular foramen (*concave arrow*). The mass abuts but does not encase the left internal carotid artery (*arrowheads*, bilaterally). Near complete absence of the posterior cortex of the left clivus is present and is suggestive of an aggressive lesion. This appearance can be compared with the normal dark cortical line of the posterior clivus on the right side (*small concave arrows*). The appearance of the right jugular foramen is normal, as the sigmoid sinus courses down toward the jugular bulb (*straight arrow*).

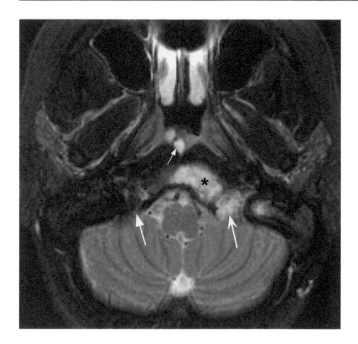

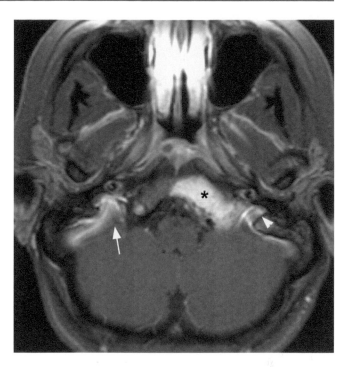

Fig. 11.23 Axial T2-weighted image with fat saturation at the same level shows that the process involving the left clivus (*) and jugular foramen (*concave arrow*) is high in signal intensity. Normal low signal is seen in the right jugular foramen (*straight arrow*). A small, bright benign-appearing cyst is incidentally noted in the nasopharynx (*small straight arrow*).

Fig. 11.24 Axial postcontrast T1-weighted image with fat saturation at the same level demonstrates intense enhancement of the mass (*). Enhancing tumor extends into the anterior aspect of the left jugular foramen and abuts the left jugular vein (*arrowhead*). The normal right sigmoid sinus and jugular bulb (*white arrow*) are shown on the right. This lesion subsequently progressed and was eventually confirmed to represent a hemangioendothelioma metastasis to the skull base.

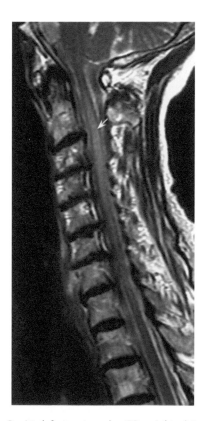

Fig. 11.25 Sagittal fast spin echo T2-weighted image demonstrates diffuse high signal intensity (*arrow*) involving the right side of the cervical spinal cord from the C-2 to approximately T-1 levels.

Case 11.5

A 58-year-old female presents with several-day onset of progressive right-sided weakness and hyperreflexia. On examination, she is also noted to have weakness of head turning to the left and right shoulder elevation (**Figs. 11.25, 11.26, 11.27, 11.28**).

Diagnosis

The patient responded to high-dose steroids. Therefore, the presumptive diagnosis is an acute demyelinating syndrome, likely acute disseminated encephalomyelitis (ADEM).

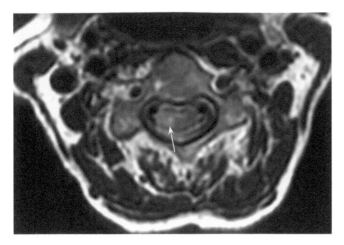

Fig. 11.26 Axial fast spin echo T2-weighted image at the C-3 level demonstrates high signal intensity (*arrow*) in the right lateral aspect of the spinal cord. The right side of the cord is mildly swollen as well.

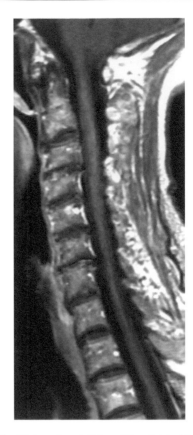

Fig. 11.27 Sagittal post-gadolinium T1-weighted image demonstrates moderate diffuse enhancement of the cervical spinal cord.

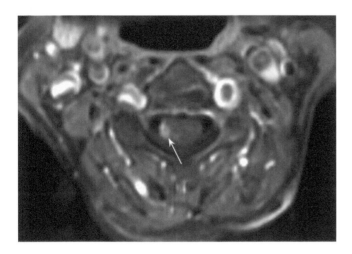

Fig. 11.28 Axial post-gadolinium T1-weighted image confirms enhancement of the right lateral aspect of the spinal cord (*arrow*). The imaging appearance is nonspecific, but inflammatory or demyelinating conditions would be most likely. Other considerations could include vasculitis or infectious myelitis, or perhaps a paraneoplastic condition. Sarcoidosis could also be considered. Clinically this patient was diagnosed with acute disseminated encephalomyelitis (ADEM).

12 Hypoglossal Nerve

Functions

- General somatic efferent (GSE). Somatic motor to all the intrinsic muscles of the tongue (longitudinal, transverse, and vertical muscle bundles) and all of the extrinsic muscles of the tongue (hyoglossus, genioglossus, styloglossus) except palatoglossus (innervated by cranial nerve [CN] X).

Anatomy

- Fibers arise from the *hypoglossal nucleus* in the posterior paramedian medulla beneath the *hypoglossal eminence* of the floor of the fourth ventricle. The hypoglossal nucleus extends nearly the entire craniocaudal extent of the medulla (**Figs. 12.1, 12.2**). Hypoglossal rootlets travel ventrolaterally within the medullary reticular formation, lateral to the medial longitudinal fasciculus and medial lemniscus, and emerge from the medulla at the preolivary (anterior lateral) sulcus between the inferior olive and the pyramid. In the premedullary cistern, the 10 to 15 small hypoglossal rootlets lie in close proximity to the intracranial vertebral artery, converge into two nerve bundles, and penetrate the dura to enter the bony hypoglossal canal (**Fig. 12.3**) inferior and medial to the jugular foramen.
- After passing through the hypoglossal canal, the hypoglossal nerve turns sharply inferiorly. It then enters and runs for several centimeters in the carotid sheath medial to CNs IX/X/XI, which have exited the jugular foramen and entered the carotid space. The hypoglossal nerve descends between the internal carotid artery (ICA) and the internal jugular vein (IJV) in the nasopharyngeal carotid space to the level of the transverse process of the atlas, where it turns forward along the lateral surface of the ICA and the external carotid artery (ECA), entering the digastric triangle of the neck above the level of the hyoid bone and deep to the posterior belly of the digastric muscle. Here it ramifies into *muscular branches* that supply most of the extrinsic muscles of the tongue (styloglossus, hyoglossus, and genioglossus) before supplying all of the intrinsic muscles of the tongue (longitudinal, transverse, and vertical muscles) (**Fig. 12.4**).
- In its course, the hypoglossal nerve travels with fibers from the nodose ganglion of the vagus nerve, postganglionic sympathetic fibers from the superior cervical ganglion, and fibers from C1 (**Fig. 12.4**). As CN XII crosses the ICA, most of the fibers from C1 separate from CN XII and course inferiorly as the *descending hypoglossal ramus* (*descendens hypoglossi*) (superior root of the ansa hypoglossi); this unites with the descending cervical ramus (inferior root of the ansa hypoglossi), which consists of fibers from C2 and C3 (**Fig. 12.4**). The *ansa hypoglossi* provides motor innervation to three infrahyoid strap muscles (sternohyoid, sternothyroid, and omohyoid). The other strap muscle (thyrohyoid) and the geniohyoid muscle are innervated by C1 fibers that initially travel

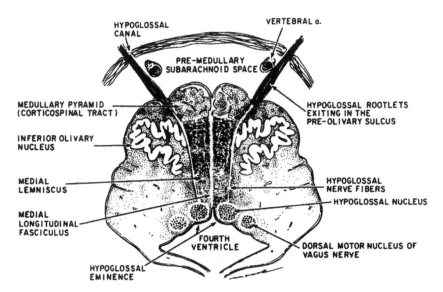

Fig. 12.1 Cross-sectional diagram of the lower medulla. The hypoglossal nucleus lies in the floor of the fourth ventricle. The slight bulge into the fourth ventricle is termed the *hypoglossal eminence*. Hypoglossal rootlets project ventrally through the medulla to emerge in the preolivary sulcus. Note the proximity of the cisternal portion of the hypoglossal nerve to the vertebral artery. (From Smoker WRK. The hypoglossal nerve. Neuroimaging Clin North Am 1993;3:193-206. Reprinted with permission.)

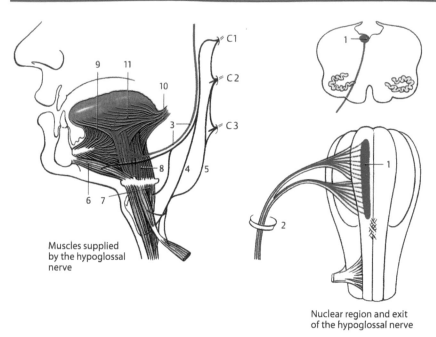

Fig. 12.2 Hypoglossal nerve. (1, nucleus of the hypoglossal nerve; 2, hypoglossal canal; 3, hypoglossal nerve; 4, descending hypoglossal ramus of cervical plexus; 5, descending cervical ramus of cervical plexus; 6, geniohyoid muscle; 7, thyrohyoid muscle; 8, hyoglossus; 9, genioglossus; 10, styloglossus; 11, intrinsic muscles of the tongue.)

Muscles supplied by the hypoglossal nerve

Nuclear region and exit of the hypoglossal nerve

with the main trunk of CN XII and are not part of the ansa (**Fig. 12.4**).

- Summary of submandibular region/strap muscle innervation (**Table 12.1**).

- Supranuclear control of CN XII is via corticobulbar fibers from the lower precentral gyrus. There is bilateral supranuclear innervation of all CN XII–innervated muscles except for the genioglossus, which is crossed and unilateral.

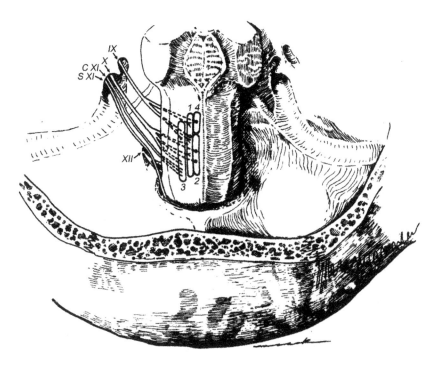

Fig. 12.3 Nuclear origins and cisternal courses of glossopharyngeal, vagus, and spinal accessory nerves. Note that the glossopharyngeal nerve traverses the more anterior part of the jugular foramen (*pars nervosa*), whereas the vagus and spinal accessory nerves pass through the posterior part (*pars vascularis*). The hypoglossal nerve is shown exiting through the more inferiorly located hypoglossal canal. (1, nucleus solitarius; 2, dorsal motor nucleus of CN X; 3, nucleus ambiguus; 4, superior salivatory nucleus; C XI, cranial root of CN XI; S XI, spinal root of CN XI.) (From Harnsberger HR. Handbook of Head and Neck Imaging (2nd ed.) St. Louis, MO: Mosby, 1995. Reprinted with permission.)

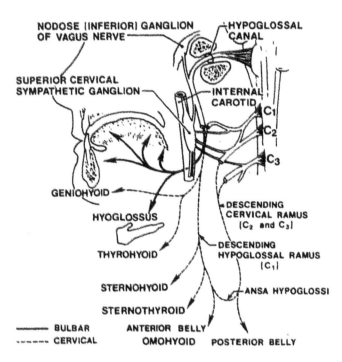

Fig. 12.4 Peripheral connections of the hypoglossal nerve. Note the communication of the hypoglossal nerve with fibers from C1, the nodose ganglion of the vagus nerve, and the superior cervical (sympathetic) ganglion. Structures supplied by the hypoglossal nerve are indicated by solid lines, whereas those supplied by fibers of cervical origin are indicated by dashed lines. The hypoglossal nerve provides motor innervation to the extrinsic (hyoglossus, styloglossus, and genioglossus) and intrinsic muscles of the tongue. Note the ansa hypoglossi, formed by the descending hypoglossal and cervical rami. See text for details. (From Smoker WRK. The hypoglossal nerve. Neuroimaging Clin North Am 1993;3:193-206. Reprinted with permission.)

Table 12.1 Summary of Tongue, Submandibular, and Strap Muscle Innervation

Muscle	Innervation
Mylohyoid	V_3
Digastric, anterior belly	V_3
Digastric, posterior belly	VII
Stylohyoid	VII
Palatoglossus	X (via pharyngeal plexus)
Styloglossus	XII
Hyoglossus	XII
Genioglossus	XII
Intrinsic tongue muscles	XII
Geniohyoid	C1 (*not* via ansa hypoglossi)
Thyrohyoid	C1 (*not* via ansa hypoglossi)
Sternohyoid	Ansa hypoglossi (C1–C3)
Sternothyroid	Ansa hypoglossi (C1–C3)
Omohyoid	Ansa hypoglossi (C1–C3)

Hypoglossal Nerve: Normal Images (Figs. 12.5, 12.6, 12.7, 12.8, 12.9)

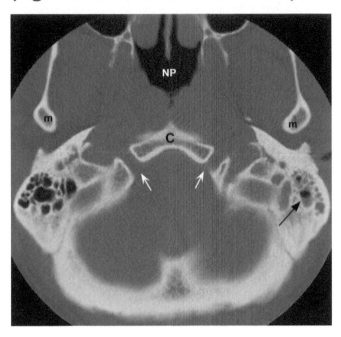

Fig. 12.5 Axial CT image in bone window at the level of the hypoglossal canals (*white arrows*). Also shown are clivus (C), nasopharyngeal airway (NP), and inferior aspect of the mandibular condyles (m). A small amount of fluid is incidentally noted in the left mastoid air cells (*black arrow*).

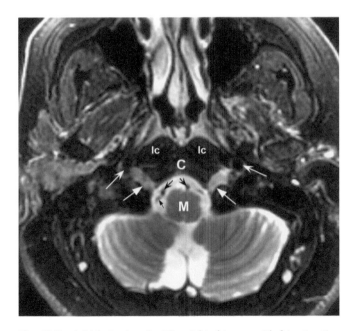

Fig. 12.6 Axial fast spin echo T2-weighted image with fat saturation at a similar level as in Fig. 12.5. Normal somewhat high signal is noted within the hypoglossal canals bilaterally (*straight white arrows*). Normal flow voids adjacent to the medulla (M) represent the vertebral arteries (*concave black arrows*). A smaller flow void (*straight black arrow*) posterolateral to the right vertebral artery represents the posterior inferior cerebellar artery (PICA) arising from the adjacent vertebral artery. Anterolateral to the hypoglossal canal are flow voids within the internal carotid arteries (*concave white arrows*). (C, clivus; lc, longus colli muscles.)

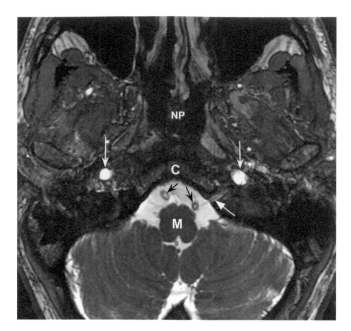

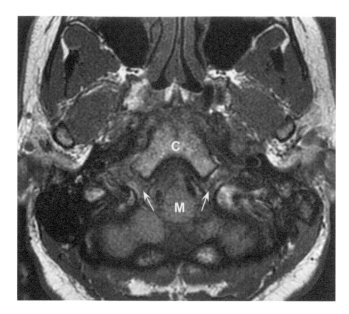

Fig. 12.7 An axial high-resolution fast imaging employing steady-state acquisition (FIESTA) image at the level of the medulla (M) demonstrates the left hypoglossal nerve as it enters the hypoglossal canal (*straight white arrow*). Normal vertebral arteries (*black arrows*) are present within the premedullary cistern. Normal T2 hyperintensity is seen within the internal carotid arteries bilaterally (*concave white arrows*). (C, clivus; NP, nasopharynx.)

Fig. 12.8 Axial T1-weighted image at the level of the medulla (M) demonstrates normal intermediate signal within the hypoglossal canals (*arrows*). (C, clivus.)

Hypoglossal Nerve Lesions

Evaluation

- Observation of the tongue at rest and with protrusion and movement is necessary. Examination of tongue movement to the left and right against resistance may also be performed.
- The key to understanding which way the tongue will deviate with lesions is to understand the normal action of the genioglossus muscle, which is to draw the root of the tongue forward and cause it to protrude. Therefore, a unilaterally weak genioglossus muscle will lead to imbalance and deviation of the tongue toward the *weak side* on protrusion.
- Supranuclear upper motor neuron (UMN) pathology affecting hypoglossal function results in paresis of the contralateral genioglossus muscle, with resulting deviation of the tongue *away from* the side of the lesion (*toward* the side of the paretic genioglossus muscle).
- Nuclear (brainstem) and unilateral lower motor nerve (LMN) lesions result in ipsilateral hemitongue paresis, atrophy, fibrillations, and fasciculations. There is deviation of the tongue *toward* the side of the lesion (again, *toward* the side of the paretic genioglossus muscle).
- *Dysarthria* is impaired speech due to abnormal neuromuscular control, manifest as abnormalities of articulation, prosody, resonance, and phonation. Particular difficulty with lingual consonants (D, T, L) is seen with hypoglossal pathology.
- Unilateral hypoglossal palsy leads to paresis, atrophy, fibrillations, and fasciculations in the affected half of the

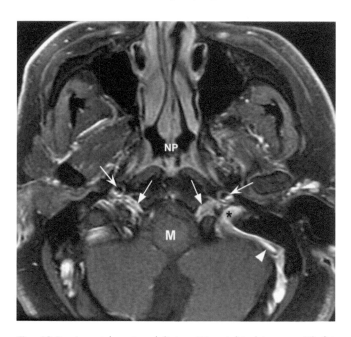

Fig. 12.9 An axial post-gadolinium T1-weighted image with fat saturation at a similar level shows normal symmetric enhancement within the hypoglossal canals (*straight arrows*), predominantly due to enhancement of normal venous structures such as the anterior condylar veins. Normal enhancement is noted within the left sigmoid sinus (*arrowhead*) extending into the internal jugular vein. The left jugular foramen (*) is shown, located posterior and lateral to the hypoglossal canal. The internal carotid arteries are seen as flow voids (*concave arrows*) anterolateral to the hypoglossal canals. (M, medulla; NP, nasopharynx.)

tongue and mild dysarthria. Bilateral lesions result in bilateral tongue atrophy, weakness, and fibrillations, and severe dysarthria and dysphagia. Oropharyngeal airway compromise may occur due to tongue flaccidity.

Types

Supranuclear Lesions

- Occur from the level of the precentral gyrus to the hypoglossal nucleus (e.g., ischemic infarction).
- UMN hypoglossal deficit (described above) is typically associated with other neurologic findings (most commonly hemiparesis/hemiplegia).
- Not usually associated with atrophy/fasciculations/fibrillations.
- *Spastic dysarthria* may result from poor supranuclear control of the tongue.
- Bilateral supranuclear lesions (e.g., *pseudobulbar palsy* from repeated infarctions) may lead to bilateral tongue paralysis and severe dysarthria.

Nuclear Lesions

- Rare to cause CN XII palsy in isolation.
- Unilateral lesions result in a unilateral LMN syndrome (described above).
- Causes of nuclear injury include the following:
  - Vascular. *Medial medullary syndrome* (Dejerine anterior bulbar syndrome), due to occlusion of vertebral or anterior spinal artery. This involves the ipsilateral pyramid, medial lemniscus, and hypoglossal nucleus, and results in ipsilateral LMN palsy of CN XII as well as contralateral hemiplegia and loss of position/vibratory sensation (with facial sparing). See Appendix A.
  - Infectious/inflammatory (e.g., infectious mononucleosis, bulbar poliomyelitis).
  - Neoplasm (e.g., brainstem glioma).
  - Demyelinating disease (e.g., multiple sclerosis [MS]).
  - Neurodegenerative disease (e.g., progressive bulbar palsy).
  - Syringobulbia.

Premedullary Subarachnoid Space and Hypoglossal Canal Lesions

- Result in unilateral LMN syndrome.
- Often involve adjacent CNs (IX, X, XI) (e.g., Collet-Sicard syndrome: IX–XII palsies).
- Causes of injury include the following:
  - Neoplasms (e.g., hypoglossal schwannoma, meningioma, skull base metastasis, extension of jugular foramen lesions such as paraganglioma. Also, nasopharyngeal carcinoma and other head and neck malignancies may extend posteriorly to the lower clivus and hypoglossal canal.).

  - Trauma (e.g., occipital condyle fracture or basal skull fracture through the hypoglossal canal).
  - Infection (e.g., skull base osteomyelitis may affect CN XII, often in association with other CN palsies).
  - Vascular (e.g., vertebral dissection or dolichoectasia).

Extracranial Lesions

- Proximal extracranial lesions may involve vessels (ICA and IJV) and other lower CNs (IX, X, XI) as they travel together in the upper carotid space.
- Lesions within the carotid space:
  - Vascular (e.g., ICA aneurysm or dissection)
  - Infectious/inflammatory (e.g., neck abscess, tuberculosis, rheumatoid arthritis)
  - Iatrogenic (e.g., IJV puncture, carotid endarterectomy, postradiation)
  - Neoplasm (e.g., squamous cell carcinoma, non-Hodgkin lymphoma, paraganglioma, schwannoma, sarcoma, metastasis)
  - Trauma (e.g., knife or gunshot wound)
- If strap muscle function is also affected, then the localization of the lesion is distal to where the hypoglossal nerve is joined by the C1 fibers extracranially. Strap muscle function is best tested by attempted downward movement of the jaw against resistance.
- Lesions within the sublingual space and tongue:
  - Neoplasm (typically squamous cell carcinoma arising from base of tongue or floor of mouth)
  - Infection (odontogenic abscess involving the sublingual space)
  - Iatrogenic (e.g., from floor of mouth surgery)

Hypoglossal Nerve: Pathologic Images

Case 12.1

A 51-year-old female presented with vertigo and dysarthria, and on examination her tongue was found to deviate to the left (**Fig. 12.10**).

Diagnosis

Cavernous malformation of dorsal medulla

Cavernous Malformation

- *Epidemiology.* Peak age of presentation is 20 to 40 years of age. Supratentorial (~70%) or infratentorial (~30%) (cerebellum, pons). Spinal cord involvement is rare. Most are sporadic, but several genes have so far been identified (*CCM1–CCM4*).
- *Clinical presentation.* Most are asymptomatic, but they can present with seizures, focal neurologic deficits (de-

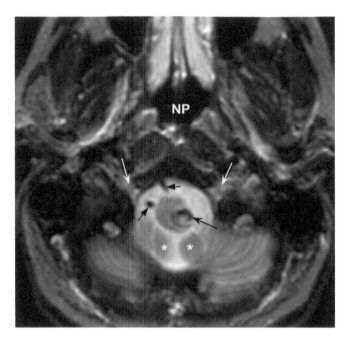

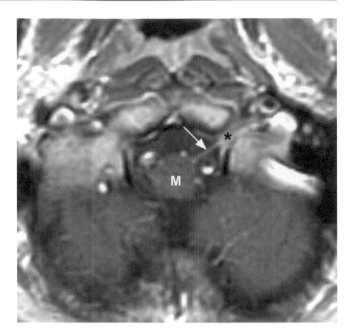

Fig. 12.10 An axial T2-weighted image through the lower skull base at level of the nasopharynx (NP), hypoglossal canals (*white concave arrows*), and cerebellar tonsils (*) demonstrates a round, somewhat heterogeneous, peripherally hypointense lesion within the left dorsolateral medulla at the approximate level of the hypoglossal nucleus and traversing hypoglossal nerve fibers. Peripheral dark signal (*black concave arrow*) around the lesion is consistent with the peripheral hemosiderin rim of a cavernous malformation. Flow voids adjacent to the medulla represent the normal vertebral arteries (*black straight arrows*). A cavernous malformation was confirmed at surgery.

Fig. 12.11 A slightly oblique axial postcontrast T1-weighted image with fat saturation at the level of the left hypoglossal canal demonstrates linear enhancement along the cisternal segment of the left hypoglossal nerve (*arrow*) as it extends from the medulla (M) to the hypoglossal canal (*). This patient was subsequently diagnosed with Lyme disease and this finding is consistent with hypoglossal neuritis.

pending on location), and hemorrhage. Risk of hemorrhage is 0.5 to 1% per year. Risk may be higher in patients with previous hemorrhages, posterior fossa lesions, and familial inheritance.

- *Imaging.* Computed tomography (CT) often negative but may demonstrate acute hemorrhage or calcification. Magnetic resonance imaging (MRI) shows characteristic *"popcorn"* lesion on T2-weighted image with heterogeneous mixed signal centrally and a dark rim of hemosiderin. May be hyperintense or isointense on T1-weighted images depending on age of blood products. Gradient-echo sequences are most sensitive for finding smaller lesions due to "blooming" effects of hemorrhage. Postcontrast images show little or no enhancement although there may be an associated developmental venous anomaly (venous angioma). Angiography (including CTA and MRA) is normal.
- *Pathology.* Multilobulated berry-like structures filled with blood of different ages. Composed of closely approximated endothelial-lined sinusoidal spaces, no feeding artery, and *multiple thin-walled vessels without intervening normal brain tissue*. Frequent calcifications.

- *Treatment.* Options include conservative management (e.g., anticonvulsant therapy for cavernous malformation that are causing seizures but that have not hemorrhaged), radiosurgery, and surgical removal.

Case 12.2

A 33-year-old HIV+ male presents with fever, stiff neck, right facial weakness, and dysarthria. On examination his tongue deviated to the left. His CD4 count is 1200, viral load is 0, and his history is notable for recent hiking (**Fig. 12.11**).

Diagnosis

Lyme disease. See Case 9.3, Chapter 9 for more information about Lyme disease.

Case 12.3

A 30-year-old female presents with progressive onset of reduced hearing, vertigo, dysarthria, and dysphagia (**Figs. 12.12, 12.13, 12.14**).

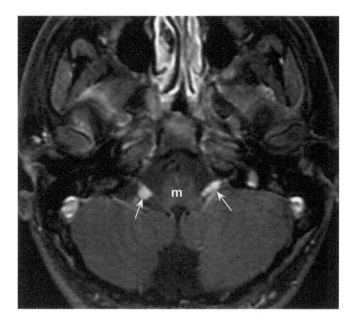

Fig. 12.12 An axial postcontrast T1-weighted image with fat saturation at the level of the medulla (m) demonstrates enhancing masses (*arrows*) along the cisternal segments of the hypoglossal nerves bilaterally.

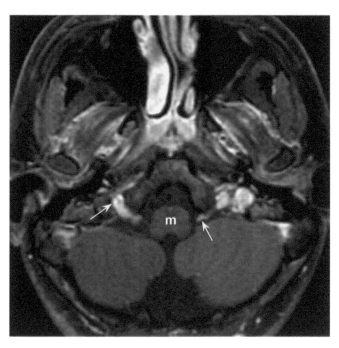

Fig. 12.13 More inferiorly, an axial postcontrast T1-weighted image with fat saturation shows the bilateral enhancing masses entering and traversing the hypoglossal canals (*arrows*). (m, medulla.)

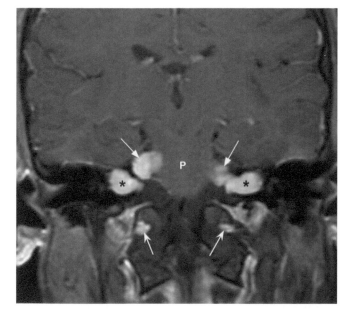

Fig. 12.14 A coronal postcontrast T1-weighted image with fat saturation through the pons (P) in the same patient shows the bilateral homogeneously enhancing hypoglossal nerve masses within the hypoglossal canals (*concave arrows*). Additional enhancing masses are seen within both internal auditory canals (*) and lateral to the pons along the trigeminal nerves (*straight arrows*). Patient has known diagnosis of NF-2 with multiple schwannomas.

Diagnosis

Bilateral CN XII schwannomas in a patient with a known diagnosis of neurofibromatosis type 2 (NF-2).

Case 12.4

A 37-year-old female presents with dysarthria. On physical examination, a mass in the nasopharynx is noted as well as a right CN XII palsy (**Fig. 12.15, 12.16**).

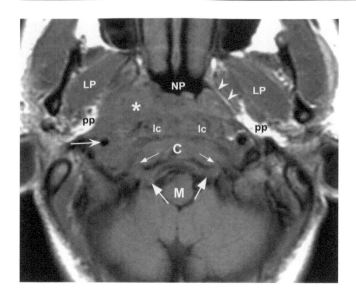

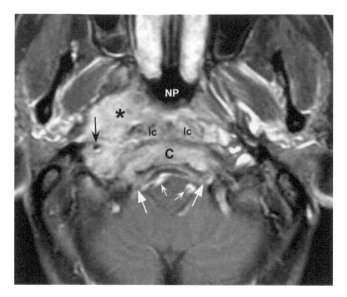

Fig. 12.15 An axial T1-weighted image through the skull base demonstrates an infiltrative soft tissue mass (*) centered in the posterolateral right nasopharynx (NP) that effaces the normal fat planes lateral and posterior to the nasopharynx. A normal fat plane is seen on the left (*arrowheads*). The partially effaced right parapharyngeal fat (pp) is indicated, as is the normal left parapharyngeal fat. The mass encases the right internal carotid artery (*concave arrow*) and extends posteriorly to invade the longus colli muscles (lc) and clivus (C). There is loss of the normal cortical bone that forms the anteromedial border of the hypoglossal canals (*small straight arrows*). The right hypoglossal canal and nerve are infiltrated and expanded by soft tissue. Abnormal soft tissue is also seen within the retroclival epidural space (*large straight arrows*) ventral to the medulla (M). Also indicated are the lateral pterygoid muscles (LP).

Fig. 12.16 An axial postcontrast T1-weighted image with fat saturation at the same level shows moderate enhancement of the infiltrative nasopharyngeal mass (*), which is again seen to invade the longus colli muscles (lc) and clivus (C) and to encase the right internal carotid artery (*black arrow*). Enhancing tissue extends into the retroclival epidural space and right hypoglossal canal and approaches the left hypoglossal canal (*white straight arrows*). The bilateral vertebral arteries are indicated (*small concave arrows*). Biopsy proved nasopharyngeal carcinoma. (NP, nasopharynx.)

Diagnosis

Nasopharyngeal carcinoma with extension into the right hypoglossal canal. See Case 5.8, Chapter 5 for more information about nasopharyngeal carcinoma.

Case 12.5

A 75-year-old female with diabetes and otitis externa presents with left facial and ear pain, difficulty swallowing, and tongue deviation to the left (**Figs. 12.17, 12.18, 12.19, 12.20, 12.21, 12.22, 12.23**).

Diagnosis

Skull base osteomyelitis affecting CN XII

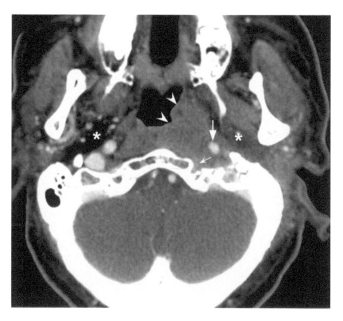

Fig. 12.17 An axial postcontrast CT image through the lower skull base shows asymmetric soft tissue swelling in the left nasopharynx, with bulging of the left lateral pharyngeal wall medially (*arrowheads*). There is preservation of the smooth mucosal contour of the nasopharyngeal surface. Fat within the parapharyngeal space (*) is effaced and infiltrated on the left and normal on the right. Abnormal soft tissue extends posteriorly on the left to encase the left internal carotid artery (*straight arrow*) and extend into the left hypoglossal canal (*concave arrow*).

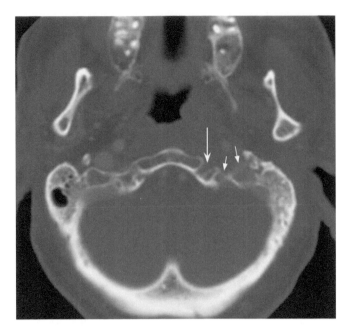

Fig. 12.18 An axial CT image at the same level in bone window demonstrates subtle erosion of the occipital bone (*small straight arrows*) lateral to the left hypoglossal canal (*concave arrow*). This can also be seen in **Fig. 12.17**, but is better assessed on the dedicated bone window.

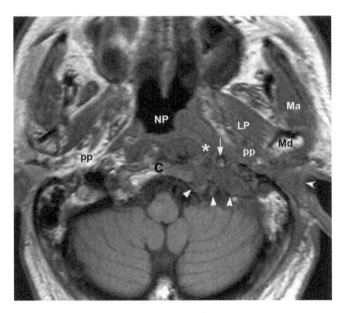

Fig. 12.19 An axial T1-weighted image at a similar level through the lower skull base and nasopharynx (NP) shows asymmetric infiltrative soft tissue (*) deep to the left nasopharyngeal mucosal surface that encases the left internal carotid artery (*straight arrow*) and effaces the left parapharyngeal fat (pp). There is extension into the skull base with intermediate signal intensity tissue replacing the normal fatty marrow of the left clivus (C). Abnormal soft tissue also extends into the left hypoglossal canal and jugular foramen (*straight arrowheads*). Soft tissue fullness is also seen posterior to the left mandibular condyle (Md) at the level of the external ear (*concave arrowhead*). (LP, lateral pterygoid muscle; Ma, masseter muscle.)

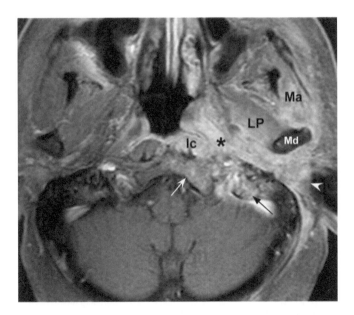

Fig. 12.20 An axial postcontrast T1-weighted image with fat-saturation at a similar level shows marked asymmetric enhancement throughout the left submucosal nasopharyngeal (*) and parapharyngeal soft tissues. There is posterior extension into the left longus colli muscle (lc) and marrow enhancement within the left clivus (*white concave arrow*) and occipitomastoid bone (*black concave arrow*). Diffuse enhancement is also seen throughout the left masticator space surrounding the mandibular condyle (Md) and involving the lateral pterygoid (LP) and masseter (Ma) muscles, as well as extending laterally into the external ear canal (*arrowhead*) and subcutaneous fat.

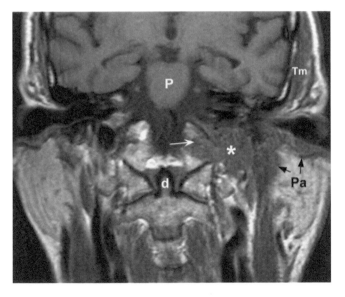

Fig. 12.21 A coronal T1-weighted image through the upper neck at the level of the odontoid (d), ventral pons (P), and hypoglossal canals (*concave arrow*) demonstrates asymmetric soft tissue (*) infiltrating the left skull base and adjacent soft tissues. Abnormal soft tissue (*black straight arrows*) is also seen medial and superior to the left parotid gland (Pa), with the superior soft tissue involving the floor of the left external auditory canal. The left temporalis muscle (Tm) in the suprazygomatic masticator space is asymmetrically thickened, consistent with edema and inflammation.

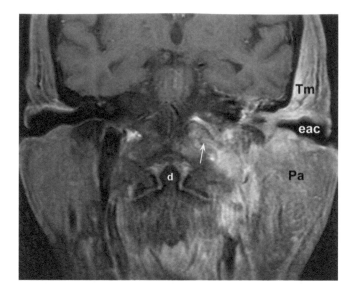

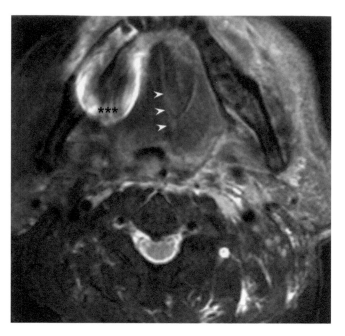

Fig. 12.22 A coronal postcontrast T1-weighted image with fat saturation at a similar level shows diffuse enhancement throughout the left upper neck and deep spaces of the left face with skull base involvement. Marrow enhancement is seen around the left hypoglossal canal (*concave arrow*). There is thickening and enhancement of tissue along the left external auditory canal, causing it to be narrow compared with the right. Enhancement and swelling of the left temporalis muscle (Tm) and enlargement and enhancement of the parotid gland are consistent with myositis and parotitis, respectively. The diffuse infiltrative nature of this process in association with the lack of a dominant mass as well as involvement of the external auditory canal are most consistent with a diagnosis of skull base osteomyelitis secondary to external otitis. (eac, external auditory canal; d, odontoid.)

Fig. 12.23 An axial T2-weighted image with fat saturation in the same patient, who clinically had a left CN XII palsy. This image shows diffuse edema with T2 hyperintensity involving the left parotid, masticator, and perivertebral spaces, as well as the subcutaneous fat on the left. A bright artifact (***) due to nonremovable dental work obscures parts of the right mandible and hemitongue. The left hemitongue is mildly hyperintense compared with the right. In addition, the lingual septum (*arrowheads*) deviates to the left, and the posterior aspect of the left hemitongue has prolapsed back into the oropharynx. These changes are consistent with subacute denervation of the left hemitongue.

Clinical Pearl

The nomenclature related to skull base osteomyelitis (SBO) can be confusing. *Otitis externa* refers to a soft tissue infection of the EAC without bony involvement. *Malignant otitis externa* has been used in the past to refer to an infection involving both the EAC and the surrounding marrow-containing spaces of the base of skull, but this term has largely been replaced by the preferred term *skull base osteomyelitis*. SBO typically originates from otitis externa in older diabetic patients, but it may also originate from sphenoid sinus disease or hematogenous sources. SBO may spread to involve the parotid gland, temporomandibular joint (TMJ), mastoid and stylomastoid foramen, and the region of the jugular foramen and/or hypoglossal canal. Common organ-isms responsible for SBO include *Pseudomonas aeruginosa* (particularly in diabetic patients), *Staphylococcus aureus*, *S. epidermidis*, *Proteus*, *Salmonella*, and *Aspergillus* (in immunocompromised patients). Clinical presentation may include otalgia, headache, otorrhea, hearing loss and/or ear fullness, and variable CN involvement. The peripheral white blood cell (WBC) count may be normal but the erythrocyte sedimentation rate (ESR) is usually markedly elevated. The mainstay of treatment is long-term antimicrobial therapy after specific microbiologic diagnosis. Surgical debridement may be required in selected cases unresponsive to antibiotic therapy or for tissue diagnosis and culture. Hyperbaric oxygen has been used as adjunctive therapy for refractory cases.

Imaging Pearl

CT and MRI typically show soft tissue infiltration of the fat-containing marrow spaces of the bones of the skull base and sometimes associated bone erosion and destruction. Skull base osteomyelitis is a marrow-space process, not an air-space process like more typical otitis media or otomastoiditis. Bone destruction may be lytic or sclerotic depending on the aggressiveness of the organism and age of the process. Subacute or chronic infections may lead to more sclerosis and hypertrophic bone reaction. The margins of the soft tissue process are often ill-defined and associated with edema and inflammatory changes. CT is the best modality for identifying osseous destruction, but MRI is far better for showing the extent of marrow space and soft tissue involvement and is often necessary to determine intracranial invasion as well as orbital and cavernous sinus involvement. MR is definitely the study of choice when SBO is being considered in the differential diagnosis. Technetium and gallium nuclear medicine scans have also been used to assess skull base involvement and can be helpful in monitoring disease activity during the course of extended antibiotic therapy.

Case 12.6

A 59-year-old female presents with a 4-month history of mild dysarthria, pulsatile tinnitus, and an audible bruit. On examination, her tongue deviates slightly to the left (**Figs. 12.24, 12.25, 12.26, 12.27**).

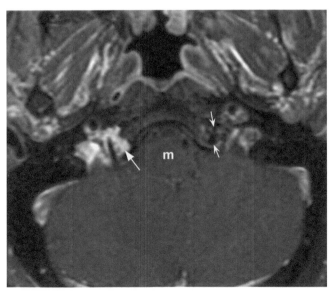

Fig. 12.25 An axial postcontrast T1-weighted image with fat saturation at the same level demonstrates asymmetry of the hypoglossal canals, but no evidence for a mass lesion on the left. Normal venous enhancement of the hypoglossal canal is seen on the right side (*straight arrow*). Within the left hypoglossal canal, multiple flow voids (*concave arrows*) are again appreciated. (m, medulla.)

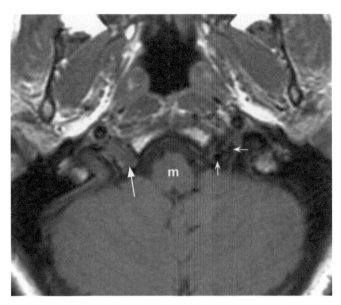

Fig. 12.24 An axial T1-weighted image at the level of the medulla (m) and hypoglossal canals (*straight arrow* on right) demonstrates heterogeneity of signal within the left hypoglossal canal as compared with homogeneous intermediate signal intensity on the right. Multiple subtle flow voids (*concave arrows*) are seen, suggesting either a vascular lesion or hypervascular mass.

Diagnosis

Dural arteriovenous fistula (dAVF) at the hypoglossal canal

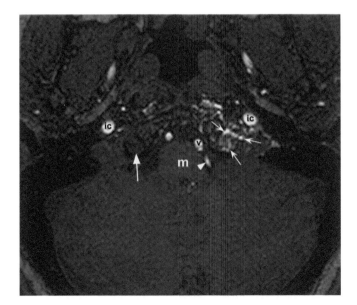

Fig. 12.26 An axial source image from a three-dimensional time-of-flight intracranial MR angiogram at a similar level shows numerous tiny vessels (*concave arrows*) within and around the left hypoglossal canal when compared with the normal right hypoglossal canal (*straight arrow*). Normal high signal due to flow-related enhancement is seen within the bilateral internal carotid arteries (ic), vertebral arteries (labeled v on the left) and left posterior inferior cerebellar artery (*arrowhead*). (m, medulla.)

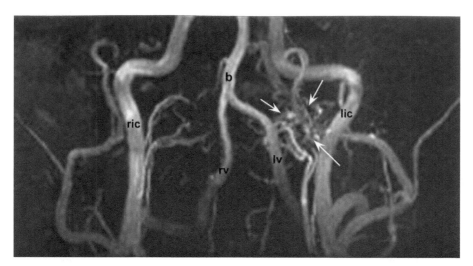

Fig. 12.27 A maximum intensity projection (MIP) image from the same intracranial MR angiogram demonstrates an abnormal cluster of vessels (*concave arrows*) projecting between the left vertebral artery (lv) and left internal carotid artery (lic) at the approximate level of the hypoglossal canal. A dural arteriovenous fistula was suspected, and was subsequently confirmed angiographically and treated endovascularly. (b, basilar artery; ric, right internal carotid artery; rv, right vertebral artery.)

Clinical Pearl

A dAVF is an abnormal direct connection between a meningeal artery and a meningeal vein or dural venous sinus. They are usually acquired although they can occur congenitally, and typically develop after venous sinus thrombosis or trauma. Peak age at presentation is 40 to 60 years of age. Transverse and sigmoid sinuses are common sites. Findings are related to site and size of the fistula as well as the occurrence of any hemorrhage but may include bruit, headache, and pulsatile tinnitus. The *Borden classification* of dAVFs groups them into three types based on venous drainage:

Type 1. Dural arterial supply drains anterograde into venous sinus.

Type 2. Dural arterial supply drains into venous sinus but high pressure in sinus (e.g., due to outflow obstruction) results in both anterograde and retrograde drainage via subarachnoid veins.

Type 3. Dural arterial supply drains only retrograde into subarachnoid veins.

The primary risk factor for hemorrhage from a dAVF is retrograde leptomeningeal/cortical venous drainage. Treatment is directed at obliteration of the fistula, either by endovascular embolization or direct surgical interruption.

Imaging Pearl

The most common sites of skull base dAVFs are the transverse sinus followed by the cavernous sinus. Unenhanced CT is usually normal unless associated with hemorrhage or venous ischemia. Enhanced CT may also be normal although larger dAVFs may show abnormal vessels, and certainly CTA may detect abnormal feeding arteries and abnormal venous sinuses and/or draining veins. Signs of remote trauma (e.g., skull fracture) may be present. On MRI, signs of venous sinus thrombosis (loss of the normal flow void and increased signal within the venous sinus on T1-weighted and/or T2-weighted images) may be the only clue, but a cluster of abnormal flow voids within or around the thrombosed venous sinus may be present and is highly suspicious for dAVF. MRA may show abnormal vessels adjacent to a thrombosed venous sinus and may show enlargement of feeding arteries such as the middle meningeal artery, meningohypophyseal trunk, or the occipital artery. MR venography may be useful to confirm venous sinus thrombosis. However, caution is advised because hypoplastic transverse or sigmoid venous sinuses are a common normal variant. Conventional digital subtraction angiography (DSA) is the "gold standard" for diagnosis of dAVF. DSA is most sensitive for picking up small lesions as well as identifying the flow characteristics of the lesion and pattern of venous drainage.

Case 12.7

A 67-year-old female presents with 1.5 years of tongue weakness and fasciculations (**Figs. 12.28, 12.29, 12.30, 12.31, 12.32, 12.33, 12.34, 12.35**).

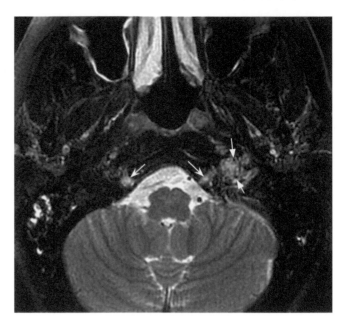

Fig. 12.29 An axial T1-weighted image at the level of the left hypoglossal canal (*straight arrow*) demonstrates asymmetric soft tissue (***) at the distal aspect of the left hypoglossal canal, posterior to the left internal carotid artery (*concave arrow*).

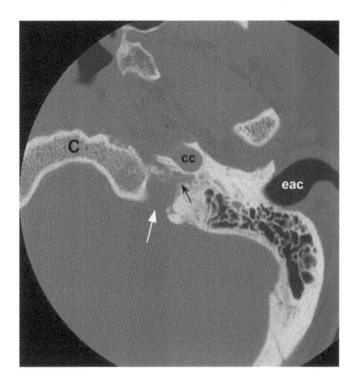

Fig. 12.28 An axial CT image in bone window through the skull base at the level of the left hypoglossal canal (*white arrow*) demonstrates irregular bony erosion (*black arrow*) along the anterolateral cortical margin of the hypoglossal canal immediately posterior to the proximal aspect of the vertical petrous carotid canal (cc), as well as expansion of the hypoglossal canal. (C, clivus; eac, external auditory canal.)

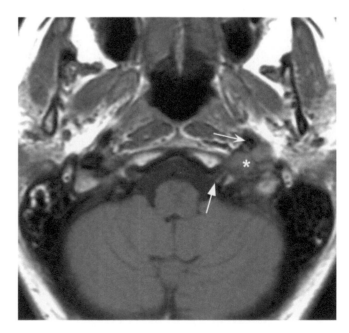

Fig. 12.30 An axial T2-weighted image with fat saturation at a similar level (hypoglossal canals, *concave arrows*) demonstrates a mildly heterogeneous T2 hyperintense soft tissue mass. In addition, scattered small flow voids (*straight arrows*) are present in and around the mass, consistent with hypervascularity of the mass.

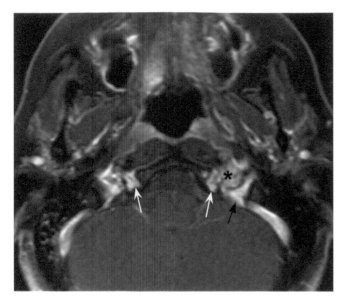

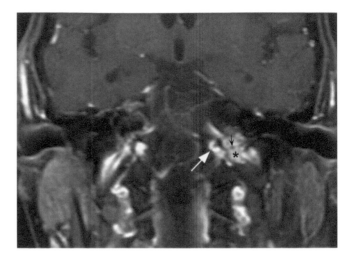

Fig. 12.32 A coronal postcontrast T1-weighted image with fat saturation shows intense enhancement of the mass (*) lateral to normal enhancement within the proximal left hypoglossal canal (*white arrow*). Flow voids are again noted within the lesion (*small black arrow*). A paraganglioma was confirmed surgically.

Fig. 12.31 An axial post-contrast T1-weighted image with fat saturation at a similar level shows intense slightly heterogeneous enhancement of this mass (*) centered at the left hypoglossal canal and just anterior to the left jugular foramen. Normal venous enhancement is seen within the bilateral hypoglossal canals (*white arrows*) and bilateral jugular foramina (*black arrow*).

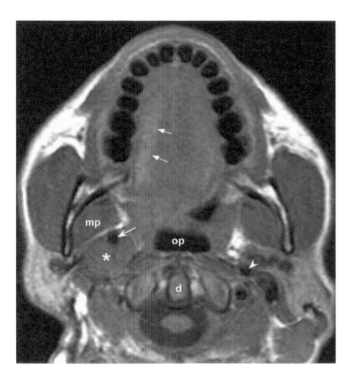

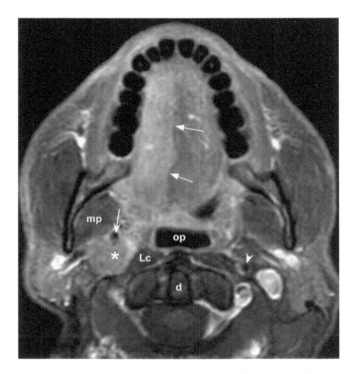

Fig. 12.33 An axial T1-weighted image just below the skull base and caudal to the hypoglossal canal at the level of the tip of the dens (d) and oropharynx (op) demonstrates a homogeneous oval soft tissue mass (*) centered within the right carotid space that displaces the right internal carotid artery (*concave arrow*) anteriorly. The mass is fairly well-defined and isointense to muscle. Fat planes around the adjacent medial pterygoid muscle (mp) are preserved. Faint hyperintensity within the right tongue (*small straight arrows*) is compatible with mild fatty replacement. Left internal carotid artery (*concave arrowhead*).

Fig. 12.34 An axial postcontrast T1-weighted image with fat saturation at the same level shows fairly intense and homogeneous enhancement of the right carotid space mass (*) that displaces the right internal carotid artery (*concave arrow*) anteriorly. The mass abuts and slightly displaces the right longus colli muscle (Lc), but no invasion into muscle or skull base is seen. The right hemitongue shows diffuse enhancement with a sharp demarcation medially (*straight arrows*). Mild lateral deviation from the midline is compatible with right CN XII dysfunction and muscle atrophy. Note the left internal carotid artery (*arrowhead*). (d, tip of dens; op, oropharynx; mp, right medial pterygoid muscle.)

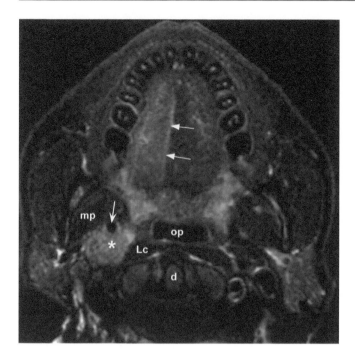

Fig. 12.35 An axial T2-weighted image with fat saturation at the same level shows a mildly hyperintense mass (*) in the right carotid space. Faint hyperintensity within the right hemitongue is compatible with mild edema. The medial margin (*straight arrows*) is sharply demarcated and the midline lingual septum is deviated laterally. Note the right internal carotid artery (*concave arrow*). (d, tip of dens; Lc, longus colli muscles; op, oropharynx; mp, right medial pterygoid muscle.)

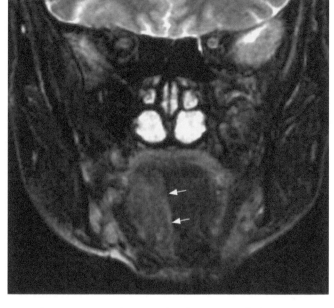

Fig. 12.36 A coronal T2-weighted image with fat saturation through mid tongue shows asymmetry of the tongue with faint hyperintensity and lateral deviation of the right hemitongue (*arrows*) compatible with mild edema and atrophy in the setting of late subacute right hypoglossal nerve denervation changes.

Diagnosis

Paraganglioma involving the hypoglossal canal. Please see Case 10.2, Chapter 10 for more information regarding paragangliomas.

Case 12.8

A 42-year-old female status post prior partial resection of a jugular foramen meningioma now presents with hemitongue weakness, atrophy, and fasciculations (**Fig. 12.36**).

Diagnosis

Residual/recurrent meningioma causing CN XII palsy and subacute denervation changes in the tongue

Case 12.9

A 69-year-old male with metastatic prostate carcinoma presents with left hemitongue weakness and leftward tongue deviation (**Figs. 12.37, 12.38, 12.39**).

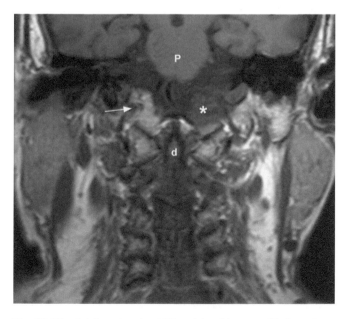

Fig. 12.37 Axial postcontrast T1-weighted image with fat saturation in the same patient shows diffuse volume loss and enhancement throughout the left hemitongue (*) with ipsilateral shift of the lingual septum consistent with subacute denervation changes in this patient with prostate carcinoma metastases.

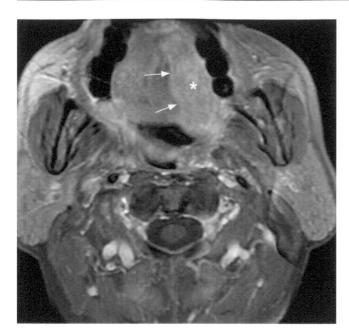

Fig. 12.38 An axial T1-weighted image at the level of the medulla (m) and nasopharynx (NP) demonstrates an infiltrative soft tissue mass (*) involving the left skull base and adjacent soft tissues and foramina. There is invasion into the left side of the clivus (C), which shows loss of normal fatty marrow signal. The mass is centered on the hypoglossal canal and extends intracranially to the posterior fossa. Note normal right hypoglossal canal (*white arrow*) for comparison.

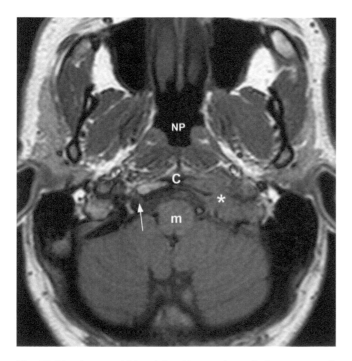

Fig. 12.39 A coronal T1-weighted image through the upper neck in the same patient demonstrates a similar appearing infiltrative soft tissue mass (*) involving the left skull base with bone marrow and soft tissue invasion at the level of the hypoglossal canal (*arrow* shows normal right side). (d, dens; P, pons.)

Diagnosis

Skull base metastasis causing left CN XII palsy and subacute denervation change in the tongue

Case 12.10

A 55-year-old female with a carotid space mass displays persistent left hemitongue weakness, atrophy, and fasciculations (**Figs. 12.40, 12.41, 12.42**).

Diagnosis

Schwannoma causing chronic denervation change in the tongue (**Table 12.2**)

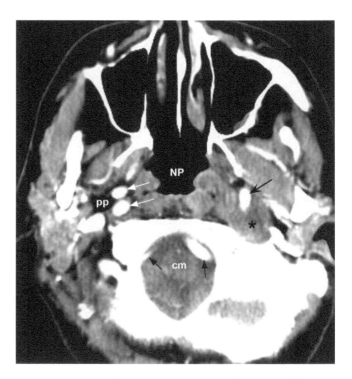

Fig. 12.40 An axial postcontrast CT image through the foramen magnum at the level of the nasopharynx (NP) demonstrates a soft tissue mass (*) anterior to the skull base and inferior to the hypoglossal canal that effaces the parapharyngeal fat and displaces the left internal carotid artery (*concave arrow*). On the right, the parapharyngeal fat (pp) appears normal though the internal carotid artery (*white arrows*) is tortuous. Normal vertebral arteries, left larger than right (*black straight arrows*), are seen within the foramen magnum at the level of the cervicomedullary junction (cm).

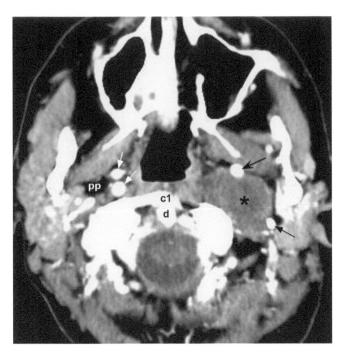 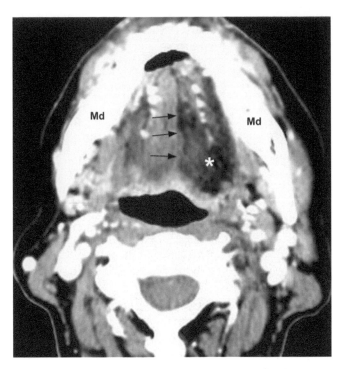

Fig. 12.41 More inferiorly at the level of the dens (d) and C-1 vertebra (c1), an axial postcontrast CT image shows a minimally enhancing, well defined, round-to-oval soft tissue mass (*) centered in the upper carotid space that displaces the left internal carotid artery (*concave arrow*) anteriorly and effaces the left parapharyngeal fat. The mass is medial to the styloid process (*black straight arrow*) and parotid gland. A tortuous right internal carotid artery (*white straight arrows*) and normal right parapharyngeal fat (pp) are also seen.

Fig. 12.42 More inferiorly at the level of the tongue and mandible (Md), an axial postcontrast CT image demonstrates asymmetric hypodensity of the tongue. There is fatty atrophy (*) of the left hemi-tongue that sharply respects the midline (*arrows*). In addition, slight deviation of the midline lingual septum to the left side is compatible with volume loss in the setting of chronic denervation change.

Table 12.2 Denervation Change: MRI Findings

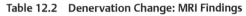

Acute/subacute	Chronic
Edema	Atrophy
T2 hyperintense	No T2 hyperintensity
Contrast enhancement	No enhancement
Minimal fatty replacement	Fatty replacement

Appendix A: The Brainstem

See Table A.1 for abbreviations used in Appendix A

The Brainstem

See **Figs. A.1, A.2, A.3**.
- Divided into midbrain, pons, and medulla.
- Continuous with the diencephalon cranially and the spinal cord caudally.
- Contains cranial nerve (CN) nuclei (except for CNs I and II), other intrinsic nuclei, ventricular system, and ascending and descending white matter tracts.
- CN I (olfactory nerve) and CN II (optic nerve) differ from other CNs in that they are really central nervous system (CNS) tracts. Both are composed of secondary sensory axons rather than primary sensory axons.
- Some white matter tracts cross multiple levels of the brainstem (midbrain, pons, and/or medulla) but each tract is listed separately at each level below.

Table A.1 Abbreviations

AICA	anterior inferior cerebellar artery
CN	cranial nerve
CNS	central nervous system
CTT	central tegmental tract
GP	globus pallidus
GPi	globus pallidus internus
GSE	general somatic efferent
GSPN	greater superficial petrosal nerve
ICP	inferior cerebellar peduncle
IO	inferior oblique
ION	inferior olivary nucleus
IR	inferior rectus
LC	locus ceruleus
LGN	lateral geniculate nucleus
LL	lateral lemniscus
LMN	lower motor neuron
LPS	levator palpebrae superioris
LR	lateral rectus
MCP	middle cerebellar peduncle
MGN	medial geniculate nucleus
ML	medial lemniscus
MLF	medial longitudinal fasciculus
MR	medial rectus
PAG	periaqueductal gray
PCA	posterior cerebral artery
PICA	posterior inferior cerebellar artery
PPRF	paramedian pontine reticular formation
RiMLF	rostral interstitial nucleus of the medial longitudinal fasciculus
RN	red nucleus
SCA	superior cerebellar artery
SCP	superior cerebellar peduncle
SN	substantia nigra
SNc	substantia nigra pars compacta
SNr	substantia nigra pars reticulata
SR	superior rectus
STN	subthalamic nucleus
STT	spinothalamic tract
SVE	special visceral efferent
TTT	trigeminothalamic tract
VA	ventral anterior
VIP	vasoactive intestinal polypeptide
VL	ventral lateral
VPL	ventral posterior lateral
VPM	ventral posterior medial

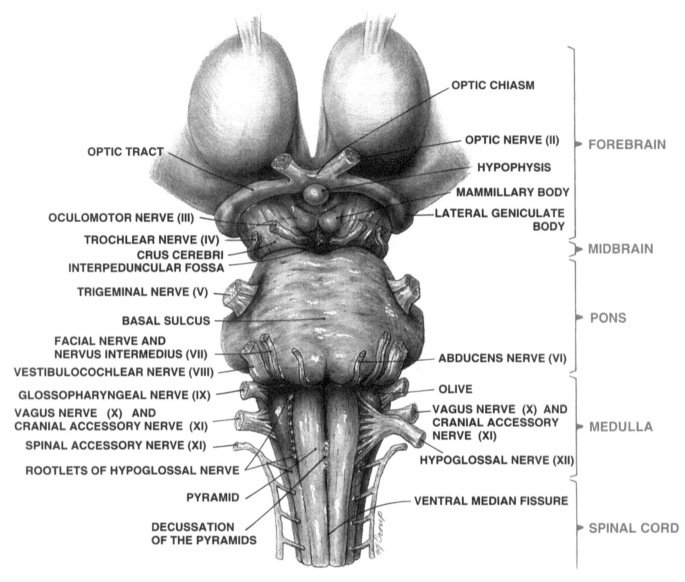

Fig. A.1 Ventral view of the brainstem (labeled). (From Manter and Gatz's Essentials of Clinical Neuroanatomy and Neurophysiology (10th ed.) by S. Gilman and S.W. Newman, Philadelphia, PA: F.A. Davis Publishers, 2003. Reprinted with permission.)

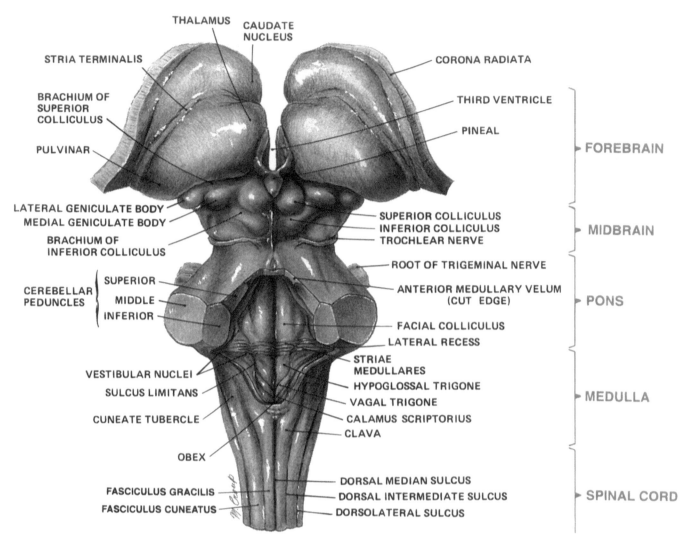

Fig. A.2 Dorsal view of the brainstem (labeled). (From Manter and Gatz's Essentials of Clinical Neuroanatomy and Neurophysiology (10th ed.) by S. Gilman and S.W. Newman, Philadelphia, PA: F.A. Davis Publishers, 2003. Reprinted with permission.)

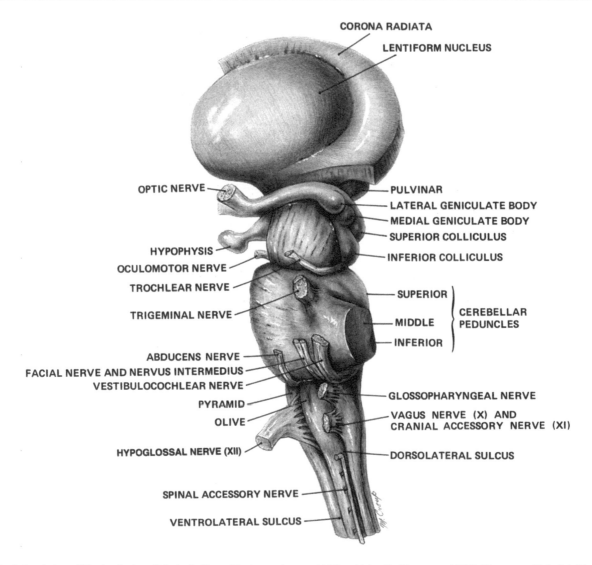

Fig. A.3 Lateral view of the brainstem (labeled). (From Manter and Gatz's Essentials of Clinical Neuroanatomy and Neurophysiology (10th ed.) by S. Gilman and S.W. Newman, Philadelphia, PA: F.A. Davis Publishers, 2003. Reprinted with permission.)

Midbrain

See **Figs. A.4, A.5**
- Also called mesencephalon
- Extends from superior to inferior colliculi
- Consists of the following:
  - *Tectum* (contains the *corpora quadrigemina*—superior and inferior colliculi)
  - *Tegmentum* (contains various nuclei, see below)
  - *Crus cerebri* (cerebral peduncles, see below)
  - *Cerebral aqueduct (aqueduct of Sylvius)*

Upper Midbrain: Level of the Superior Colliculus

See **Figs. A.4, A.5**.

Nuclei

- *Superior colliculus.* The *superior colliculus* is the rostral part of the tectum and is a laminated nucleus with the superficial layers connected to the visual system and the deep layers connected to the muscles for head and eye movements. *Input* from the visual system including the retina (*retinocollicular tract*), lateral geniculate nucleus (LGN), and occipital cortex enters via *brachium of the superior colliculus. Input* also from more caudal areas including brainstem nuclei and spinal cord (via *spinotectal tract* that travels with spinothalamic tract). *Output* to the thalamus (pulvinar and LGN via *tectothalamic tract*), paramedian pontine reticular formation (PPRF, horizontal gaze center), rostral interstitial nucleus of the MLF (RiMLF, vertical gaze center), reticular formation, and spinal cord (via *tectospinal tract*). Functions in visual reflexes and object tracking. Unilateral *damage* causes contralateral visual field neglect and impaired tracking, but no deficit in eye movements. *Stimulation* causes *contralateral conjugate deviation* (despite a lack of direct projections to the extraocular muscles) by (1) stimulating the RiMLF to excite the ipsilateral CN III; and (2) stimulating the PPRF to excite the contralateral CN VI and RiMLF.
- *Oculomotor nuclear complex* is a V-shaped group of nuclei just ventral to the aqueduct of Sylvius. Nerve roots exit in a paramedian location in the interpeduncular fossa. The nuclear complex includes (see also Chapter 3)
  - Lateral subnucleus. Supplies ipsilateral IO, IR, and MR muscles.
  - Medial subnucleus. Supplies contralateral SR muscle (via decussating axons).

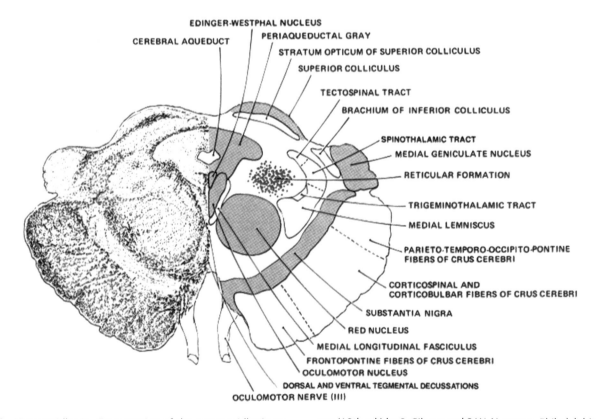

Fig. A.4 Upper midbrain. Cross-section of the upper midbrain at the level of the superior colliculus and red nucleus. (From Manter and Gatz's Essentials of Clinical Neuroanatomy and Neurophysiol-ogy (10th ed.) by S. Gilman and S.W. Newman, Philadelphia, PA: F.A. Davis Publishers, 2003. Reprinted with permission.)

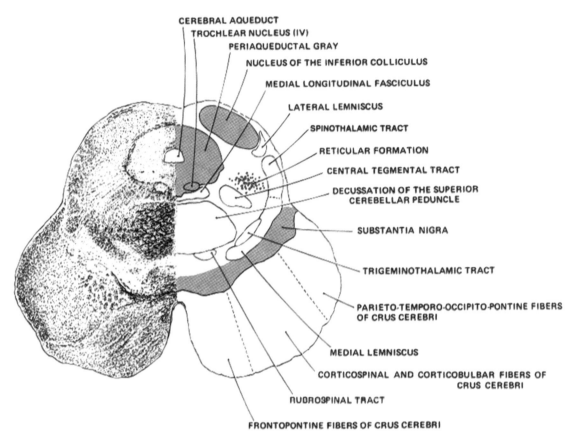

CEREBRAL AQUEDUCT
TROCHLEAR NUCLEUS (IV)
PERIAQUEDUCTAL GRAY
NUCLEUS OF THE INFERIOR COLLICULUS
MEDIAL LONGITUDINAL FASCICULUS
LATERAL LEMNISCUS
SPINOTHALAMIC TRACT
RETICULAR FORMATION
CENTRAL TEGMENTAL TRACT
DECUSSATION OF THE SUPERIOR
CEREBELLAR PEDUNCLE
SUBSTANTIA NIGRA
TRIGEMINOTHALAMIC TRACT
PARIETO-TEMPORO-OCCIPITO-PONTINE FIBERS
OF CRUS CEREBRI
MEDIAL LEMNISCUS
CORTICOSPINAL AND CORTICOBULBAR FIBERS OF
CRUS CEREBRI
RUBROSPINAL TRACT
FRONTOPONTINE FIBERS OF CRUS CEREBRI

Fig. A.5 Lower midbrain. Cross-section of the lower midbrain at the level of the inferior colliculus and decussation of the superior cerebellar peduncles. (From Manter and Gatz's Essentials of Clinical Neuroanatomy and Neurophysiology (10th ed.) by S. Gilman and S.W. Newman, Philadelphia, PA: F.A. Davis Publishers, 2003. Reprinted with permission.)

- ○ Central subnucleus. Supplies bilateral LPS.
- ○ Edinger-Westphal subnucleus. Preganglionic parasympathetic innervation to Sphincter Pupillae and ciliary muscles.
- • *Accessory oculomotor nuclei* and structures include the RiMLF, the interstitial nucleus of Cajal, nucleus of Darkshevich, the pretectal region and the posterior commissure.
- • *Red nucleus* (RN). Reddish due to high iron content. Functions to maintain *flexor* tone (especially in upper extremities).
  - ○ *Input* from (1) deep cerebellar nuclei (dentate nucleus and nucleus interpositus)—fibers exit the cerebellum via superior cerebellar peduncle (SCP) and cross to contralateral side in the midbrain to reach the RN; (2) cerebral cortex via *corticorubral* fibers from precentral, premotor, supplementary motor area, motor cortex; (3) superior colliculus via *tectorubral* tract; and (4) globus pallidus internus (GPi) via *pallidorubral* tract.
  - ○ *Output* to (1) contralateral cervical spinal cord via *rubrospinal tract*; (2) contralateral interposed nuclei, facial nucleus, medulla, and spinal cord via crossed *ventral tegmental tract*; and (3) ipsilateral inferior

olivary nucleus (ION) via uncrossed *central tegmental tract* (CTT).
- ○ Fibers of the oculomotor nerve and SCP pass directly through the RN.
- ○ *Triangle of Guillain-Mollaret* is the projection from RN to ipsilateral ION via CTT, from ION to contralateral cerebellar cortex via inferior cerebellar peduncle (ICP), to dentate nucleus, then via SCP to contralateral RN. *Lesion of the triangle produces palatal myoclonus clinically and hypertrophic olivary degeneration on magnetic resonance imaging (MRI) scans.*
- ○ Stimulation elicits increased tone in contralateral flexors and decreased tone in contralateral extensors.
- ○ Injury to RN can lead to changes in muscle tone and tremor ("rubral tremor").
- ○ *Substantia nigra* (SN) (Latin, "black substance" from melanin pigmentation). Located between crus cerebri and midbrain tegmentum and extends from globus pallidus rostrally to pons caudally.
- ○ SN *pars compacta* (SNc). Dorsal (dark) zone, comprising large dopaminergic neurons.
  - ▪ *Input* from other basal ganglia nuclei (e.g., subthalamic nucleus [STN]), brainstem (e.g., pedunculopontine nucleus).

- *Output* to striatum ("nigrostriatal" dopaminergic pathway).
  - SN *pars reticulata* (SNr). Ventral (pale) zone, contains GABAergic (γ-aminobutyric acid-containing) neurons.
    - *Input* from cerebral cortex, striatum (caudate/putamen), globus pallidus (GP), and STN.
    - *Output* to VA and VL thalamus, superior colliculus, and pedunculopontine nucleus.
  - *Parkinson's disease* is associated with degeneration of the nigrostriatal dopaminergic pathway and has four cardinal clinical signs: tremor, rigidity, bradykinesia, and postural instability.
- *Periaqueductal gray* (PAG) is a group of nuclei variously involved with central *analgesia*, anxiety, vocalization, and head movements. Contains a large number of peptidergic neurons (including VIP, enkephalin, cholecystokinin). Connections to hypothalamus, septal area, entorhinal cortex, hippocampus, cerebellum, reticular formation, locus ceruleus (LC), raphe nuclei of pons and medulla.

Tracts

- *Crus cerebri.* Contain descending white matter tracts. The central two thirds contains corticospinal and corticobulbar tracts. The medial and lateral ends are corticopontine with frontopontine medial and parieto-temporo-occipitopontine laterally. One million of the 20 million fibers are corticospinal.
- *Dentatorubrothalamic tract.* Contains ascending fibers from the contralateral dentate nucleus of the cerebellum that give off collaterals to the RN before reaching their primary target—the VL thalamus. Involved in coordination of movement and other cerebellar functions.
- *Brachium of superior colliculus.* Transmits fibers from optic tract (*retinocollicular tract*) and corticotectal fibers to the superior colliculus and rostrally projecting fibers from the superior colliculus (*tectothalamic tract*).
- *Spinothalamic tract (STT).* Conveys pain/temperature information derived from contralateral spinal cord to the reticular formation and thalamic VPL. *Spinotectal tract* runs in close apposition to STT.
- *Trigeminothalamic tract (TTT).* Conveys fine touch and pain/temperature information from the face (from spinal trigeminal and principal sensory nuclei) to thalamic VPM. Divided into two tracts, *dorsal* (uncrossed) and *ventral* (crossed; see Chapter 5).
- *Tectospinal tract.* Originates in the superior colliculus, crosses in the midbrain *dorsal tegmental decussation*, and terminates on lower motor neurons in cervical spinal cord. Involved in visual reflexes (e.g., turning the head toward an auditory stimulus).
- *Medial lemniscus (ML).* Conveys contralateral fine touch/proprioception/vibration from the nucleus gracilis and nucleus cuneatus (see Medulla, below) to the VPL nucleus of thalamus (second part of "dorsal column–medial lemniscus pathway").

- *Brachium of inferior colliculus.* Conveys tonotopic auditory information from the inferior colliculus to the medial geniculate nucleus (MGN) of thalamus.
- *Medial longitudinal fasciculus (MLF).* Conveys ascending and descending fibers from various brainstem nuclei (including PPRF, superior colliculus, vestibular nuclei, pontine reticular formation, interstitial nucleus of Cajal). Ascending fibers include fibers from PPRF to contralateral oculomotor nucleus complex for control of horizontal eye movements. Descending fibers terminate in the cervical spinal cord and are involved in coordination of head, neck, and eye movements.
- *Central tegmental tract (CTT).* Contains ascending fibers from the medullary reticular formation that terminate in the thalamus and descending fibers from midbrain regions that terminate in the ION.
- *Habenulointerpeduncular tract* (fasciculus retroflexus of Meynert). Conveys fibers from the habenular nuclei (epithalamus) to the interpeduncular nucleus and midbrain reticular formation.

Lower Midbrain: Level of the Inferior Colliculus

See **Fig. A.5.**

Nuclei

- *Inferior colliculus.* The *inferior colliculus* receives auditory input via the *lateral lemniscus* (LL), contains a tonotopic representation of auditory information and projects via the *brachium of the inferior colliculus* to the *medial geniculate nucleus* (MGN) of the thalamus, which in turns projects to the primary auditory cortex (transverse temporal gyrus of Heschl) (see Chapter 8).
- *Trochlear nucleus.* The *trochlear nucleus* lies inferior to the oculomotor nuclear complex, dorsal to the MLF, and ventrolateral to the cerebral aqueduct. Trochlear nerve *fascicles* course posteroinferiorly around the cerebral aqueduct to *decussate in the superior medullary velum* of the midbrain and exit the contralateral side of the dorsal midbrain just below the inferior colliculus (see Chapter 4 and **Figs. 4.1, 4.2,** and **4.3**).
- *Mesencephalic nucleus of trigeminal (CN V).* Located immediately lateral to the PAG. Extends from principal sensory nucleus (in pons) cranially to superior colliculus (in midbrain). Contains the *primary sensory neurons* (i.e., there is no synapse in the trigeminal ganglion) involved in proprioception of head muscles (see Chapter 5).
- *Interpeduncular nucleus.* Located just dorsal to the interpeduncular fossa. Input is from habenular nucleus via habenulointerpeduncular tract (fasciculus retroflexus of Meynert) and there is *diffuse output* with cholinergic fibers to various parts of the CNS.

- *Pedunculopontine nucleus.* Located in the lateral tegmentum ventral to the inferior colliculus. Input is from cortex, GPi, SNr. Output is to thalamus and SNc. A *major source of cholinergic output.* Involved with control of locomotion, stimulation causes walking movements.
- The inferior portion of SN and PAG also lie at this level.

Tracts

- Crus cerebri
- Trigeminothalamic tract (TTT)
- Medial lemniscus (ML)
- Spinothalamic tract (STT)
- Lateral lemniscus (LL). Conveys auditory information from the cochlear nucleus to the inferior colliculus (see Chapter 8).
- Rubrospinal tract. Carries fibers from RN to contralateral cervical spinal cord. Involved with maintenance of flexor tone in the upper extremities.
- Medial longitudinal fasciculus (MLF)
- Central tegmental tract (CTT)
- Decussation of the SCP. Fibers of the SCP cross at this level (e.g., dentatorubrothalamic tract fibers).
- Tectospinal tract

Midbrain Vascular Supply

- Paramedian perforators from the PCA include thalamoperforators to thalamus and peduncular arteries (to medial peduncles and midbrain tegmentum, CN III, RN, SN).
- *Quadrigeminal arteries* from the PCA supply superior and inferior colliculi.
- SCA sends branches to peduncles and SCP before supplying superior cerebellum.
- Posterior choroidal arteries supply peduncles, lateral superior colliculi, thalamus, choroid plexus of the third ventricle.
- Anterior choroidal arteries help supply peduncles.

Midbrain Syndromes

- *Weber syndrome.* Lesion of cerebral peduncle damaging pyramidal fibers and nerve CN III, leading to contralateral hemiplegia and ipsilateral oculomotor paresis (with parasympathetic paresis, dilated pupil).
- *Claude syndrome.* Lesion of midbrain tegmentum, RN, SCP, CN III with ipsilateral CN III palsy, contralateral ataxia, tremor.
- *Benedikt syndrome (Weber + Claude).* Lesion of midbrain tegmentum damaging RN, SCP, CN III, and pyramidal tracts leading to ipsilateral oculomotor paresis (with dilated pupil), and contralateral ataxia, tremor, and hemiplegia.

- *Nothnagel syndrome.* Lesion of midbrain tectum, SCPs, CN III. Bilateral or unilateral CN III palsy, gaze paralysis, cerebellar ataxia.
- *Parinaud syndrome.* "Dorsal mesencephalic syndrome" or "Sylvian aqueduct syndrome." It is due to lesion of dorsal rostral midbrain by hydrocephalus or pineal tumors. Includes some or all of the following signs:
  - Paralysis of conjugate upward gaze
  - Light-near dissociation (with mydriasis)
  - Convergence-retraction nystagmus (*nystagmus retractorius*) on upward gaze
  - Pathologic lid retraction (Collier sign)
  - Lid lag
- *Top of the basilar syndrome.* Occlusion of rostral basilar artery results in infarction of midbrain, thalamus, portions of temporal and occipital lobes; may also occur with giant basilar tip aneurysms. Variably includes
  - Disorders of eye movements: for example, unilateral or bilateral paralysis of upward or downward gaze
  - Pupillary abnormalities
  - Behavioral abnormalities
  - Visual defects (hemianopsia, cortical blindness, Balint syndrome)
  - Motor and sensory deficits

Pons

See **Figs. A.6, A.7**
- Pons = bridge (Latin).
- Extends from inferior colliculi/cerebral peduncles rostrally to stria medullaris/pontomedullary sulcus caudally.
- Dorsal part is pontine *tegmentum*; ventral part is *basis pontis.*
- Aqueduct has enlarged into the fourth ventricle at this level.

Upper Pons (Level of the Principal Sensory and Motor Nuclei of CN V)

See **Fig. A.6**.

Nuclei

- *Mesencephalic nucleus of trigeminal* (CN V). Extends from principal sensory nucleus (in pons) cranially to superior colliculus (in midbrain) (see Chapter 5). Dorsal to motor and main sensory nuclei at this level.
- *Motor and principal sensory nuclei of trigeminal* (CN V). Motor medial, sensory lateral in pontine tegmentum. Fibers carrying fine touch and pressure synapse in the principal sensory nucleus and then ascend in the *trigeminal lemniscus,* which crosses to the opposite side of the brainstem and the smaller *dorsal trigeminothalamic tract* (uncrossed), both of which terminate in the VPM tha-

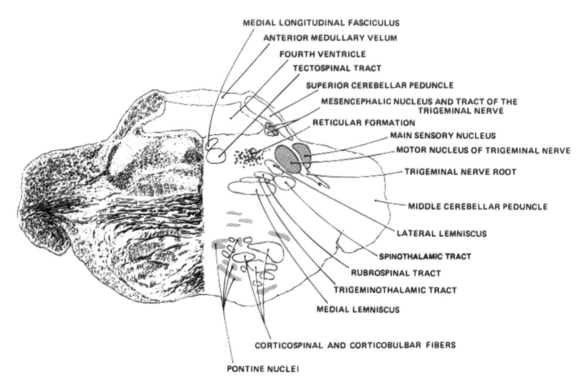

MEDIAL LONGITUDINAL FASCICULUS
ANTERIOR MEDULLARY VELUM
FOURTH VENTRICLE
TECTOSPINAL TRACT
SUPERIOR CEREBELLAR PEDUNCLE
MESENCEPHALIC NUCLEUS AND TRACT OF THE TRIGEMINAL NERVE
RETICULAR FORMATION
MAIN SENSORY NUCLEUS
MOTOR NUCLEUS OF TRIGEMINAL NERVE
TRIGEMINAL NERVE ROOT
MIDDLE CEREBELLAR PEDUNCLE
LATERAL LEMNISCUS
SPINOTHALAMIC TRACT
RUBROSPINAL TRACT
TRIGEMINOTHALAMIC TRACT
MEDIAL LEMNISCUS
CORTICOSPINAL AND CORTICOBULBAR FIBERS
PONTINE NUCLEI

Fig. A.6 The upper pons. Cross-section of the upper pons at the level of the main (principal) sensory and motor nuclei of CN V. (From Manter and Gatz's Essentials of Clinical Neuroanatomy and Neuro-physiology (10th ed.) by S. Gilman and S.W. Newman, Philadelphia, PA: F.A. Davis Publishers, 2003. Reprinted with permission.)

lamic nucleus. Motor nucleus of CN V sends motor root, which leaves the pons and ultimately joins the *mandibular nerve* (see Chapter 5).
- *Paramedian pontine reticular formation (PPRF).* (See Reticular Formation.)

Tracts

- Medial longitudinal fasciculus (MLF)
- Medial lemniscus (ML)
- Corticospinal, corticobulbar, corticopontine fibers
- Spinothalamic tract (STT)
- Trigeminothalamic tract (TTT)
- Tectospinal tract
- Central tegmental tract (CTT)
- Rubrospinal tract
- Lateral lemniscus (LL)
- Middle cerebellar peduncle
- Superior cerebellar peduncle

Lower Pons (Level of the Nuclei of CN VI and VII)

See **Fig. A.7**.

Nuclei

- *Spinal trigeminal nucleus* (CNs V, VII, IX, X). Extends from principal sensory nucleus (in pons) caudally all the way to C2 (cervical spinal cord), where it merges with the substantia gelatinosa (pain-related lamina in the spinal cord). Receives input from CNs V, VII, IX, and X. Fiber carrying pain and temperature (and crude touch as well) descend via the *spinal trigeminal tract,* synapse in the spinal trigeminal nucleus, then cross via *ventral trigeminothalamic tract* to ascend to the VPM thalamic nucleus (see Chapter 5).
- *Abducens nucleus (CN VI).* Lies in dorsal pontine tegmentum just ventral to the fourth ventricle (separated from floor of the fourth ventricle by genu of facial nerve) (see also Chapter 6, **Fig. 6.1**). *Fascicles* course ventrally through the pons and through the ML medial to facial nerve fascicles to emerge at the pontomedullary junction just lateral to the pyramid.
- *Facial nucleus (CN VII).* Lies in caudal pontine tegmentum anterolateral to CN VI nucleus, sends axons dorsally toward the fourth ventricle that loops around the CN VI nucleus (forming the genu of the facial nerve), and then travel ventrolaterally to emerge from the pontomedullary junction between CN VI and CN VIII (see Chapter 7, **Fig. 7.1**).

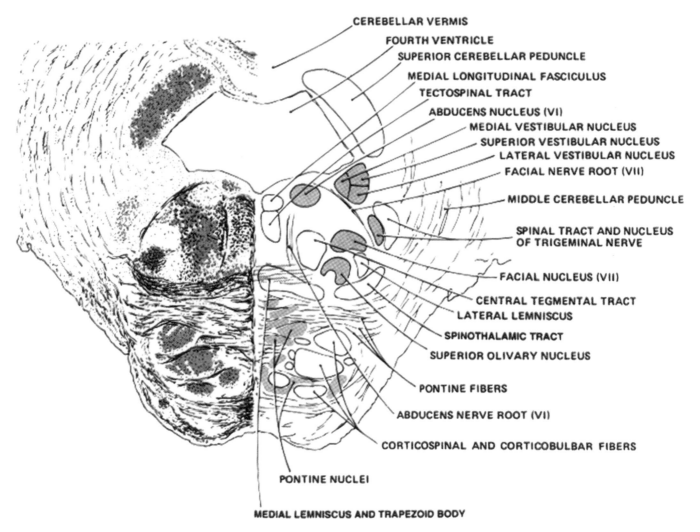

CEREBELLAR VERMIS
FOURTH VENTRICLE
SUPERIOR CEREBELLAR PEDUNCLE
MEDIAL LONGITUDINAL FASCICULUS
TECTOSPINAL TRACT
ABDUCENS NUCLEUS (VI)
MEDIAL VESTIBULAR NUCLEUS
SUPERIOR VESTIBULAR NUCLEUS
LATERAL VESTIBULAR NUCLEUS
FACIAL NERVE ROOT (VII)
MIDDLE CEREBELLAR PEDUNCLE
SPINAL TRACT AND NUCLEUS
OF TRIGEMINAL NERVE
FACIAL NUCLEUS (VII)
CENTRAL TEGMENTAL TRACT
LATERAL LEMNISCUS
SPINOTHALAMIC TRACT
SUPERIOR OLIVARY NUCLEUS
PONTINE FIBERS
ABDUCENS NERVE ROOT (VI)
CORTICOSPINAL AND CORTICOBULBAR FIBERS
PONTINE NUCLEI
MEDIAL LEMNISCUS AND TRAPEZOID BODY

Fig. A.7   The lower pons. Cross-section of the lower pons at the level of the nuclei of CN VI and VII. (From Manter and Gatz's Essentials of Clinical Neuroanatomy and Neurophysiology (10th ed.) by S. Gilman and S.W. Newman, Philadelphia, PA: F.A. Davis Publishers, 2003. Reprinted with permission.)

- *Superior salivatory nucleus* and *lacrimal nucleus (CN VII).* Lie medial to the facial nucleus. Send preganglionic parasympathetic axons to the nervus intermedius to (1) the *greater superficial petrosal nerve* (GSPN) to the *pterygopalatine ganglion* to the lacrimal gland (for lacrimation) and the mucosa of the nose and mouth (palatal and nasal glands); and (2) the *chorda tympani* nerve that joins with the lingual nerve (CN V$_3$) to the *submandibular ganglion* to the submandibular and sublingual glands for salivation.
- *Superior and lateral vestibular nuclei* (CN VIII). Vestibular nuclei all straddle the pontomedullary junction (see Medulla for inferior and medial vestibular nuclei). *Superior vestibular nucleus* (of Bechterew) involved with vestibulo-ocular reflexes. *Lateral vestibular nucleus* (Deiters' nucleus) involved with postural control, gives rise to the *lateral vestibulospinal tract.*
- Auditory nuclei: *dorsal* and *ventral cochlear nuclei* (CN VIII), *nucleus of the lateral lemniscus, superior olivary nuclear complex.* Auditory information via the cochlear nerves enters the brainstem at the pontomedullary junction to synapse in the ventral and dorsal cochlear nuclei. The *trapezoid body* connects ventral cochlear nuclei to the contralateral superior olivary nuclear complex. Cochlear nuclei are also connected to the inferior colliculi via the *lateral lemniscus.* See Chapter 8 for details.
- PPRF (see Reticular Formation).

Tracts

- Medial longitudinal fasciculus (MLF)
- Medial lemniscus (ML)
- Corticospinal, corticobulbar, corticopontine fibers
- Spinothalamic tract (STT)
- Spinal trigeminal tract (CNs V, VII, IX, and X)
- Tectospinal tract
- Central tegmental tract (CTT)

- Rubrospinal tract
- Auditory tracts: lateral lemniscus (LL), trapezoid body
- Middle cerebellar peduncle (MCP)
- Superior cerebellar peduncle (SCP)

Reticular Formation

- From Latin *reticulum,* "netlike structure"
- Area of interspersed small nuclei and fibers that forms the central core of the brainstem tegmentum
- Located in midbrain, pons and medulla
- Involved with the following:
  ○ Motor control (e.g., muscle tone controlled by *reticulospinal tracts*)
  ○ Sensory control (e.g., pain)
  ○ Visceral control (e.g., respiration and blood pressure)
  ○ Consciousness (sleep-wake cycle and control of arousal by *ascending reticular activating system*)
- Bilaterally symmetric and divided into three zones arranged in medial to lateral sequence:
  1. *Raphe nuclei* (from Greek *raphe,* "seam"). Adjacent to midline. Have extensive connections including the *ventral tegmental tract* to the medial forebrain bundle to the hypothalamus, striatum, thalamus, amygdala, hippocampus, cortex, and olfactory bulb. Use serotonin, cholecystokinin and enkephalin as neurotransmitters. Involved in sleep-wake, arousal, mood and aggression and provide endogenous analgesia via descending connections to spinal cord (*substantia gelatinosa*).
  2. *Medial zone.* Source of long ascending and descending projections from the reticular formation. These differ in pons versus medulla:
     - *Pontine reticular formation* sends ipsilateral *medial reticulospinal tract* to the LMNs of the spinal cord (runs next to MLF). Involved with *maintenance of extensor tone.*
     - *Medullary reticular formation* (especially *gigantocellular reticular nucleus,* named for the large cells therein) sends bilateral *lateral reticulospinal tract* to the LMNs of the spinal cord. Involved with *inhibition of extensor tone.*
     - Both pontine and medullary reticular formation receive descending fibers from the cortex, basal ganglia, RN, and SN via the *central tegmental tract* and send ascending fibers also via the CTT to the thalamic intralaminar nuclei for arousal. The intralaminar nuclei in turn project to widespread areas of the cortex. This entire system involved with cortical arousal is termed the *ascending reticular activating system.*
     - *Paramedian pontine reticular formation* (PPRF) (horizontal gaze center). Extends from pontomesencephalic junction to the abducens nucleus. Receives impulses from frontal eye fields and coordinates horizontal saccades.
       - *Locus ceruleus.* Pigmented (melanin) and uses norepinephrine as neurotransmitter with wide projections. Controls cortical activation and paradoxical (rapid eye movement) sleep.
  3. *Lateral zone.* Particularly prominent in caudal pons and rostral medulla. Together with the medial zone, concerned with CN reflexes and visceral functions. Includes the following centers:
     - Pedunculopontine nucleus
     - Pontine pneumotaxic center
     - Medullary respiratory centers (respiratory control)
     - Medullary pressor and depressor areas (blood pressure control)
     - Bulbar pressor area is the main control and the depressor area is in the rostral medulla/caudal pons.

Cerebellar Nuclei and Peduncles

- *Deep cerebellar nuclei.* Four paired nuclei. From medial to lateral: fastigial, globose, emboliform, dentate (mnemonic: feel good each day).
  ○ *Fastigial nucleus.* In the midline roof (*fastigium* = roof) of the fourth ventricle and sends fibers to the vestibular system bilaterally. Associated with the *vestibulocerebellum* (archicerebellum). Input is from the flocculonodular lobe and vermis. Output via ICP to vestibular nuclei (*cerebellovestibular pathway*). Assists equilibrium, stance, gait. Lesions may cause abasia, truncal ataxia, scanning speech, and hypotonia.
  ○ *Globose and emboliform nuclei.* Together called the *nucleus interpositus,* involved with muscle tone. Associated with the *spinocerebellum* (paleocerebellum). Input is from paravermian zone cerebellar cortex. Output via SCP to contralateral RN. Assists segmental reflexes, postural stability, and ipsilateral limb movements. Lesions may cause titubation, dysdiadochokinesis, action tremor, dysmetria, appendicular ataxia, and hypotonia.
  ○ *Dentate nucleus.* Largest and most lateral. Associated with *cerebrocerebellum* (neocerebellum). Input from cerebellar cortex. Output via SCP to contralateral RN and VL thalamus. Assists in coordination/fine dexterity. Lesion may cause difficulty in initiating/terminating movements, decomposition of movement, intention (terminal) tremor, and incoordination.
- Afferent fibers to the cerebellum enter mainly through the MCP and ICP, and outnumber efferent fibers 40:1. Efferent fibers exit mainly from the deep cerebellar nuclei and most leave through SCP.
- *Superior cerebellar peduncle.* Forms lateral wall of fourth ventricle. Contains afferent and efferent fibers.

- Afferent fibers (to cerebellum) include the following:
  - *Ventral spinocerebellar tract.* Conveys "efference copy" of motor commands and exteroceptive and proprioceptive information for the lower extremities. Initial cell bodies are "spinal border cells" in the anterior and intermediate horns. Tract ascends bilaterally, enters SCPs bilaterally, and ends in the spinocerebellum (fastigial and interposed nuclei). Ventral spinocerebellar tract input allows the cerebellum to monitor spinal circuit operation.
  - *Tectocerebellar tract.* Arises in superior and inferior colliculi, carries auditory and visual information.
  - *Trigeminocerebellar tract.* Carries proprioceptive fibers from mesencephalon and sensory information from the principal sensory nucleus of CN V.
- Efferent fibers (from cerebellum) (*brachium conjunctivum*) include the following:
  - *Dentatorubral tract.* Output to contralateral RN, primarily from nucleus interpositus. *Lesion causes appendicular ataxia.*
  - *Dentatothalamic tract.* Larger than dentatorubral tract. Output from dentate nucleus (primarily), passes through or around contralateral RN to terminate in contralateral thalamic VL and VPL. *Lesion causes intention tremor.*
  - *Uncinate fasciculus (bundle of Russell).* Output from fastigial nucleus to contralateral vestibular nuclei and reticular formation.
- *Middle cerebellar peduncle (brachium pontis).* Contains only afferent fibers. Largest of the three peduncles. Cerebral cortex (including motor, premotor, and sensory cortices) sends fibers to ipsilateral pons then via pontocerebellar tract to contralateral cerebellar hemisphere (corticopontocerebellar pathway). These fibers terminate as *mossy fibers.*
- *Inferior cerebellar peduncle* is made up of *restiform body* and *juxtarestiform body*. Contains afferent and efferent fibers.
  - Restiform body (afferent fibers).
    - *Dorsal spinocerebellar tract.* Proprioceptive and exteroceptive information from the lower extremity joints, Golgi tendon organs and muscle spindles synapses on neurons in the dorsal nucleus of Clarke (in Clarke column, T1-L2 spinal cord). Fibers from these neurons form the dorsal spinocerebellar tract and ascend ipsilaterally via the ICP as mossy fibers to terminate in the cerebellar cortex of the spinocerebellum (fastigial and interposed nuclei).
    - *Cuneocerebellar tract.* Upper extremity equivalent to dorsal spinocerebellar tract. Conveys proprioception of upper extremity and neck in fasciculus cuneatus but synapses in the accessory cuneate nucleus in the caudal medulla above the cuneate nucleus and then enters the ipsilateral ICP to reach spinocerebellum (like the dorsal spinocerebellar tract).
    - *Rostral spinocerebellar tract.* Upper extremity equivalent to the ventral spinocerebellar tract. Provides ipsilateral internal feedback and enters the inferior cerebellar peduncle.
    - *Olivocerebellar tract.* Carries somatosensory information from contralateral IO. Terminates as *climbing fibers* directly on Purkinje cell dendrites.
    - *Reticulocerebellar tract.* From lateral reticular and paramedian nuclei of medulla to cerebellar vermis.
  - Juxtarestiform body (afferent and efferent fibers from vestibular system). Medial to the restiform body. It contains *vestibulocerebellar* and *cerebellovestibular* tracts.

Pons: Vascular Supply

- Paramedian perforators from basilar artery supply medial basal pons (pontine nuclei, corticospinal fibers, ML). Short circumferential branches from basilar artery supply ventrolateral basis pontis. Long circumferential arteries supply the rest of the pons, including the following. SCA supplies rostral pons, brachium pontis, dorsal reticular formation. AICA supplies lateral tegmentum of lower two thirds of pons and ventrolateral cerebellum. Internal auditory artery (branch of AICA) supplies facial (VII) and cochlear (VIII) nerves.

Pontine Syndromes

- Ventral pontine syndromes.
  - *Millard-Gubler syndrome.* Unilateral lesion of ventrocaudal pons affecting corticospinal tract and CN VI and CN VII with contralateral hemiplegia, ipsilateral LR paresis and facial paresis.
  - *Pure motor hemiparesis.* Unilateral lesion of corticospinal tracts in basis pontis.
  - *Locked-in syndrome.* Bilateral ventral pontine lesions (deefferented state). Quadriplegia (corticospinal tract), aphonia (corticobulbar fibers), and occasionally horizontal ophthalmoplegia due to involvement of bilateral CN VI. Reticular formation not injured thus patient is fully awake. Patients communicate with vertical eye movements and blinking.
- Dorsal pontine syndromes.
  - *Foville syndrome.* Lesion of pontine tegmentum in caudal one third of pons. Contralateral hemiplegia, ipsilateral facial palsy (CN VII), and paresis of horizontal eye movements (PPRF).
- *Lateral inferior pontine syndrome.* Due to *AICA* occlusion (also called AICA syndrome, ventral cerebellar infarct). It causes ipsilateral nystagmus, vertigo, nausea/vomiting (involvement of vestibular nuclei), facial paralysis (CN VII), paresis of conjugate gaze (PPRF), deafness and tinnitus (CN VIII), ataxia, decreased facial sensation (spinal trigeminal nucleus/tract), contralateral decreased pain/

temperature in the body (lateral spinothalamic tract), ipsilateral Horner syndrome (oculosympathetic fibers).

- *Lateral superior pontine syndrome.* Due to *SCA* occlusion (also called SCA syndrome, dorsal cerebellar infarct). It causes ipsilateral ataxia and intention tremor (SCP/dentate nucleus), vertigo, nausea/vomiting (involvement of vestibular nuclei), nystagmus (MLF and cerebellum), paresis of conjugate gaze, Horner syndrome (oculosympathetic fibers), contralateral decreased pain/temperature in the face and body (lateral spinothalamic tract), decreased proprioception in lower more than upper extremities, partial deafness, contralateral trochlear (CN IV) palsy.

Medulla

See **Figs. A.8, A.9, A.10**.

- Also called "medulla oblongata"
- Extends from stria medullaris/pontomedullary sulcus rostrally to spinomedullary junction caudally

Upper Medulla

See **Fig. A.8**.

Nuclei

- *Spinal trigeminal nucleus* (CNs V, VII, IX, X).
- *Medial and inferior vestibular nuclei* (*CN VIII*). Vestibular nuclei all straddle the pontomedullary junction (see Pons for superior and lateral vestibular nuclei). *Medial vestibular nucleus* (of Schwalbe) is the largest of the vestibular nuclei and sends crossed fibers to all extraocular nerve nuclei and to the cerebellum. Source of the *medial vestibulospinal tract*

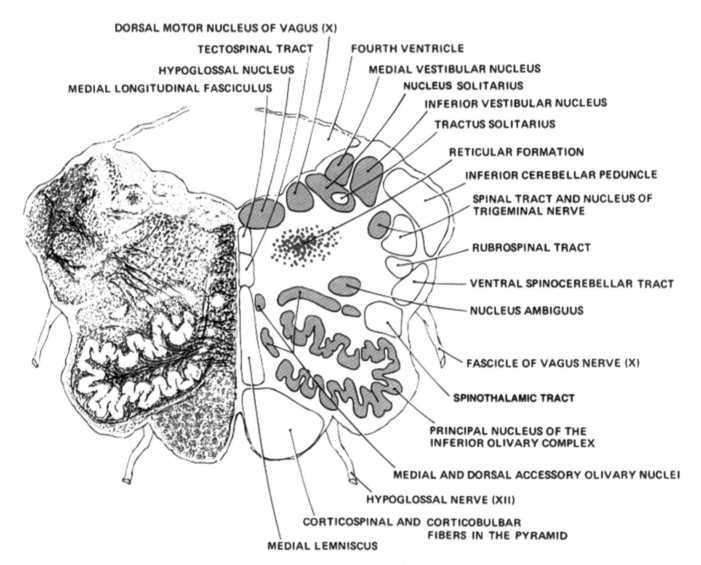

Fig. A.8   The upper medulla. Cross-section of the upper medulla. (From Manter and Gatz's Essentials of Clinical Neuroanatomy and Neurophysiology (10th ed.) by S. Gilman and S.W. Newman, Philadelphia, PA: F.A. Davis Publishers, 2003. Reprinted with permission.)

(involved in adjusting head position in space, runs with the MLF). *Inferior vestibular nucleus* integrates input from the vestibular system and the vestibulocerebellum (flocculonodular lobe). See Chapter 8 for details.

- *Dorsal motor nucleus of vagus (CN X).* Source of preganglionic parasympathetic outflow for the vagus nerve, located in the floor of the fourth ventricle in the *vagal trigone* lateral to the hypoglossal nucleus. See Chapter 10 for details.
- *Nucleus solitarius (CNs VII, IX, X)* (also sometimes called nucleus of the solitary tract). Located lateral to the dorsal motor nucleus of CN X. Rostral nucleus solitarius is gustatory (taste) with input mainly from CN VII (geniculate ganglion) and CN IX (petrosal ganglion) (but also CN X). Caudal nucleus solitarius mainly for visceral sensation (carotid body and carotid sinus from CN IX, and visceral sensation from CN X). See Chapter 10 for details.
- *Nucleus ambiguus* (CN IX, X, bulbar XI). Located in medullary reticular formation medial to spinal trigeminal nucleus. Source of SVE (branchial motor) outflow for CNs IX, X, and XI. See Chapters 9 through 11 for details.
- *Inferior salivatory nucleus (CN IX).* Located in rostral medulla (superior salivatory nucleus located in caudal

pons). Provides preganglionic parasympathetic innervation to CN IX to the otic ganglion for parotid salivation. See Chapter 9 for details.
- *Hypoglossal nucleus* (XII). Located in the paramedian medulla beneath the *hypoglossal trigone* in the floor of the fourth ventricle, extends nearly the entire length of the medulla. Source of somatic motor (GSE) outflow for the hypoglossal nerve. See Chapter 12 for details.
- *Nucleus prepositus hypoglossi.* Immediately rostral to the hypoglossal nucleus. Thought to function as a neural integrator for gaze holding. Projects directly to the oculomotor nucleus.
- *Inferior olivary complex, accessory nucleus of the inferior olive, and medial and dorsal accessory olivary nuclei.* Input to inferior olivary complex via CTT (from RN—rubroolivary tract, PAG, midbrain tegmentum), cortex (via corticoolivary tract), spinal cord (spinoolivary tract), cerebellum (cerebelloolivary tract). *Output:* Principal olivary nucleus sends efferent fibers to the cerebellar hemispheres; accessory olivary nuclei primarily send fibers to the vermis. Olivocerebellar fibers cross and then join ICPs (they make up the bulk of the ICP) and in the cerebellar cortex they become *climbing fibers* to reach Purkinje cells.

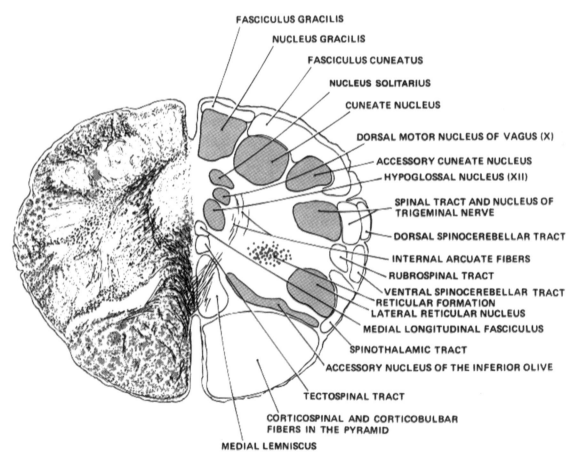

FASCICULUS GRACILIS
NUCLEUS GRACILIS
FASCICULUS CUNEATUS
NUCLEUS SOLITARIUS
CUNEATE NUCLEUS
DORSAL MOTOR NUCLEUS OF VAGUS (X)
ACCESSORY CUNEATE NUCLEUS
HYPOGLOSSAL NUCLEUS (XII)
SPINAL TRACT AND NUCLEUS OF TRIGEMINAL NERVE
DORSAL SPINOCEREBELLAR TRACT
INTERNAL ARCUATE FIBERS
RUBROSPINAL TRACT
VENTRAL SPINOCEREBELLAR TRACT
RETICULAR FORMATION
LATERAL RETICULAR NUCLEUS
MEDIAL LONGITUDINAL FASCICULUS
SPINOTHALAMIC TRACT
ACCESSORY NUCLEUS OF THE INFERIOR OLIVE
TECTOSPINAL TRACT
CORTICOSPINAL AND CORTICOBULBAR FIBERS IN THE PYRAMID
MEDIAL LEMNISCUS

Fig. A.9 The lower medulla. Cross-section of the lower medulla at the level of the decussation of the internal arcuate fibers forming the medial lemniscus. (From Manter and Gatz's Essentials of Clinical Neuroanatomy and Neurophysiology (10th ed.) by S. Gilman and S.W. Newman, Philadelphia, PA: F.A. Davis Publishers, 2003. Reprinted with permission.)

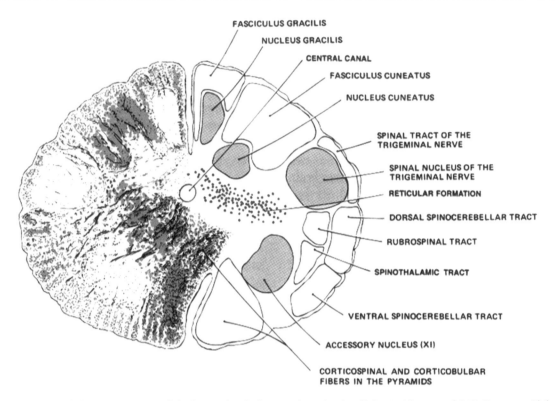

Fig. A.10 The lowest medulla. Cross-section of the lowest level of the medulla, through the decussation of the pyramids. (From Manter and Gatz's Essentials of Clinical Neuroanatomy and Neurophysi- ology (10th ed.) by S. Gilman and S.W. Newman, Philadelphia, PA: F.A. Davis Publishers, 2003. Reprinted with permission.)

Tracts

- Corticospinal tract (pyramidal tract)
- Medial lemniscus (ML)
- Medial longitudinal fasciculus (MLF)
- Ventral spinocerebellar tract (to SCP)
- Rubrospinal tract
- Tectospinal tract
- Spinothalamic tract (STT)
- Spinal trigeminal tract (CNs V, VII, IX, X)
- Tractus solitarius (solitary tract) (CNs VII, IX, X)
- Inferior cerebellar peduncle
- *Dorsal longitudinal fasciculus.* Contains ascending and descending fibers between the dorsal motor nucleus of CN X, reticular formation, intermediolateral gray column and sacral autonomic nuclei of the spinal cord and the hypothalamus. It is associated with autonomic/visceral responses.

Lower Medulla

See **Fig. A.9**.

Nuclei

- *Nucleus solitarius (CNs VII, IX, X).*
- *Dorsal motor nucleus of vagus (CN X).*

- *Hypoglossal nucleus (CN XII).*
- *Spinal trigeminal nucleus (CNs V, VII, IX, X).*
- *Nucleus gracilis.* Dorsal columns transmit ascending fine touch/proprioception/vibration information to the *nucleus gracilis* (lower extremities) and *nucleus cuneatus* (upper extremities). Postsynaptic fibers from these nuclei cross as the *internal arcuate fibers* to ascend as the *medial lemniscus* to the thalamus (VPL nucleus) and from there to somatosensory cortex.
- *Nucleus cuneatus.*
- *Accessory cuneate nucleus.* Lateral and rostral to the cuneate nucleus. Serves a similar function to the Clarke column in the thorax. Origin of fibers (*cuneocerebellar tract*, which joins the ICP) that are the upper extremity equivalent of the dorsal spinocerebellar tract.
- *Lateral reticular nucleus.* Part of the medullary reticular formation (see Reticular Formation). Receives fibers from the spinal cord (spinoreticular) and RN (rubrobulbar) and projects via ICP to cerebellum.
- *Accessory nucleus of the inferior olive.*

Tracts

- Corticospinal tract (pyramidal tract)
- Medial lemniscus (ML)
- Medial longitudinal fasciculus (MLF)

- Ventral spinocerebellar tract (to SCP)
- Dorsal spinocerebellar tract (to ICP)
- Medial and lateral reticulospinal tracts
- Medial and lateral vestibulospinal tracts
- Rubrospinal tract
- Tectospinal tract
- Spinothalamic tract (STT)
- Spinal trigeminal tract (CNs V, VII, IX, X)
- Dorsal longitudinal fasciculus
- Fasciculus gracilis
- Fasciculus cuneatus
- *Spino-olivary tract.* Conveys somatosensory information to the accessory olivary nuclei and thence to the cerebellum.

Lowest Medulla

See **Fig. A.10**.

Nuclei

- *Nucleus gracilis*
- *Nucleus cuneatus*
- *Spinal trigeminal nucleus (CNs V, VII, IX, X)*
- *Accessory nucleus (CN XI).* It supplies branchial motor (SVE) innervation for CN XI (see Chapter 11 for details).

Tracts

- Corticospinal tract (pyramidal tract)
- Medial longitudinal fasciculus (MLF)
- Ventral spinocerebellar tract (to SCP)
- Dorsal spinocerebellar tract (to ICP)
- Medial and lateral reticulospinal tracts
- Medial and lateral vestibulospinal tracts
- Rubrospinal tract
- Tectospinal tract
- Spinothalamic tract (STT)
- Spinal trigeminal tract (CNs V, VII, IX, X)
- Spinoolivary tract

- Dorsal longitudinal fasciculus
- Fasciculus gracilis
- Fasciculus cuneatus

Medulla Vascular Supply

- Paramedian medulla (hypoglossal nucleus, MLF, ML, pyramids, medial inferior olive) supplied by vertebral artery and anterior spinal artery
- Lateral portion of medulla supplied by vertebral artery or PICA.

Medullary Syndromes

- *Medial medullary syndrome* (Dejerine anterior bulbar syndrome). Occlusion of anterior spinal artery or parent vertebral artery resulting in ipsilateral tongue paresis/atrophy/fibrillation (CN XII), contralateral hemiplegia with sparing of face (pyramids), and contralateral loss of proprioception/vibration (ML).
- *Lateral medullary syndrome* (Wallenberg syndrome). Occlusion of intracranial vertebral artery or PICA resulting in ipsilateral facial hypalgesia and thermoanesthesia (spinal CN V nucleus), contralateral trunk and extremity hypalgesia and thermoanesthesia (STT), ipsilateral vocal cord paralysis, dysphagia, dysarthria (nucleus ambiguus), ipsilateral Horner syndrome (due to interruption of descending sympathetic fibers), vertigo, nausea, vomiting (CN VIII), ipsilateral cerebellar signs/symptoms (ICP, cerebellum), and sometimes hiccups and diplopia. Oculomotor abnormalities including dysfunction of ocular alignment (skew deviation due to damage to vestibular nuclei), nystagmus, smooth pursuit and gaze-holding abnormalities, and abnormalities of saccades (saccadic dysmetria) may also be observed.
- *Hiccups* (singultus). May be a component of the lateral medullary syndrome. Can also occur with posterior fossa masses, medullary masses or lesions, uremia. Inhibited by elevated PCO_2.

Appendix B: The Pupil

Autonomic Innervation

- *Sympathetic innervation.* First-order neuron is ipsilateral from posterolateral hypothalamus via *hypothalamospinal pathway* in lateral tegmentum of brainstem to intermediolateral gray matter at levels C8 to T3 (synapse #1 occurs here). Second-order neuron (preganglionic) is from C8 to T3 cells to sympathetic chain over lung apex and under subclavian artery to *superior cervical ganglion* (SCG) (synapse #2 occurs here). Third-order neuron (postganglionic): sudomotor and vasoconstrictor fibers to the face go via external carotid artery (ECA) branches, other postganglionic sympathetics go via the internal carotid artery (ICA) to join CN V_1 (via long ciliary nerves) to the orbit to the dilator pupillae muscle, with a separate branch via the ophthalmic artery to Müller muscle of eyelid.
- *Parasympathetic innervation.* Edinger-Westphal subnucleus in rostral portion of oculomotor nuclear complex to CN III (periphery of nerve) to inferior division to ciliary ganglion (synapse) (near the apex of the cone of extraocular muscles) to six to 10 *short ciliary nerves* that travel with branches of CN V_1 to travel forward between choroid and sclera to reach ciliary body and iris, control sphincter pupillae muscle to cause pupillary constriction and ciliary muscles to cause lens accommodation. Involved in *near reflex* (miosis, accommodation, convergence).

The Pupillary Reflex

See **Fig. B.1**.
- *Afferent* arc is CN II with optic tract collaterals in *retinopretectal tract* to pretectal nucleus, synapse and disperse *bilaterally* via crossing in posterior commissure (*pretectooculomotor tracts*), and travel ventral to the cerebral aqueduct to end in bilateral Edinger-Westphal nuclei. *Efferent* arc is CN III (Edinger-Westphal subnucleus) to sphincter pupillae.

Pupillary Dysfunction

Anisocoria

- Fifteen to 30% of population have 0.4 mm or greater of simple anisocoria (pupils react normally).
- *Marcus-Gunn pupil.* Also known as *relative afferent pupillary defect* (RAPD), signifies asymmetric optic nerve or chiasmatic lesion.

Sympathetic Dysfunction

- Oculosympathetic paralysis results in *Horner syndrome* (miosis, ptosis due to paralysis of Müller muscle, anhidrosis of forehead, and apparent enophthalmos).
- Results from interruption of
  - descending uncrossed hypothalamospinal pathway in tegmentum of brainstem or cervical cord;
  - preganglionic sympathetic fibers at any point from origin in intermediolateral cell column of C8 to T3 and the superior cervical ganglion; or
  - postganglionic sympathetic fibers on the carotid artery
- Common causes:
  - Tumor or inflammation of cervical lymph nodes
  - Cervical trauma or chest tubes placed high in chest
  - Carotid artery dissection
  - Tumors of the proximal brachial plexus
  - Lesions in the first and second thoracic spinal segments
  - Infarcts/lesions in lateral medulla (Wallenberg syndrome)
  - Idiopathic/hereditary
- Anhidrosis of forehead inconstant after postganglionic lesions (sympathetics following ECA should compensate).
- *Heterochromia iridis* (different iris colors) may signify congenital or acquired Horner syndrome.
- Dilatation lag (slow dilation after lights turned out in smaller pupil) indicative of Horner syndrome.
- Central (preganglionic) Horner syndrome most commonly follows brainstem vascular lesions (e.g., Wallenberg syndrome).
- A *Pancoast tumor* involves the sympathetic chain at the apex of the lung.
- *Oculosympathetic spasm* refers to pupillary dilation brought on by elevation/stretch of arm or leg in patient with C3 to C6 lesions.

Parasympathetic Dysfunction

- If one pupil (usually the larger one) reacts poorly to light then there are four possibilities:
  1. Damage to parasympathetic outflow via Edinger-Westphal nucleus to CN III.
  2. Damage to ciliary ganglion or short ciliary nerves, resulting in a *tonic pupil. Adie tonic pupil* due to degeneration of the ciliary ganglion and postganglionic parasympathetic fibers; may be unilateral or bilateral, female predominance, age 20 to 40 years. Causes my-

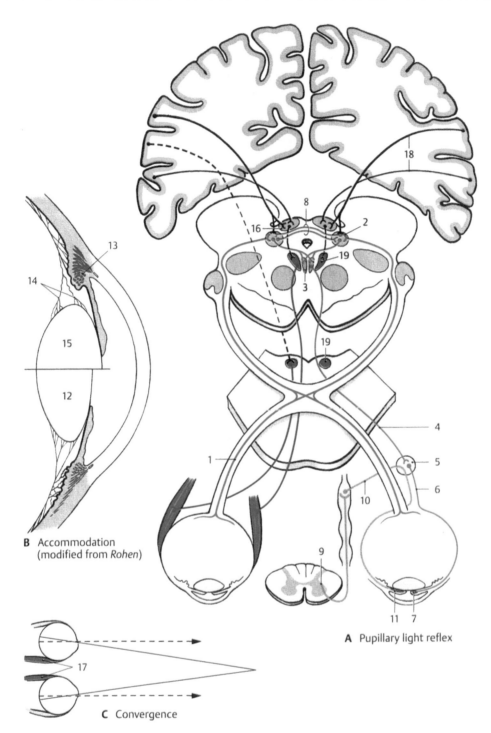

B Accommodation
(modified from *Rohen*)

A Pupillary light reflex

C Convergence

Fig. B.1 Pupillary light reflex, accommodation and convergence pathways. (1, optic nerve; 2, pretectal nucleus; 3, Edinger-Westphal nucleus; 4, preganglionic parasympathetic fibers from the Edinger-Westphal nucleus; 5, ciliary ganglion; 6, postganglionic parasympathetic fibers (short ciliary nerves); 7, sphincter pupillae muscle; 8, epithalamic commissure; 9, ciliospinal center; 10, postganglionic sympathetic fibers; 11, dilator pupillae muscle; 12, lens; 13, ciliary muscle; 14, zonular fibers; 15, lens rounded after ciliary muscle contraction; 16, superior colliculus; 17, medial rectus muscle; 18, corticofugal fibers to superior colliculus; 19, oculomotor nucleus.)

driasis and blurry vision with pupils *that accommodate (constrict) as part of the near reflex but do not react to light stimulation* ("light-near dissociation," also seen with syphilis and Parinaud syndrome). May be associated with corneal hypesthesia and depressed deep tendon reflexes (*Holmes-Adie syndrome*).

3. Damage to the iris due to ischemia, trauma, or an inflammatory process.

4. Mydriasis induced by parasympatholytic drugs (e.g., atropine, scopolamine).

Other Pupillary Abnormalities

- *Pontine lesion.* Produces *pinpoint pupils* due to unblocked parasympathetic input and loss of sympathetic input from the hypothalamus to the superior cervical ganglion.
- *Argyll-Robertson pupil.* Syphilitic pupil that accommodates but does not react (light-near dissociation). Lesion may be in the midbrain. Pupil is small, irregular, and does not dilate with mydriatics.
- *Light-near dissociation.* Seen with pinealoma, multiple sclerosis (MS), diabetes, Argyll-Robertson pupil, Parinaud syndrome.
- *Flynn phenomenon.* Paradoxical constriction of pupils to darkness (can occur with congenital achromatopsia, optic atrophy).
- *Episodic anisocoria.*
- *Traumatic iridoplegia* (common cause of pupillary dilatation).

Appendix C: Parasympathetic Ganglia

Ciliary Ganglion

See **Fig. C.1**.
- Preganglionic parasympathetic innervation supplied by the *Edinger-Westphal nucleus* in the rostral portion of the oculomotor nuclear complex.
- Preganglionic parasympathetics travel with the inferior division of CN III and terminate in the ciliary ganglion. Postganglionic fibers form six to 10 *short ciliary nerves* that travel with the *nasociliary nerve* (of CN V$_1$) forward between choroid and sclera to reach the ciliary body and iris. These control the *sphincter pupillae* muscle to cause pupillary constriction (miosis) and the *ciliary muscles* to cause lens accommodation (also see **Fig. 3.5**).

Pterygopalatine Ganglion

See **Fig. C.1**.
- Preganglionic parasympathetic innervation supplied by the *superior salivatory nucleus* and associated *lacrimal nucleus* in dorsal pons.
- Preganglionic parasympathetics travel with the *nervus intermedius* of CN VII into the internal auditory canal and then join the GSPN at the geniculate ganglion in the temporal bone.
- The GSPN (parasympathetic + sensory) exits the petrous temporal bone via the greater petrosal foramen to enter the middle fossa and pass down to the pterygoid canal (vidian canal), where it joins with the *deep petrosal*

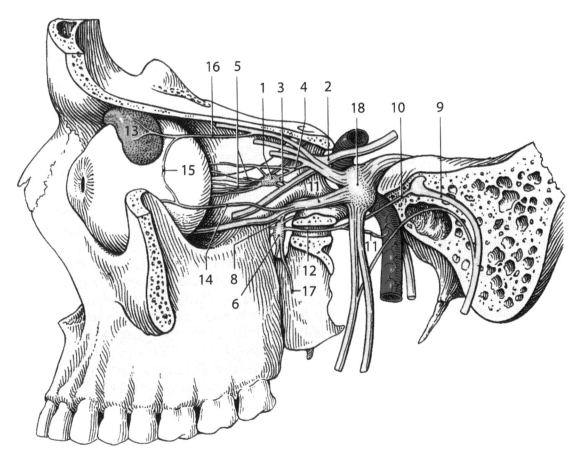

Fig. C.1 Ciliary and pterygopalatine ganglia. (1, ciliary ganglion; 2, oculomotor nerve; 3, parasympathetic component of CN III; 4, nasociliary nerve; 5, short ciliary nerves; 6, pterygopalatine ganglion; 7, maxillary nerve [CN V$_2$]; 8, ganglionic branches from CN V$_2$ to pterygopalatine ganglion; 9, facial nerve [labyrinthine segment]; 10, GSPN; 11, deep petrosal nerve; 12, nerve of the pterygoid canal [vidian nerve]; 13, lacrimal gland; 14, zygomatic nerve; 15, anastomosis between zygomatic nerve and lacrimal nerve [carrying secretomotor parasympathetic fibers from pterygopalatine ganglion]; 16, lacrimal nerve; 17, palatine nerve; 18, trigeminal ganglion.)

nerve (sympathetic fibers from ICA plexus) to form the *nerve of the pterygoid canal (vidian nerve)*. This nerve (parasympathetic + sympathetic + sensory) reaches to the pterygopalatine fossa where the pterygopalatine ganglion is suspended from a branch of CN V$_2$ (pterygopalatine nerve). The *parasympathetics* synapse in the pterygopalatine ganglion.

- Postganglionic parasympathetics then travel with zygomatic nerve (branch of CN V$_2$) into the inferior orbital fissure to join the lacrimal nerve (branch of CN V$_1$) and innervate the lacrimal gland (for lacrimation). Other postganglionic parasympathetics travel with CN V$_2$ branches (nasal and palatine nerves) to the oral and nasal mucosa (nasal and palatal glands).
- The GSPN also carries GSA (somatic sensory) fibers from the external ear to the geniculate ganglion (cell bodies) to nervus intermedius to spinal trigeminal tract and spinal trigeminal nucleus.

Otic Ganglion

See **Fig. C.2**.

- Preganglionic parasympathetic innervation is supplied by the *inferior salivatory nucleus* in rostral medulla (at superior pole of rostral CN X nucleus).
- Preganglionic parasympathetics travel with CN IX and join the tympanic nerve into the tympanic plexus, which gives rise to the lesser superficial petrosal nerve (LSPN). The LSPN reenters the cranium through a small canal in the petrous temporal bone lateral to the canal for the GSPN, then travels back out through the foramen ovale where the parasympathetics synapse in the *otic ganglion* (which sits below the foramen ovale surrounding a branch of CN V$_3$).
- Postganglionic parasympathetics travel with the auriculotemporal nerve (branch of CN V$_3$) to the parotid gland to cause salivation and vasodilation.

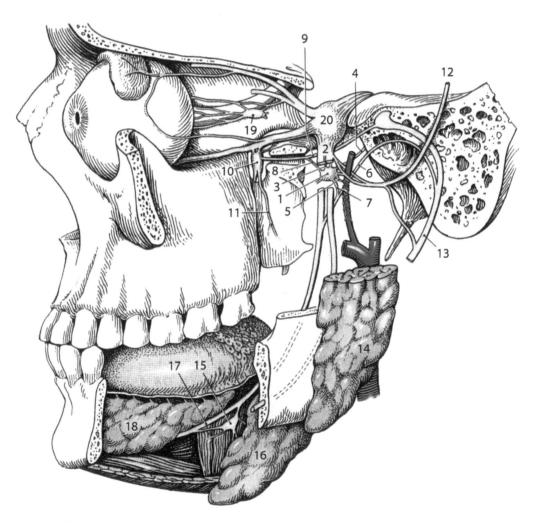

Fig. C.2 Otic and submandibular ganglia. (1, otic ganglion; 2, mandibular nerve [CN V$_3$]; 3, sensorimotor roots [of CN V$_3$]; 4, LSPN; 5, sympathetic fibers [from plexus on middle meningeal artery]; 6, chorda tympani; 7, communicating branch between chorda tympani and otic ganglion; 8, communicating branch between otic ganglion and GSPN; 9, GSPN; 10, pterygopalatine ganglion; 11, palatine nerves; 12, auriculotemporal nerve; 13, facial nerve; 14, parotid gland; 15, submandibular ganglion; 16, submandibular gland; 17, lingual nerve; 18, sublingual gland; 19, ciliary ganglion; 20, trigeminal ganglion.)

Submandibular Ganglion

See **Fig. C.2**.

- Preganglionic parasympathetic innervation is supplied by the *superior salivatory nucleus* in dorsal pons.
- Preganglionic parasympathetics travel with the nervus intermedius of CN VII into the internal auditory canal and through the temporal bone where they join the chorda tympani nerve.
- The chorda tympani (parasympathetic and taste) runs across the inner surface of the eardrum in the middle ear medial to the tympanic membrane, and exits the cranium via a part of the petrotympanic fissure known as the *canal of Huguier* to join the lingual branch of CN V_3 1 cm below the foramen ovale to travel to the submandibular ganglion. Preganglionic parasympathetics synapse in the submandibular ganglion, which is suspended from the lingual nerve (branch of CN V_3).
- Postganglionic parasympathetics are distributed to the submandibular and sublingual glands (salivation).
- The chorda tympani also carries gustatory afferents from the anterior two thirds of the tongue to geniculate ganglion (cell bodies) to the nervus intermedius to the rostral portion of the nucleus solitarius (also called "gustatory nucleus") in the medulla.

Appendix D: Cranial Nerve Reflexes

Table D.1   Cranial Nerve Reflexes

Function/Reflex	Anatomic Basis
Emotional response to odors	CN I to medial olfactory stria to septal area/subcallosal gyrus
Salivation with odors	CN I to lateral olfactory stria to piriform cortex to amygdala then via stria terminalis to hypothalamus then to superior and inferior salivatory nuclei (medulla)
Accelerated peristalsis and increased gastric secretion with odors ("cephalic" phase of digestion or "gastrocolic" reflex)	CN I to lateral olfactory stria to piriform cortex to amygdala, then via stria terminalis to hypothalamus, then to dorsal motor nucleus of CN X (medulla) to CN X to GI tract
Pupillary light reflex	CN II to retinopretectal tract to pretectum then via pretectooculomotor tract to bilateral Edinger-Westphal nuclei to CN III (parasympathetic) to ciliary ganglion to sphincter pupillae muscle
Light-induced circadian rhythms	CN II to retinohypothalamic tract to suprachiasmatic nucleus (SCN) of hypothalamus
"Near reflex"	1. *Pupillary constriction (miosis)*—via bilateral Edinger-Westphal nuclei to CN III (parasympathetic) to ciliary ganglion to sphincter pupillae muscle
	2. *Lens accommodation*—via bilateral Edinger-Westphal nuclei to CN III (parasympathetic) to ciliary ganglion to ciliary mm. (contraction causes lens to bulge, increasing diopter power)
	3. *Ocular convergence*—via superior colliculus to bilateral CN III (medial rectus)
Corneal reflex	CN V$_1$ to principal sensory nucleus of CN V to CN VII to orbicularis oculi
Jaw jerk (masseter reflex)	CN V$_3$ sensory to mesencephalic nucleus of CN V to motor nucleus of CN V to masseter and temporalis
Tearing	CN V$_1$ to superior salivatory nucleus (medulla) to GSPN parasympathetics (initially in nervus intermedius) to pterygopalatine ganglion to lacrimal gland and mucosa of nose and mouth (palatal and nasal glands)
Crying	Limbic system to hypothalamus to superior salivatory nucleus and lacrimal nucleus (medulla) to GSPN parasympathetics (initially in nervus intermedius) to pterygopalatine ganglion to lacrimal gland and mucosa of nose and mouth (palatal and nasal glands)
Salivation with taste stimulation	Anterior two thirds of tongue to chorda tympani nerve (of CN VII) to geniculate ganglion to rostral nucleus solitarius to superior and inferior salivatory nuclei OR posterior one third of tongue to CN IX to rostral nucleus solitarius to superior and inferior salivatory nuclei
Salivation	Superior salivatory nucleus to chorda tympani parasympathetics to submandibular ganglion to submandibular and sublingual glands. Inferior salivatory nucleus to CN IX parasympathetics via tympanic nerve (Jacobson's nerve) to LSPN to otic ganglion to parotid gland.
Sneezing	CN V sensory to the nucleus ambiguus to the respiratory center of the reticular formation, phrenic nerves, and intercostal muscles
Acoustic reflexes	Mediated by CN VIII (cochlear nerve) to spiral ganglion to ventral cochlear nucleus to *superior olivary complex* to (1) both motor CN VII nuclei to the stapedius muscles to decrease amplitude of sound waves by reducing ossicle movement; and (2) both motor CN V nuclei to the tensor tympani muscles to decrease sensitivity of tympanic membrane by pulling it taut. Reflex activated during loud sounds to protect cochlea and during speech production to decrease hearing of one's own speech.
Vestibuloocular reflex (VOR)	(Keeps visual image still by compensating for horizontal eye movements.) Left head movement increases activity in left horizontal semicircular canal to CN VIII (vestibular nerve) to superior and medial vestibular nuclei to contralateral CN VI (stimulate right lateral rectus) and via medial longitudinal fasciculus to ipsilateral CN III (stimulate left medial rectus)
Gag reflex	CN IX sensory to caudal nucleus solitarius to nucleus ambiguus to CN X to pharyngeal muscles
Cough reflex	CN X sensory (usually larynx, trachea, or bronchial tree) to caudal nucleus solitarius to medullary respiratory center for forced expiration and to nucleus ambiguus to CN X to muscles of larynx and pharynx for cough
Vomiting reflex	CN X sensory to caudal nucleus solitarius to nucleus ambiguus to CN X to close glottis and also to reticulospinal tract to cause contraction of diaphragm and abdominal muscles. May be stimulated also by increased intracranial pressure and by emetics stimulating the area postrema of caudal medulla

Index

Note: Page numbers followed by *f* and *t* indicate figures and tables, respectively. Boxed text is indicated by *b*. I preceding a page number indicates the Introduction.